Pharmacological and Psychosocial Treatment in Schizophrenia

Third Edition

T0251663

Pharmacological and Psychosocial Treatments in Schizophrenia

Third Edition

Edited by

David J. Castle MSc DLSHTM MD FRCPsych MRCPsych FRANZCP
St Vincent's Health and the University of Melbourne,
Fitzroy, Victoria, Australia

David L. Copolov PhD FRACP FRANZCP
Monash University,
Clayton, Victoria, Australia

Til Wykes MPhil PhD
Centre for Recovery in Severe Psychosis,
Institute of Psychiatry, King's College London, London, UK

Kim T. Mueser PhD
Dartmouth Medical School,
Hanover, New Hempshire, USA
NH Center for Psychiatric Rehabilitation,
Boston University, Boston, Massachusetts, USA

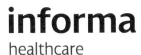

A CIP record for this book is available from the British Library.
Library of Congress Cataloging-in-Publication Data available on application
Cover art © 2012 Ingi

ISBN-10: 1-84214-534-7
ISBN-13: 978-1-84214-534-0
eISBN: 978-1-84214-535-7

Orders may be sent to: Informa Healthcare, Sheepen Place, Colchester, Essex CO3 3LP, UK
Telephone: +44 (0)20 7017 6682
Email: Books@Informa.com
Informa Healthcare Website: informahealthcarebooks.com
Informa website: www.informa.com

For corporate sales please contact: CorporateBooksIHC@informa.com
For foreign rights please contact: RightsIHC@informa.com
For reprint permissions please contact: PermissionsIHC@informa.com

Typeset by Exeter Premedia Services Pvt Ltd, Chennai, India
Printed and bound in Great Britain by MPG Books Ltd, Bodmin

Artist's Commentary on "Little Voices" Cover Art

A young woman, who is having her morning cup of tea and wearing her slippers, is hearing voices. (Hearing voices can happen during the most mundane moments...)

Her voices have scarlet lips, indicating they are false, seductive and treacherous. The young woman's head is huge, depicting how largely distorted her cognition is.

Her cat, an intuitive animal, is startled by the situation.

Ingi

Contents

Contributors

Diane Agoro
Institute of Psychiatry, King's College London,
London, UK

Deirdre Alderton
Fremantle Hospital,
South Metropolitan Health Region, Fremantle,
Western Australia, Australia

Christine Barrowclough
University of Manchester, Manchester, UK

Morris D. Bell
VA Connecticut Healthcare System,
West Haven, Connecticut, USA
Department of Psychiatry, Yale University
School of Medicine, West Haven,
Connecticut, USA

Peter Bosanac
Department of Psychiatry, St Vincent's Health
and the University of Melbourne, Fitzroy,
Victoria, Australia

Tom Burns
Department of Psychiatry, University of
Oxford, Oxford, UK

David J. Castle
St Vincent's Health and the University of
Melbourne, Fitzroy, Victoria, Australia

Jimmy Choi
VA Connecticut Healthcare System, West
Haven, Connecticut, USA
Department of Psychiatry, Yale University
School of Medicine, West Haven,
Connecticut, USA

Amanda Collins Messman
Central Iowa VA Health Care System,
Des Moines, Iowa, USA

David L. Copolov
Monash University, Clayton, Victoria, Australia

Marc Corbière
Department of Rehabilitation, University of
Sherbrooke, Quebec, Canada CAPRIT
(Centre d'Action en Prévention et Réadaptation
de l'Incapacité au Travail), Montreal, Quebec,
Canada

Richard Drake
University of Manchester, Manchester, UK

Chris Fassnidge
Institute of Psychiatry, King's College London,
London, UK

Paul B. Fitzgerald
Alfred Psychiatry Research Centre, The Alfred
Hospital, Melbourne, Victoria, Australia
Monash University School of Psychology,
Psychiatry and Psychological Medicine,
Melbourne, Victoria, Australia

Shirley M. Glynn
Department of Psychiatry and Biobehavioral
Sciences, University of California, Los Angeles,
California, USA
Semel Institute of Neuroscience and Human
Behavior, University of California, Los Angeles,
California, USA
VA Greater Los Angeles Healthcare System, Los
Angeles, California, USA

Peter Hayward
Institute of Psychiatry, King's College London, London, UK

Wynne James
Drug and Alcohol Office, Government of Western Australia, Perth, Western Australia, Australia

Robert W. Johnson
Fulton State Hospital, Fulton, Missouri, USA

Natalie Knoesen
St Vincent's Mental Health, St Vincent's Hospital, Melbourne, Victoria, Australia

Jayashri Kulkarni
Alfred Psychiatry Research Centre, The Alfred Hospital, Melbourne, Victoria, Australia
Monash University School of Psychology, Psychiatry and Psychological Medicine, Melbourne, Victoria, Australia

Nicola Lautenschlager
St Vincent's Aged Psychiatry Service, University of Melbourne, Melbourne, Victoria, Australia

Tania Lecomte
Department of Psychology, University of Montreal, Quebec, Canada
Fernand Seguin Research Centre, Montreal, Quebec, Canada

Shon Lewis
University of Manchester, Manchester, UK

Anna Lui
VA Greater Los Angeles Healthcare System, Los Angeles, California, USA

Evelina Medin
Centre for Recovery in Severe Psychosis, Institute of Psychiatry, King's College London, London, UK

Kim T. Mueser
Dartmouth Medical School, Hanover, New Hampshire, USA
NH Center for Psychiatric Rehabilitation, Boston University, Boston, Massachusetts, USA

Paul E. Mullen
Monash University, Fairfield, Victoria, Australia

John W. Newcomer
Psychology and Medicine, Washington University School of Medicine, St Louis, Missouri, USA

Ginger E. Nicol
Department of Psychiatry, Washington University, St Louis, Missouri, USA

Jeffrey R. Nolting
Fulton State Hospital, Fulton, Missouri, USA

Urban Ösby
Department of Molecular Medicine and Surgery, Neurogenetics Unit, Karolinska Institutet, Stockholm, Sweden

Peter Rabins
Johns Hopkins University, Baltimore, Maryland, USA

Alison Ram
Institute of Psychiatry, King's College London,London, UK

Mary V. Seeman
University of Toronto, Toronto, Ontario, Canada
Department of Psychiatry, Institute of Medical Science, Toronto, Ontario, Canada

William D. Spaulding
University of Nebraska, Lincoln, Nebraska, USA

Craig Steel
Charlie Waller Institute of Evidence-Based Psychological Treatments, University of Reading, Reading, UK

Danny H. Sullivan
Victorian Institute of Forensic Mental Health, Melbourne, Victoria, Australia
Department of Psychological Medicine, Monash University, Clayton, Victoria, Australia

Sarah Swan
Institute of Psychiatry, King's College London, London, UK

Rumina Taylor
Institute of Psychiatry, King's College London, London, UK

Nga Tran
St Vincent's Mental Health, St Vincent's Hospital, Melbourne, Victoria, Australia

India Webb
Centre for Recovery in Severe Psychosis, Institute of Psychiatry, King's College London, London, UK

Til Wykes
Centre for Recovery in Severe Psychosis, Institute of Psychiatry, King's College London, London, UK

Foreword to the First Edition

Treating patients with severe and persistent mental illnesses such as schizophrenia is not for the faint of heart. There are many reasons for this cautionary view including the fact that these illnesses are severe, recurrent, debilitating, and often, if not usually, lifelong. They are also poorly understood by scientists in terms of their etiology and pathophysiology, by lay persons in terms of their level of recognition and understanding of the symptoms and nature of mental illness, and by most clinicians with the exception of those who are trained and experienced in their care and management. Moreover, the patients themselves often lack awareness of their illness and they either are not motivated or deny the need for treatment.

Despite these numerous and significant obstacles, the body of knowledge and repertoire of therapeutic modalities for the treatment of schizophrenia is prodigious. This is fortuitous as patients with schizophrenia suffer from multiple kinds of morbidity and disabilities, and thus often need different treatments. Patients experience a spectrum of symptoms including psychosis (positive symptoms), and disturbances in drive, interest, affect, and impoverishment of thought and speech (collectively known as negative symptoms) and also may incur mood symptoms of depression, anxiety, or excitement. In addition, at some point in the course of their illness, they sustain impairments in their cognition and functional capacity. They also exhibit disproportionately high rates of suicide, substance abuse, and violent or aggressive behaviors. Finally, the impact of the illness is not limited to the patients themselves. The consequences of the illness have devastating effects on the family and ultimately on the community at large which all too frequently is required to assume some level of responsibility for persons with mental illness.

The revised edition of *Pharmacological and Psychosocial Treatments in Schizophrenia* edited by David Castle, David Copolov, and Til Wykes provides a thoughtful, comprehensive, and state-of-the-art guide for the clinical management of patients with severe and persistent mental illness. It is clear to anyone who works with such patients that although medication is an essential component of treatment, by itself it is insufficient. Thus, this well-conceived volume begins with psychopharmacological management but then immediately proceeds to discuss methods for the psychological management of psychosis before considering other pathological dimensions of the illness (management of negative symptoms, cognitive dysfunction in schizophrenia, and depression and anxiety in schizophrenia), and clinical complications of the illness (substance abuse comorbidity in schizoprhenia; management of acute arousal in schizophrenia). The final three chapters address the prevalent and challenging problems of promoting adherence to treatment, work, and recovery and family intervention in schizophrenia.

The beauty of this work lies in its pragmatic and fundamental selection of topics and their natural combination in this concise, lucid, and straightforward volume. The seemingly effortless composition of this book makes the integration of pharmacological and psychosocial therapies appear seamless and natural. Would that this were the case in mental healthcare systems and general clinical practice. Regrettably this is the exception with limited and fragmentary therapeutic services being the rule of what usually exists in mental healthcare settings. To paraphrase the divine plea "from your mouth to God's ears," one might say that for comprehensive and integrated treatment for patients with severe and persistent mental illness "from the mouths of Castle, Copolov, and Wykes to the ears of all mental healthcare providers."

Jeffrey A. Lieberman MD
University of North Carolina School of Medicine,
Chapel Hill, North Carolina,
USA

Foreword to the Second Edition

It has been a welcome trend in recent years to see the emergence of specialist books on schizophrenia. This condition is so complex and, although major treatment breakthroughs are still elusive, the field is moving at a pace that is hard for the specialist—let alone the busy general psychiatrist—to keep up with treatment developments. In a relatively short time, there has been a shift in treatment focus with growing emphasis now on psychiatric and medical comorbidities, and on improving functionality. Additionally, there is a greater need to define and measure these outcomes, whether these relate to risky behaviors or more generally to broader functional outcomes of work performance and socialization.

Accordingly, I was delighted to see the next version of this book. The second edition of *Pharmacological and Psychological Treatments in Schizophrenia* will serve as an authoritative source on schizophrenia for mental health clinicians, particularly since it has been updated to include new chapters directly pertinent to the most current issues in schizophrenia research and therapeutics.

The latest text reflects advances in both pharmacological and psychosocial treatments of schizophrenia. From lifestyle issues to clinical rating scales, and even to the delivery of care for women with schizophrenia, the textbook covers the clinical essentials of schizophrenia in a balanced and remarkably comprehensive manner. As a departmental chairman, I am particularly pleased to see that every effort has been made to include the very latest key publications while also citing references to seminal papers on schizophrenia in the chapters. Given the scope of this text, this balance is no small task and the editors (Drs Castle, Copolov, Wykes, and Mueser) and contributing authors are to be congratulated.

Recognized experts, with the guidance and oversight of the editors, have contributed clinically relevant chapters. It is evident that each contributor has carefully ensured that his or her chapter is complete and the editors have been careful in their role of delivering a well-integrated textbook. This is exemplified best in the chapters on cognitive dysfunction in schizophrenia (chap. 4) and enhancing socialization (chap. 12), although this approach is evident throughout the text.

While my own research focus is on the medication treatment of schizophrenia, I was very pleased to see excellent contributions on facets of vocational and social impairments of this illness as well as the emphasis on psychiatric and medical comorbidities. These are practical and contain clinically pertinent new material. The textbook is well weighted with respect to psychological and somatic therapies, a key consideration for trainees. Having two chapters dedicated to acute agitation and then violence and the forensic aspects of schizophrenia makes a lot of sense since this is such an important and complex focus in management today. As a point of observation, the reader may also wish to keep an eye on emerging medication augmentation studies for refractory schizophrenia. This is covered briefly in the chapter on treatment-resistant schizophrenia and is always an area of innovation (even if the evidence base is weakly confined to mainly small clinical trials). A chapter on recovery and consumerism should make its way into the third edition, though that may be some time off as this version is so current that it will likely have a substantial "shelf-life."

Drs Castle, Copolov, Wykes, and Mueser and the contributing authors have done an excellent job in providing a comprehensive clinically pertinent text that hopefully with wide distribution will raise the understanding of the modern day treatment of schizophrenia.

Peter F. Buckley MD
Department of Psychiatry,
Medical College of Georgia,
Augusta, GA, USA

Foreword to the Third Edition

Schizophrenia is a complex disorder which requires a comprehensive approach to treatment, encompassing excellent psychopharmacology as well as psychological treatments and interventions aimed at limiting social disability. Treatments need to be appropriate to the developmental and illness stage of the individual, and be appropriate for their particular psychosocial context.

I am very pleased to recommend this updated, revised, and expanded new edition of what has been an extremely popular book; it continues to provide a succinct and clinically relevant overview of pharmacological and psychosocial interventions for individuals with schizophrenia and related disorders. The major need areas for pharmacologic and psychosocial treatments are reviewed, including psychotic symptoms (both positive and negative); cognitive symptoms (a particular focus, given the apparent primacy of these symptoms in determining disability in schizophrenia); comorbid symptoms such as depression and anxiety; general health issues; lifestyle issues; violence in schizophrenia, with guidelines about risk assessment; and programs specifically to improve adherence with treatment. New to this edition is material on further specific patient groups such as the elderly and an appraisal of models of care and community treatment. All chapters have been brought up to date, with recent important advances highlighted and appropriately referenced.

Each chapter is self-contained, yet there is extensive cross-referencing between chapters that gives an overall coherence to the book. Although the various chapter authors bring their own viewpoints to the material at hand, there is little redundancy between chapters and the overall messages are clearly delivered. Practical tips, fact boxes and summary tables assist the reader in negotiating what is a wealth of material.

This book should be a ready reference for all clinicians involved in the care of people with schizophrenia. The editors and their world-renowned contributors should be commended on what is a most practical and clinically focused book. I hope other readers learned as much as I did from it.

Professor Sir Robin M. Murray MD DSc FRCP FRCPsych FMedSci FRS
Institute of Psychiatry,
King's College London,
London, UK

Acknowledgments

A number of individuals gave helpful advice regarding various chapters of this book, at varying stages of production. We thank these people, who include Shon Lewis (Manchester, UK), Peter Norrie (ACT, Australia), Josh Geffen (Brisbane, Australia), Dan Lubman (Melbourne, Australia), Allan White (Newcastle, Australia), Christine Culhane (Melbourne, Australia), John Farhall (Melbourne, Australia), Julie Lord (Melbourne, Australia), and John Fielding (Melbourne, Australia). For administrative support, we thank, in particular Mary Veljanovska.

chapter 1

Psychopharmacological management of schizophrenia

David J. Castle, Nga Tran, and Deirdre Alderton

It is now well established that antipsychotic medications are one of the mainstays of treatment for psychotic disorders. This has been shown to be the case for both acute management and maintenance treatment aimed at reducing relapse (1). This chapter concentrates on the pharmacological aspects of the initial and ongoing treatment of psychosis (the management of acute behavioral disturbance in psychosis is covered in chap. 8).

Historical background

The discovery of the calming effects of chlorpromazine in the 1950s set the modern pharmacological management of psychotic disorders in motion. Further antipsychotics were soon developed, based on the notion that it was the dopamine D2 blockade in the brain that mediated the antipsychotic effects. Haloperidol was the "cleanest" D2 blocker of all these earlier agents and became the benchmark against which other agents were measured.

One of the drawbacks of the older, so-called typical antipsychotics is their greater propensity to produce extrapyramidal side effects (EPSEs) such as parkinsonism, dystonias, and akathisia, and the longer-term problem of tardive dyskinesia (TD) (Table 1.1) (2). It was thus with great interest that the atypical antipsychotic (AAP) clozapine was welcomed to the marketplace in the mid-1960s. Clozapine was noted to be a potent antipsychotic with minimal propensity to EPSE/TD and particular efficacy in so-called treatment-resistant cases. However, the limitations of clozapine, notably its propensity to cause a potentially fatal agranulocytosis in around 1% of patients, led to its withdrawal in a number of countries in the 1970s (it was reintroduced in the late 1980s, with strict hematological monitoring controls), and the race was on to develop "clozapine-like" drugs that did not cause blood dyscrasias.

Table 1.1 Extrapyramidal side effects (EPSEs) of antipsychotic drugs

Type of ESPE	Clinical features
Parkinsonism	Mask-like facies
	Muscle rigidity ("cog-wheeling")
	"pill-rolling" tremor
	shuffling gait; festination; retropulsion
	diminished arm swing
Dystonia	Acute: Involuntary sustained spasm of muscles, notably head and neck (e.g., facial grimacing, protrusion of tongues, opisthotonus, oculogyric crisis); may be painful
	Chronic: Sustained involuntary spasm of skeletal muscles, resulting in abnormal posture (e.g., trunk)
Akathisia	Subjective feeling of "inner restlessness," with a drive to move;
	Objective: frequent changes of posture, inability to sit still, constant walking
Tardive Dyskinesia	Orobuccofaciolingual: abnormal involuntary movements of face tongue and lips with chewing movements, tongue movement, puckering of lips, grimacing;
	May be associated truncal movements, and choreoathetoid movements of the extremities

Based on the belief that the atypicality of clozapine was a consequence of its high ratio of serotonin (5HT2): dopamine D2 receptor occupancy, the pharmaceutical industry produced risperidone, which mimicked that particular pharmacological property of clozapine. This product was the first novel AAP to be marketed, and showed a relatively benign side-effect profile compared with haloperidol, though EPSEs still occurred at higher doses (3). Subsequent novel atypicals include olanzapine, quetiapine, zotepine, sertindole, ziprasidone, amisulpride, aripiprazole, and paliperidone. Most recently, three new AAPs were approved by the U.S. Food and Drug Administration (FDA): iloperidone, asenapine, and lurasidone for the treatment of acute schizophrenia in adults. Asenapine is also approved for the maintenance of schizophrenia and as monotherapy or as an adjunct to lithium or valproate for the treatment of bipolar manic or mixed episodes. Iloperidone and asenapine are dosed twice daily in contrast to lurasidone, which is dosed once daily with food. Incidence of sedation and/or somnolence has been reported with each medication, and it is clearly dose related for lurasidone. Iloperidone is essentially free of EPSEs or akathisia, whereas dose-related akathisia has been reported with asenapine and lurasidone. Preliminary studies indicate that they are similar in efficacy to currently approved drugs with some added potential safety benefits. Future practical effectiveness studies of their benefit/ risk profile compared with established antipsychotics will greatly broaden the scope of AAPs and improve the expectations of psychopharmacological treatment for schizophrenia.

Other newer antipsychotics such as perospirone, bifeprunox, and cariprazine require further evaluation to establish their role in the psychiatric armamentarium.

Three large pragmatic clinical studies focusing on the effectiveness of typical antipsychotics and AAPs in the "real world" were evaluated recently. Both the Clinical Antipsychotic Trials of Intervention Effectiveness (CATIE) (1) and the Cost Utility of the Latest Antipsychotic Drugs in Schizophrenia (CUtLASS) (4) studies compared typical antipsychotics to AAPs in people with multi-episode schizophrenia, whereas the European First-Episode Schizophrenia Trial (EUFEST) (5) compared haloperidol to multiple AAPs in people with first-episode schizophrenia. Results from these studies suggest that there are limited positive symptom efficacy differences (except, possibly, for olanzapine) between the typical and atypical groups (4–6), especially for those patients who experience adequate symptom control and minimal side effects with a typical agent. Considerations of the choice of antipsychotic medication should be made on the basis of individual preference, prior treatment response, side-effect experience, adherence history, relevant medical history and risk factors, individual medication side-effect profile, and long-term treatment planning.

Typical antipsychotics

There are various definitions of typical and AAPs. Here, typical antipsychotics are considered to be those drugs that tend (at antipsychotic doses) to produce EPSEs. Table 1.2 shows the main typical agents, by class, and their side effects— it should be noted that not all these agents are available in some countries.

The most potent D2 blockers, notably those without intrinsic anticholinergic properties (e.g., haloperidol) are most likely to cause EPSEs though these effects can occur with higher doses of any of these agents. Other side effects of the typical antipsychotics also tend to be a reflection of receptor binding. For example, those agents with potent H1 blockade tend to be sedating; those with peripheral anticholinergic (muscarinic) effects have a propensity to cause dry mouth, constipation, urinary retention, and blurring of vision; those with α-adrenergic blockade can cause problematic postural hypotension. Other potential effects of these agents include weight gain, hyperprolactinemia (which can result in sexual dysfunction and galactorrhea), and lowering of the seizure threshold.

Table 1.2 Typical antipsychotics (oral)

Drug	Adult oral max. dose mg/day	Half-life hours	Antichol-inergic	Cardiac	EPSE	Hypo-tension	Sedation	Minor O/D	Weight gain	Prolactin	Procon-vulsant
Phenothiazines											
Chlorpromazine	1000	16–30	++	++	++	+++	+++	+++	+++	+++	+++
Levomepromazine (methotrimeprazine)	1000	16–78	+++	++	++	+++	+++	+++	?	+++	++
Promazine	800	–	++	++	+	++	++	+	?	+++	+++
Thioridazine	600	9–30	++	+++	+	+++	++	+++	?	+++	+++
Pericyazine	300	–	+	+++	+	++	++	+	++	+++	+
Fluphenazine	20	13–58	0	++	+++	+	+	+	+	+++	+++
Perphenazine	24	9–21	0	++	++	+	+	++	+++	+++	+++
Trifluoperazine	20	13	0	+++	++	++	+	++	?	+++	+
Butyrophenones											
Benperidol	1.5	–	?	?	?	+	++	?	?	+++	+
Haloperidol	30	12–36	++	++	+++	+	+	+	+	+++	+
Thioxanthines											
Flupenthixol	18	26–36	++	0	++	0	+	+	+	++	+
Zuclopenthixol	150	12–28	++	+	+++	+	++	++	?	++	0
Diphenylbutylpiperidine											
Pimozide	20	29–55	+	+++	++	++	+	+	0	+++	+
Substituted Benzamides											
Sulpiride	2400	–	+	0	+	0	+	+	+	++	0

+++ = Marked effect; ++ = Moderate effect; += Mild effect; 0 = Little or nothing reported; ? = No information available.

Source: Adapted from Ref. 125.

There are other particular side effects of certain agents that might influence prescribing habits. For a comprehensive list of particular side effects see Ref. (7). Of particular concern is the effect some antipsychotics have on cardiac conduction, notably prolongation of the QTc interval, with the potential for sudden death. Pimozide has long been identified in this regard, especially at high doses, and electrocardiogram monitoring is required. More recently, concern about thioridazine has led to restriction of its use in many countries and the oral form of droperidol has been withdrawn with restrictions placed on the use of the parenteral form in some countries. Other side effects are less dangerous but also affect prescribing. For example, chlorpromazine results in a photosensitivity that makes its use in sunny climes problematic, while thioridazine at high doses over prolonged usage can result in retinitis pigmentosa.

Atypical antipsychotics

A number of agents have now been developed that demonstrate antipsychotic efficacy at doses that do not usually result in EPSEs. These agents are often referred to as either novel or AAPs. To avoid confusion with clozapine, which is the archetypal AAP, these agents are henceforward referred to as novel atypicals; when clozapine is grouped with them they are jointly referred to as atypicals. It should be emphasized, however, that this group contains a number of drug types, with differences in receptor-binding profiles, different side effects, and possibly differential efficacies against particular symptoms in different patients. The main current drugs in this group, along with side effects, are shown in Table 1.3; again, not all drugs are available in all countries. It should be noted that a usual dose range is provided for each agent: this is on the basis of the literature and clinical experience, and does not preclude the use of lower or higher doses in some patients; for example low doses are often used in the elderly and higher doses in partial responders. As always, judgment about dosing is based on clinical response and side-effect burden.

It is still unclear as to which drug would be most beneficial for each individual patient, and often clinical trial and error guides therapeutic interventions. Certainly, efficacy against positive psychotic symptoms seems to be similar between agents; clozapine has some advantage for negative symptoms ((3) and chap. 3) while amisulpride at low dose (50–300 mg per day) has some benefit for negative symptoms (8); asenapine has also been shown to ameliorate negative symptoms in short- and long-term trials (see below). In clinical practice, it is the side-effect profile that probably plays the main role in the drug choice: for example, sedation and weight gain with olanzapine; the problems of EPSEs at high doses and raised prolactin levels with risperidone/paliperidone; and the potential for cardiac conduction problems with ziprasidone and sertindole might mitigate against the use of each of these agents for particular patients. Specific concern has been raised by the propensity of the

Table 1.3 Atypical antipsychotics

Drug	Usual adult oral dose mg/day (see text)	Half-life hours	Anticholinergic	Cardiac	EPSE	Hypotension	Sedation	Minor O/D	Weight Gain	Prolactin elevation	Proconvulsant[a]
Amisulpride	1200	12	++	0	+	0	0	0	+	++	+
Aripiprazole	15–30	75 (31–146)	0	+	0	0	0	?	+	0	0
Asenapine	10–20	6[b]	0	?	+	+	++	?	+	?	?
Clozapine	300–500	4–12	++	+++	0	+	+++	?	+++	0	+++
Olanzapine	10–20	30 (21–54)	+	0	0	0	++	?	+++	+	+
Paliperidone	6–12	23	0	0	0	+	+	0	+	++	0
Quetiapine	300–450	7	+	0	0	+	+	+	+	+	+
Risperidone	2–6	20–30	+	0	0	+	0	0	+	++	0
Sertindole	20	55–90	0	++	0	++	0	0	++	0	0
Ziprasidone	80–160	7	0	++	0	0	0	?	0	0	0
Zotepine	150–300	14–24	++	++	+	++	+	?	?	?	?

+++ = Marked effect; ++ = Moderate effect; + = Mild effect; +/– = Minimal effect at usual therapeutic doses; 0 = Little or nothing reported; ? = No information available.

[a]Dose-dependent effect; [b]Biphasic half-life: 6 h for the first 18 h, then terminal half-life is 23 h.

Source: Adapted from Ref. 125.

dibenzodiazepines in particular, to cause weight gain, diabetes, and dyslipid-emia (chap. 6). In patients with additional risk factors for these outcomes, aripiprazole or ziprasidone might have particular benefits. Stahl (3) provides useful clinical pearls of wisdom about these agents. We now provide a brief review of the most recent of the AAPs.

Aripiprazole's partial agonist activity at dopamine D2 receptors stabilizes the dopamine system while avoiding the hypodopaminergia that may limit the tolerability of currently available antipsychotics. *Bifeprunox*, similar to aripip-razole, is a partial D2 receptor agonist while also exhibiting little efficacy at 5-HT2A, 5-HT2C, or noradrenaline receptors (9). Findings from a short-term study suggest that bifeprunox is safe and well tolerated by patients with an acute exacerbation of schizophrenia (10). However, despite it having minimal propensity to increase serum prolactin (11) or cause weight gain or EPSEs (12), it did not receive approval from the FDA as it demonstrated less efficacy than comparator antipsychotics, was too activating, had a slow titration, and caused nausea and vomiting (13).

Paliperidone is the active metabolite of risperidone, thus has a similar 5-HT2A/D2 antagonism profile as risperidone. It is a D2 and 5-HT2A antago-nist formulated as an osmotic controlled release oral delivery system (OROS) to reduce fluctuations in plasma levels and remove the need for dosage titra-tion (14). Paliperidone undergoes limited hepatic metabolism and this may reduce the potential for drug interactions (15). Paliperidone has been shown to be as effective as olanzapine (16) and more efficacious than quetiapine (17) in short-term studies. There are some long-term results suggesting paliperi-done's efficacy in preventing relapse (18–20). Paliperidone pharmacokinetic profiles, both in the sustained-release and long-acting formulations obviate the need for titration and are associated with improved tolerability.

Iloperidone, a new D2/5-HT2A antagonist structurally related to risperidone with better efficacy and less extrapyramidal symptoms than D2 antagonist antipsychotics has recently been approved by the FDA for the treatment of schizophrenia in the United States. The oral formulation has demonstrated efficacy in reducing symptoms of acute schizophrenia at fixed daily doses ranging from 12 to 24 mg; therapeutic response and adverse events such as dizziness, somnolence, and dry mouth appear to be dose dependent. Iloperi-done is administered twice daily and should be titrated slowly (12 mg/day over a 4-day period) (21,22) in order to minimize problems associated with α1 adrenergic antagonism, such as postural hypotension. Akathisia is rare but prolongation of QTc interval is comparable to that of haloperidol and ziprasi-done (23,24), which may be of concern. Iloperidone doses should be adjusted when concomitantly coadministered with potent CYP2D6 and CYP3A4 inhib-itors, and similarly in poor or extensively metabolized subjects. From limited efficacy studies, it appears that iloperidone is relatively well tolerated once titrated to a therapeutic level; however, further comparisons with other avail-able agents are needed.

Asenapine is a newer AAP with affinity for D2, 5-HT 2A, 5-HT 2C, and $\alpha1/\alpha2$ adrenergic receptors along with relatively low affinity for H1 and negligible affinity for muscarinic receptors. It has a chemical structure related to mirtazapine (a tetracyclic antidepressant) with antagonist actions at 5-HT2C and $\alpha2$ receptors, suggesting potential antidepressant properties (but additional research is required to determine this). Results from a pivotal phase II trial (25) suggested that asenapine 5 mg twice daily was superior to risperidone 3 mg twice a day and placebo in acute schizophrenia and was as well tolerated as placebo (double-blind, three-arm, fixed asenapine dose, 6-week, placebo and risperidone controlled trial); there was apparent particular efficacy for negative symptoms, though this effect requires further evaluation. Kane et al. (26) demonstrated that asenapine was more effective than placebo in preventing relapse of schizophrenia after long-term treatment (a 26-week double-blind placebo-controlled trial followed 26 weeks of open label treatment). Transient somnolence, akathisia, and oral hypoesthesia were among the most common side effects, while the incidence of other common side-effects (compared to many AAPs) such as weight gain, hyperprolactinemia, and alterations in glucose and lipid profiles, has generally been low (25,27,28). Asenapine is administered sublingually for rapid absorption through the oral mucosa. Its bioavailability reduces from 35% to less than 2% if swallowed so no drinking or eating for 10 minutes is allowed following sublingual administration. Coadministration of asenapine with known CYP1A2 inhibitors such as fluvoxamine can alter the metabolism of asenapine, although concomitant smoking during administration does not alter the pharmacokinetics of asenapine (29).

Lurasidone is a powerful antagonist of D2 and 5-HT2A receptors with high affinity for 5-HT7 and 5-HT1A receptors, compatible with favorable effects on cognitive function and an antidepressant action. It has minimal affinity for D1, D3, 5-HT2C and $\alpha1/\alpha2$-adrenergic receptors and no affinity for H1 or M1 receptors, suggesting a good tolerability profile. Lurasidone is administered once daily with at least 350 calories of food in order to optimize bioavailability. Lurasidone's efficacy within the dose range of 40–120 mg/day was established in four 6-week controlled studies of adults with schizophrenia. Doses above 80 mg/day did not appear to confer added benefit and may be associated with dose-related adverse side effects such as somnolence and akathisia (30,31). Coadministration with powerful CYP3A4 inhibitors or inducers is contraindicated (32). Phase 2 studies suggest that lurasidone has no significant increase in QTc prolongation with minimal risk of hyperprolactinemia and the metabolic syndrome.

Treatment approaches to early episode psychosis

The management of patients with early psychosis is multifaceted and is discussed in detail in chapter 17. Here we address only the pharmacological aspects of care. The AAPs have gained ascendancy in the pharmacological management of early episode psychosis and are promoted by most clinicians as the drugs of first choice in such patients. Box 1.1 provides a summary of general approaches for the management of early episode psychosis. Although there are no consistently established significant differences in short-term efficacy between typical and AAPs in early psychosis, there is a significant and predictable difference in adverse side effects between each agent (33). Figure 1.1 shows a treatment algorithm for a patient in their first episode of illness: it should be noted that novel atypical agents are promoted first line and if one atypical fails or produces intolerable side effects, then a trial of at least one other different novel atypical is suggested before reverting to either a typical agent or clozapine. In some countries, notably France, amisulpride is used as a first-line treatment for many patients and has a low side-effect burden, although hyperprolactinemia is relatively common and EPSEs can occur at higher doses (Table 1.3). Antipsychotic-induced weight gain is three to four times more common in younger, first-episode patients and its impact on the user should not be underestimated. Some clinicians believe that typical agents are more potent with lower risks of weight gain and metabolic side effects than most atypicals for some patients and will use these before clozapine; others believe that the particular benefits, notably greater improvement in negative symptom scores (34) that can accrue with clozapine treatment should sway clinicians to use this agent earlier in treatment (35). In the recent European First Episode Schizophrenia Trial (EUFEST), 498 patients with schizophreniform disorder or first-episode schizophrenia were randomized to open-label of either low dose haloperidol (1–4 mg/day), or one of four AAPs: amisulpride, olanzapine, quetiapine, or ziprasidone and followed over a 1-year period. There was overall equivalent efficacy across agents, and notably low dose haloperidol or AAP s had equivalence in improving cognitive function, but treatment discontinuation was the greatest for haloperidol compared with the other four AAPs.

Box 1.1   Summary of general approaches for the management of early episode psychosis.

Early intervention is associated with significant symptom reduction

Minimize deterioration

Reduce stigma from symptoms, aiming for complete remission

Consider patient preference as high priority and use the lowest effective antipsychotic dose to establish treatment acceptance and reduce the severity of side effects

Provide adequate duration of treatment and optimum long-term dosing

Monitor treatment and manage side effects appropriately

Minimize obvious side effects that might make the patient appear abnormal: extrapyramidal side effects, which reduce compliance and engagement

Exclude organic cause

Initial medication-free period of at least 48 hours, if possible

First-line treatment: low dose of atypical antipsychotic

Risperidone 1–2 mg daily
Olanzapine 5–10 mg daily
Aripiprazole 10–15 mg daily
Quetiapine 300–600 mg daily
Ziprasidone 80–120 mg daily
Amisulpride 400–600 mg daily
Paliperidone 3–6 mg daily

Good response

Partial or little response after 2–4 weeks

Continue for 12 months. Withdraw gradually after this, with careful monitoring

Good response

Increase dose *:

Risperidone 2–4 mg daily
Olanzapine 10–20 mg daily
Aripiprazole 15–30 mg daily
Quetiapine 600–800 mg daily
Ziprasidone 120–160 mg daily
Amisulpride 600–800 mg daily
Paliperidone 6–9 mg daily
Continue for at least 3–6 weeks

Partial or little response

Alternative atypical antipsychotic

Augmentation
Sodium valproate (serum level >50 micromol/L)
Lithium (serum level 0.5–1.0 mmol/L)
(if schizoaffective presentation)

Partial or little response after further 6–8 weeks

Consider trial of 'typical' agent or clozapine

Figure 1.1   Treatment guidelines: early episode psychosis.

Treatment of relapse of psychosis

For patients who are established on a typical antipsychotic and who experience a relapse of psychosis, a suggested treatment algorithm is presented in Figure 1.2. The rationale is that if the prior agent was effective and well tolerated, then that agent should be reinstituted. Having said this, many clinicians would consider relapse as an opportunity to change to an AAP. Certainly, if the patient was either inadequately controlled or experienced EPSEs or TD on the typical agent, a change to an atypical should be considered. It is also important to ascertain the cause of the relapse; if it was due to nonadherence to medication then this would need to be investigated, and if side effects were a contributing factor this would sway one to change to an AAP. A systematic review and meta-analysis of randomized-controlled trials (RCTs) (36) revealed that rates of relapse and overall treatment failure were moderately but significantly lower with AAPs.

Treatment resistance and the place of clozapine

In terms of response to medication, the criteria for treatment resistance in schizophrenia usually include at least two failed treatment trials with antipsychotics from at least two different classes (37,38). The domains usually assessed are psychotic symptoms but given the scope of symptoms and disabilities associated with schizophrenia, it is important to look at the individual in a holistic manner, including associated symptoms such as depression and anxiety, as well as relationships, social and occupational functioning, and overall quality of life. Here, attention is given to the role of medication in treatment resistance. First, the role of clozapine is considered and then pharmacological augmentation strategies. The reader is referred to other chapters in this book for broader psychological and social aspects of the treatment of persistent symptoms and disabilities in schizophrenia. Chapter 18 discusses a comprehensive approach to a patient with treatment resistant schizophrenia.

As discussed above, clozapine was the first AAP in that it does not cause EPSEs at therapeutic doses and is associated with an apparently negligible rate of TD. It also appears to have particular benefits in the treatment of patients who have failed to respond to other antipsychotics, that is, those who are considered to be treatment resistant (39). Indeed, a recent review from the World Psychiatric Association Section on Pharmacopsychiatry, utilizing data from 1600 RCTs in the treatment of schizophrenia, concluded that clozapine is more efficacious than other antipsychotics in treatment-refractory schizophrenia (40). There is also some evidence to suggest that clozapine has particular efficacy against the negative symptoms of schizophrenia and might enhance some domains of cognitive function (chaps. 3 and 4). Clozapine's particular place in the management of treatment-resistant patients has been

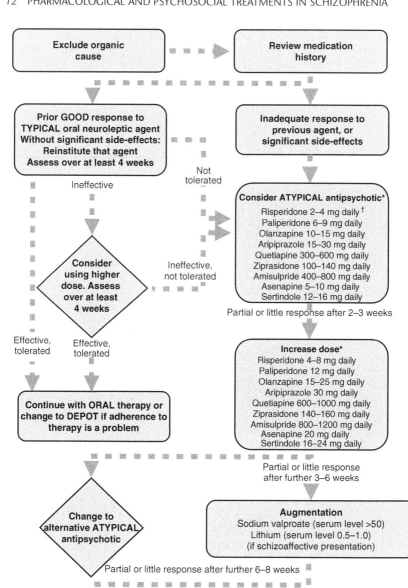

Figure 1.2 *Treatment guidelines: relapse or exacerbation of schizophrenia.*

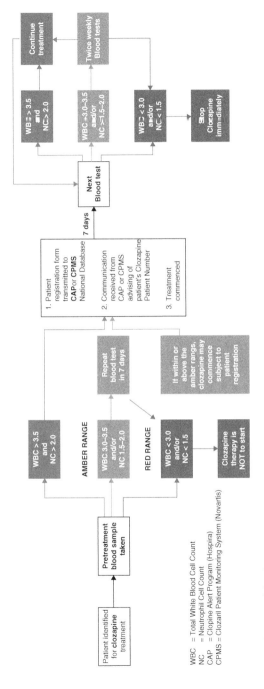

Figure 1.3   Flow chart for treatment commencement and maintenance on clozapine.

WBC = Total White Blood Cell Count
NC   = Neutrophil Cell Count
CAP = Clopine Alert Program (Hospira)
CPMS = Clozaril Patient Monitoring System (Novartis)

Notes for the use of clozapine

1. All patients must be registered with either the CAP or CPMS National Database.

2. All patients must have blood tests at least weekly for 18 weeks, then at least every four weeks thereafter.

3. Extra blood tests, immediately and twice weekly, are required if symptoms of infection are observed e.g. sore throat and mouth ulcers.

4. If treatment is stopped for non-haematological reasons, patients on weekly monitoring should continue blood-monitoring atleast weekly for four weeks: patients on monthly monitoring should have one further blood count four weeks after ceasing treatment.

5. Only medical officers and pharmacists registered with the CAP or CPMS Databases may prescribe and dispense clozapine.

6. For further information please refer to the CAP (Hospira) or CPMS (Novartis) Protocol. *N.B.Protocol details may vary in different countries.Check with national clozapine registration centre prior to prescribing.*

underscored by the recent CATIE trial (41). In that study, patients who received clozapine after discontinuation of two previous antipsychotics were less likely to discontinue treatment due to inadequate therapeutic response, than patients who received quetiapine, risperidone or olanzapine. In addition, there is clinical evidence suggesting that clozapine may be useful for those at high risk of suicide or aggression (42,43).

Clozapine does, however, produce a number of side effects that limit its use. Most dangerous of these is agranulocytosis, which can be fatal. This potential hazard is addressed by blood monitoring, as outlined in Figure 1.3 (note that monitoring regulations differ between countries, but the principles remain the same). Other side effects include sedation, weight gain, sialorrhea and lowering of the seizure threshold, which can result in convulsions, expressly at high doses. Hypotension, tachycardia, and cardiac conduction abnormalities can also occur (44). It should be noted that some or all of these last-mentioned effects can occur to a greater or lesser extent with many other antipsychotics (Tables 1.2, 1.3, 1.4). There is also a risk, albeit low, of potentially fatal myocarditis (45) and cardiomyopathy (46) for which some centres have introduced regular cardiac monitoring for patients on clozapine (47,48).

Furthermore, patients who discontinue clozapine abruptly often experience a withdrawal reaction, in part mediated by cholinergic rebound (49) and in part due to rapid displacement of clozapine from dopamine receptors (50). There is also clinical evidence that once patients have discontinued clozapine and relapsed, their chance of responding to rechallenge with clozapine is reduced. Because of these factors, patients on clozapine should be accepting of treatment and their close cooperation with the treating team is important. A suggested process for engagement and monitoring of patients of clozapine has been published (44). In cases where there is an inadequate response to clozapine, a number of augmentation strategies might be considered.

Augmentation strategies

Another approach to treatment resistance is augmentation with another psychotropic agent. Whilst often applied in clinical practice, there is still a very limited research database on such strategies, and these interventions are usually guided by clinical intuition and experience. One issue that is particularly controversial is the use of typical and atypical agents together. This is perhaps most common in people who are on a typical depot medication and an oral atypical. While an anathema to pharmacological purists, and not to be promoted in most cases, some patients do seem to benefit from such combinations and withdrawal of either agent can result in relapse. Many clinicians use other combinations of antipsychotics. In treatment-resistant patients, the combination of clozapine and a relatively specific, "tight" D2-binding AAP, such as risperidone (51–54), sulpiride (55), or amisulpride (56,57) has gained some popularity on the basis of both efficacy and that the complementarity of

Table 1.4 Depot antipsychotics – relative Side –effects

Drug	Adult max. dose	Half-life	Time to steady state	Anticholinergic	Cardiac	EPSE	Hypotension	Sedation
Fluphenazine	100 mg 2/52	14–100 days	6–12 wk	++	++	+++	+	++
Flupenthixol	400 mg 1/52	17 days	10–12 wk	+++	+/-	++	-/-	+
Fluspirilene	20 mg 1/52	7–9 days	5–6 wk	+	+	++	++	++
Haloperidol	300 mg 4/52	18–21 days	10–12 wk	+	++	+++	+	++
Olanzapine pamoate	300 mg 2/52	30 days	12 wk	+	0	0	0	++
Paliperidone palmitate	150 mg 4/52	25–49 days	16–20 wk	0	0	+	+	+
Pipothiazine	200 mg 4/52	14–21 days	8–12 wk	++	++	++	+	+
Risperidone consta	50 mg 2/52	4–6 days	6–8 wk	0	0	+	+	+
Zuclopenthixol	600 mg 1/52	17–21 days	10–12 wk	++	+	+++	+	++

+++ = Marked effect; ++ = Moderate effect; + = Mild effect; +/- = Minimal effect at usual therapeutic doses; 0 = Little or nothing reported; ? = No information available.

Source: Adapted from Ref. 125.

receptor blockade profile reduces common clozapine side effects such as seda-tion, weight gain, and other metabolic problems; there is, however, a risk of other side effects evolving with the addition of the new agent and these need to be monitored (58).

A Cochrane review by Cipriani (59) implied that the evidence against ris-peridone, sulpiride, ziprasidone, or quetiapine augmentation are not robust enough to warrant any conclusion about the relative merits of these combina-tions; whereas a review by Wang et al. (55) concluded there was some support (albeit not definitive) for the combination of clozapine plus sulpiride being more effective than clozapine alone. Clozapine augmentation with aripipra-zole can lead to weight loss or at least halt further weight gain without causing clinical deterioration (60,61). Overall, there is scant evidence of efficacy and safety regarding adjunctive psychopharmacological treatment for clozapine-resistant patients. The evidence supporting clozapine augmentation is limited by the small sample size of clinical trials, the heterogeneity of outcome mea-sures, and methodological designs (62). Barbui's meta-analysis showed the open studies favored clozapine combination in both long- and short-term tri-als, while the blinded studies demonstrated no advantage for clozapine com-binations of either duration (63).

Another fairly common strategy is to augment with a *mood stabilizer*, usu-ally lithium, carbamazepine, or sodium valproate, especially in individuals who show an affective component to their illness. Lithium can increase the neurotoxicity of antipsychotics, notably clozapine, and thus its use in com-bination requires caution. Carbamazepine can be problematic as it induces the metabolism of a number of hepatic enzymes, thus affecting levels of other drugs; it is relatively contraindicated with clozapine, due to the pro-pensity to bone marrow suppression. Furthermore, Cochrane reviews of lithium (64), valproate, (65) and carbamazepine (66) could find no clear evi-dence of efficacy as adjunctive agents. Clozapine augmentation with lamotrigine has been suggested to be useful in enhancing efficacy (67), but study outcomes are not unequivocal, in part at least due to differences in design and inclusion criteria (68); further well-designed studies would be valuable.

Evidence that the addition of *antidepressants* to antipsychotics is useful for enduring negative symptoms is equivocal (58). SSRIs such as citalopram (69), fluvoxamine (70), or fluoxetine (71) when combined with typical antipsy-chotics have shown some improvement in negative symptoms, but again not all studies concur. A study comparing mirtazapine with placebo in addition to haloperidol in patients with stable schizophrenia but prominent negative symptoms showed a significant reduction (43%) in negative symptoms in the mirtazapine group with no significant effect on depressive symptoms (72). A replication study failed to show any significant improvement in PANSS scores or any of the secondary outcome measures at any stage during the 6-week trial (73). Care needs to be taken with some combinations, for example with fluvoxamine and clozapine—the former causes elevations in the serum levels of the latter due to CYP1A2 inhibition. Also, some tricyclics have been associated with an exacerbation of psychotic symptoms in some individuals. Other augmentation strategies have also been investigated, with mixed results: those targeting negative symptoms are outlined in chapter 3 and those aiming to enhance cognition are in chapter 4.

Electroconvulsive therapy (ECT) has also been used in treatment-resistant cases, in combination with antipsychotics, and there is some evidence for additional benefits in terms of antipsychotic effects as well as prevention of relapse (74,75). A recent retrospective chart review, by Levy-Rueff and colleagues of 19 patients with schizophrenia or schizoaffective disorder nonresponsive or only partially responsive to pharmacological agents, showed improvements in mood, delusions, anorexia, and suicidal ideation, with ECT (76).

Switching antipsychotics

Reasons for considering a change in antipsychotics include symptom response and side-effect burden. Any change carries with it the possibility of relapse, and patients and their families should be fully informed of this before any such changeover is instituted. Close monitoring of mental state is also required during this phase. Ultimately, the decision about switching depends upon the following:

- Efficacy of current medication, in treating both positive and negative symptoms
- Side effects being experienced—emergent TD is particularly worrisome in patients on typical agents
- Clinical judgment
- Patient preference

In general, a slow crossover over 2–6 weeks is best tolerated, especially if:

- switching from a high dose to a high dose agent;
- changing from a "loose" D2-binding agent, such as clozapine or quetiapine; and/or
- the side-effect/receptor-binding profiles of the two agents are markedly different (Tables 1.2, 1.3, 1.4).

Box 1.2 outlines specific problems that might be encountered in switching and the suggested strategies to deal with these.

In patients on depots, the usual strategy is to commence the new agent in the place of the depot at the time that the next depot was due.

Box 1.2 Problems with switching antipsychotics.

The new agent is not effective or has insufficient tolerability: Since antipsychotic efficacy may take some time, do not abandon the new agent too quickly. In addition, side effects tend to be worse initially; hence, try to deal with them in the short term rather than abandon the new agent too soon. Showing patients the schematic below can assist in the educational process in this regard

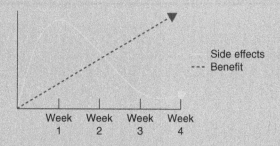

Cholinergic rebound: Flu-like symptoms with malaise, agitation, anxiety, insomnia, and GI upset can occur if switching from agent with high M1 binding (e.g., clozapine) to one with a low M1 binding (e.g., risperidone, amisulpride, aripiprazole). Slow crossover is required and use of short-term anticholinergic such as benztropine or benzhexol is recommended

"Rebound" psychosis or extrapyramidal side effects: More likely to occur if switching from "loosely bound" agent such as clozapine or quetiapine and normally occurs quicker than would expect from true psychotic relapse. Cross-titrate slowly and symptomatic treatment with beta-blocker or benzodiazepine is warranted

"Rebound insomnia": More likely if changing from more sedating agents (olanzapine, clozapine) to less sedating agents (risperidone, amisulpride, aripiprazole). Administration of the new medication in the morning rather than the evening and short-term hypnotic such as zopiclone is acceptable

The place of depot antipsychotics

As detailed in chapter 10, adherence among patients with schizophrenia and related disorders is often suboptimal, for a number of complex and inter-related reasons. Addressing adherence concerns requires multifaceted strategies, as outlined in chapter 10. Depot formulations of antipsychotics might be part of these strategies. Depot preparations can also provide a convenient alternative to taking multiple daily oral doses of antipsychotics and some patients simply prefer them. Depots are formulated either in an oily base (typical antipsychotics), an aqueous solution containing the active agent in a matrix of glycolic acid

Box 1.3 Choosing appropriate antipsychotic agents for patients at high risk for metabolic problems.

Antipsychotics with a low propensity for weight gain should be initiated for patients
  With diabetes
  At high risk for diabetes
  Treated with other medications that may increase metabolic risks (e.g., depo-provera, valproate, lithium)
Clozapine, olanzapine have highest risk of weight gain, diabetes, dyslipidemia
Risperidone, paliperidone, quetiapine have intermediate risk
Aripiprazole, amisulpride, ziprasidone, asenapine appear to have lowest risk

Box 1.4 Strategies for patients who develop features of the metabolic syndrome while on antipsychotics.

Education about healthy diet and lifestyle
Instituting a specific dietary and exercise program
Switching to an antipsychotic that has not been associated with significant weight gain or diabetes
Addition of a medication to prevent weight gain or promote weight loss (e.g., metformin)
Referring to specialised services, where appropriate

(risperidone), or in an aqueous nanosuspension (paliperidone), which should be injected deep into the deltoid or gluteal muscle. These formulations are effective for 1–4 weeks, depending on the constitution and the individual. The main depot formulations are detailed in Table 1.4. Although a meta-analysis by Adams et al. (77) concluded that there is little difference between the different typical depot formulations in terms of efficacy and side effects, some patients do seem to benefit and/or tolerate particular agents better than others, and failure of response and/or intolerable side effects of one depot should not preclude the trial of another.

Risperdal-consta, the first long-acting AAP injection became available in 2003. Several short- and long-term studies have provided evidence for its safety and efficacy. A 12-week placebo-controlled trial of acute patients by Kane and colleagues (78) showed good symptom improvement and a low incidence of side effects. In addition, a separate 1-year double-blind study of two

Box 1.5 Guidelines for dealing with complications of treatment of patients with schizophrenia.

Agitation

Add short-term oral benzodiazepine e.g., clonazepam 1–2 mg or diazepam 5–10 mg or lorazepam 1–2.5 mg

Arousal/acute behavioural disturbance

Specific strategies as outlined in chapter 8

Insomnia

Add short-term oral benzodiazepine e.g., temazepam 10–20 mg; clonazepam 1–2 mg; diazepam 5–10 mg; or hypnotic e.g., zopiclone 7.5 mg

Acute dystonic reaction

Add anticholinergic agent e.g., benztropine 2 mg intramuscularly or intravenously, up to a maximum of 6 mg in 24 h

Chronic Parkinsonism

Add regular oral anticholinergic agent e.g., benztropine 1–2 mg/day, benzhexol 2 mg tds, biperiden 1–2 mg tds

Akathisia

Reduce dose of antipsychotic if possible. If still present add propranolol 10 mg bd, an anticholinergic, clonidine 50–100 mcg bd, mirtazepine 15–30 mg nocte, or a benzodiazepine

Neuroleptic malignant syndrome

After this syndrome has occurred and been treated consider atypical antipsychotic (AAP) or clozapine; monitor closely

Tardive dyskinesia

Consider changing to novel AAP or clozapine

Persistent negative symptoms (chap. 3)

Determine whether due to primary (deficit) symptoms, or to secondary negative symptoms (e.g., response to positive symptoms, medication induced or due to depression)

If secondary ensure optimal treatment of positive symptoms and/or underlying depression, consider changing to AAP

If primary consider change to low-dose amisulpride (reasonable evidence in deficit syndrome), asenapine (some evidence of efficacy) or clozapine (good evidence for efficacy)

Intervening persistent depression

Add antidepressant e.g., SSRI

Continual nonadherence (chap. 10)

Establish reasons for nonadherence. Educate patient and family about rationale for ongoing treatment. Educate patient about side effects of antipsychotic medication and treat these vigorously. Treat any underlying depression. Consider role for AAP. If justified, consider depot antipsychotic

Illicit substance use

Counselling and specific measures (chap. 6). Clozapine might have a particular role doses (25 mg and 50 mg) of long-acting risperidone injection by Simpson (79) also showed low relapse and rehospitalization rates.

Olanzapine pamoate is a long-acting depot preparation of olanzapine. When administered intramuscularly, it has an elimination half-life of approximately 30 days, allowing it to be given at 2- or 4-weekly intervals. Olanzapine pamoate depot injection has shown comparable efficacy to oral olanzapine in several studies (80). However, during its clinical trials a post-injection delirium sedation syndrome was observed in about 1% of patients, possibly due to inadvertent intravascular injection of a portion of the dose; symptoms included excessive sedation, confusion, dizziness, and altered speech. As a result, a risk management plan is mandatory in order to reduce such adverse events; it must be administered by qualified personnel in settings where a post-injection observation period or 2–3 hours by medical personnel is available (81–83).

Paliperidone palmitate depot utilizes the "NanoCrystal" technology whereby the active nanoparticles of paliperidone are slowly released into the systemic circulation. It is available as prefilled syringes embracing a wide dose range (25, 50, 75, 100, and 150 mg eq.), and requires no refrigeration, reconstitution, or oral antipsychotic supplementation. It can be initiated the day after discontinuing previous oral antipsychotic treatment but requires loading dose strategies of two deltoid injections administered 1 week apart to achieve therapeutic concentration rapidly (84). Upon administration, the release of paliperidone starts as early as day 1, reaches maximum plasma concentration at day 13 and lasts for as long as 126 days (85). In patients switching from other depots (including long-acting risperidone and olanzapine), paliperidone palmitate dosing should be initiated at the time of what would have been the next scheduled injection of the previous depot, and continued monthly thereafter (84,86). Paliperidone palmitate treatment is generally well tolerated across the dose range (25–150 mg eq.) and efficacious in improving the symptoms of acute exacerbation of schizophrenia (randomized, double-blind, placebo-controlled trials of 9–13 weeks' duration) (87–90). As maintenance therapy, paliperidone palmitate (25–100 mg eq.) has been shown to be significantly more effective than placebo in delaying the time to first relapse in stable schizophrenia patients (91,92).

What is also not often appreciated is that some of the typical depots take up to 3 months to reach a steady state (93). Various strategies might be employed to address this problem, including a reduced dose interval (e.g., weekly for 4 weeks, then fortnightly) or (more usually and more safely) supplementation with an oral agent during this phase. Long-acting injectable risperidone, on the other hand, has no significant drug release for the first 3–4 weeks, with a peak at 4–6 weeks; with repeated injection every 2 weeks, steady state levels are usually reached by weeks 6 to 8 (94). Thus, oral cover is needed for the first 3–4 weeks, and tapered over weeks 4–5. Olanzapine and paliperidone depots, in contrast, do not require oral supplementation.

Complications of antipsychotic treatment and how to deal with them

The main side effects of the antipsychotic agents in current use are shown in Tables 1.2, 1.3, 1.4. These side effects can be very debilitating for the patient and can lead to nonadherence. Thus, patients should be warned about the possibility of side effects, and every effort should be made to recognize and treat side effects as soon as they appear.

As discussed in chapter 6, an association between *metabolic side effects* and antipsychotics, particularly AAPs, is well publicised (4–6,95–97). Antipsychotic-induced weight gain has been suggested as an important modifiable contributor to the high rates of obesity in this population. Importantly, patients who experience antipsychotic-induced weight increases exhibit elevated rates of morbidity and reduced treatment compliance, even if the psychopharmacological treatment is effective (98). Antipsychotic drug affinities for H1, D2, 5-HT2C, 5-HT1A, $\alpha 1$, and $\alpha 3$ adrenergic receptors are most closely linked to increased weight gain (99,100). The CATIE study found that patients treated with olanzapine had significantly higher levels of glycosylated hemoglobin and blood glucose than those treated with perphenazine, quetiapine, risperidone, or ziprasidone (6,98). In addition, clozapine, olanzapine, and to a lesser extent, quetiapine are associated with elevations in triglyceride and total cholesterol levels, whereas risperidone, aripiprazole, and asenapine have minimal or no effect on these lipid parameters (25,101,102). It should be underlined that low potency typical antipsychotics including chlorpromazine also showed a comparatively high risk of inducing weight gain (103). Table 1.5 shows relative risks of common side effects from the use of antipsychotics.

Findings from both short- and long-term studies of bifeprunox showed a mean reduction of up to 24% in fasting triglyceride levels and of 8% in fasting total cholesterol levels (104–106); thus, the intrinsic metabolic activity of bifeprunox deserves further exploration. Pharmacological treatments such as metformin and topiramate (107) have been tried to reverse or prevent antipsychotic-induced weight gain. Preliminary evidence from a recent systematic review showed that metformin therapy is safe and effective in abrogating weight gain, and also improves insulin sensitivity, abnormal glucose metabolism and HbA1c in both adult and adolescent patients taking AAPs (108–110). It should be considered in patients with additional risk factors such as personal or family history of metabolic dysfunction (96).

As discussed in chapter 6, rates of *tobacco addiction* in individuals with psychiatric disorders continue to remain alarmingly high despite substantial decreases in smoking in the general population. A recent meta-analysis review by De Leon (111) reported that the rate of smoking in people with schizophrenia was at least five times higher than the general population. Kao and colleagues (112) also revealed that smokers with schizophrenia had higher rates

Table 1.5   Relative risks of common side effects among antipsychotics

Side effects	*Relative risks* *High ----→ low*
EPSEs	High potency typical antipsychotics > medium potency typical antipsychotics = risperidone = paliperidone = amisulpride > low potency typical antipsychotics = asenapine > olanzapine = ziprasidone > quetiapine > clozapine
Weight gain	Clozapine = olanzapine > low potency typical antipsychotics > risperidone = paliperidone = quetiapine > medium potency typical antipsychotics > asenapine > high potency typical antipsychotics = amisulpride = aripiprazole = ziprasidone
Hyperprolactinemia/sexual side effects	Risperidone = paliperidone = amisulpride = high potency typical antipsychotics > olanzapine > ziprasidone = asenapine > quetiapine = clozapine > aripiprazole
QTc prolongation	Thioridazine > ziprasidone > quetiapine = risperidone = paliperidone = amisulpride = olanzapine = haloperidol ≥ clozapine Aripiprazole, asenapine do not appreciably prolong QTc interval[a]

[a]Asenapine and amisulpride data added by current authors based on clinical experience.
Source: Adapted from Ref. 33.

of hospitalization, lifetime suicide attempts, antipsychotic treatment side effects, psychopathology, impulsivity, depression, anxiety, and suicidal risk than nonsmokers with schizophrenia. In terms of pharmacological approaches to nicotine addiction, different forms of nicotine replacement therapy (NRT) and bupropion are the usual first-line treatments. Data from well-designed RCTs suggested that bupropion SR, with or without NRT, can be a helpful tool for establishing short-term abstinence within the context of a supportive environment (113–118). Bupropion has the potential to cause mood dysregulation in some patients and this has to be borne in mind. Varenicline is a specific partial agonist of the α4-α2 nicotinic acetylcholine receptor (119) and a full agonist at the α7 receptor; it has proven efficacy in increasing abstinence rates among cigarette smokers (120). It stimulates the release of sufficient dopamine to reduce craving and withdrawal while simultaneously acting as a partial antagonist, thereby blocking the binding of nicotine to the receptors and consequently the reinforcing effects of nicotine intake (121), and reducing the likelihood of relapse. There is some risk of serious neuropsychiatric events including changes in behavior, hostility, agitation, depressed mood, and suicidal thoughts or actions, based on postmarketing reports, while a recent meta-analysis by Singh et al. (122) raised concerns about the potential for an increased risk of serious adverse cardiovascular events associated with varenicline. Having said this, the authors' experience is that varenicline can be safely used in patients with schizophrenia, as long as careful monitoring of mental state is in place; we suggest it being used only if NRT has failed. As always, the patient needs to be fully informed regarding risks and benefits with any smoking cessation strategies and the nonpharmacological interventions provided.

Hyperprolactinemia is a side effect of a number of antipsychotics, as discussed earlier. It can be associated with reproductive dysfunction and hypogonadism in both male and female patients. In women, it can result in galactorrhea and or menstrual disturbance such as oligomenorrhea or amenorrhoea. In men, hyperprolactinemia can cause loss of libido and erectile dysfunction as a result of testosterone deficiency (123). Long-term consequences of hypogonadism include premature bone loss which may lead to osteoporosis and increased risk of minimal trauma fracture. Baseline and regular monitoring of prolactin plasma level is recommended for patients who are taking those high-risk antipsychotic medications. Switching to a prolactin-sparing agent should be considered as the initial treatment choice for patients with antipsychotic-induced hyperprolactinemia. Sex steroid replacement and dopamine agonists may also be used as treatment of secondary hypogonadism and the resultant bone loss, as discussed by Inder and Castle (123).

Another particularly dangerous, though rare, side effect is *neuroleptic malignant syndrome,* usually associated with high doses of typical antipsychotics in an aroused patient, though it has also been reported with low doses and with atypical agents (124). The syndrome is characterized by muscle rigidity, pyrexia, autonomic instability, and alteration in consciousness; blood tests show an elevated white cell count and a raised creatine phosphokinase level (124). Immediate withdrawal of the antipsychotic agent and treatment, either supportive or with bromocriptine and/or dantrolene, is required (124).

Conclusions

Schizophrenia remains a prevalent and highly disabling problem and comorbidities are common among this patient group, which can contribute to early mortality and a poorer quality of life. AAPs mostly provide good symptom control with a lower propensity to motor side effects than many of the older agents. The emergence of metabolic disorders which have resulted from antipsychotic treatment requires a coordinated, multidisciplinary management approach to ensure the optimal care of these patients. Despite recent advances in psycho-pharmacological treatment, there remain a number of important barriers to improve the individualized treatment for persons with schizophrenia and optimizing their opportunity for recovery from the illness. Pharmacological treatment remains only one part of what should be a comprehensive biopsychosocial approach to the management of people with this group of conditions. Other chapters in this book address these components of care.

References

1. Leiberman JA, Stroup TS, McEvoy JP, et al. Effectiveness of antipsychotic drugs in patients with chronic schizophrenia. NEJM 2005; 353: 1209–23.
2. Miyamoto S, Duncan GE, Marx CE, et al. Treatment of Schizophrenia: a critical review of pharmacology and mode of action of antipsychotic. Mol Psychiatry 2005; 10: 79–104.
3. Stahl SM. Selecting an atypical antipsychotic by combining clinical experience with guidelines from clinical trials. J Clin Psychiatry 1999; 60: 31–41.
4. Jones PB, Barnes TR, Davies L, et al. Randomized controlled trial of the effect on Quality of Life of second- vs first-generation antipsychotic drugs in schizophrenia: cost Utility of the Latest Antipsychotic Drugs in Schizophrenia Study (CUtLASS 1). Arch Gen Psychiatry 2006; 63: 1079–87.
5. Kahn RS, Fleischhacker WW, Boter H, et al. Effectiveness of antipsychotic drugs in first-episode schizophrenia and schizophreniform disorder: an open randomised clinical trial. Lancet 2008; 371: 1085–97.
6. Lieberman JA, Stroup TS, McEvoy JP, et al. Effectiveness of antipsychotic drugs in patients with chronic schizophrenia. N Engl J Med 2005; 353: 1209–23.
7. Virani AS, Bezchlibnyk-Butler KZ, Jeffries JJ, Procyshyn RM. Clinical Handbook of Psychotropic Drugs. Seatle: Hogrefe & Huber Publishers, 2011.
8. Leucht S, Pitschel-Walz G, Engel RR, Kissling W. Amisulpride, an unusual 'atypical' antipsychotic: a meta-analysis of randomized controlled trials. Am J Psychiatry 2002; 159: 180–90.
9. Newman-Tancredi A, Cussac D, Depoortere R. Neuropharmacological profile of bifeprunox: merits and limitations in comparison with other third-generation antipsychotics. Curr Opin Investig Drugs 2007; 8: 539–54.
10. Casey DE, Sands EE, Heisterberg J, Yang HM. Efficacy and safety of bifeprunox in patients with an acute exacerbation of schizophrenia: results from a randomized, double-blind, placebo-controlled, multicenter, dose-finding study. Psychopharmacology (Berl) 2008; 200: 317–31.
11. Cosi C, Carilla-Durand E, Assie MB, et al. Partial agonist properties of the antipsychotics SSR181507, aripiprazole and bifeprunox at dopamine D2 receptors: G protein activation and prolactin release. Eur J Pharmacol 2006; 535: 135–44.
12. Bishara D, Taylor D. Upcoming agents for the treatment of schizophrenia: mechanism of action, efficacy and tolerability. Drugs 2008; 68: 2269–92.
13. Stahl SM, Mignon L. Antipsychotics: Treating Psychosis, Mania and Depression. 2nd edn. New York: Cambridge University Press, 2010.
14. Conley R, Gupta SK, Sathyan G. Clinical spectrum of the osmotic-controlled release oral delivery system (OROS), an advanced oral delivery form. Curr Med Res Opin 2006; 22: 1879–92.
15. Spina E, Cavallaro R. The pharmacology and safety of paliperidone extended-release in the treatment of schizophrenia. Expert Opin Drug Saf 2007; 6: 651–62.

16. Marder SR, Kramer M, Ford L, et al. Efficacy and safety of paliperidone extended-release tablets: results of a 6-week, randomized, placebo-controlled study. Biol Psychiatry 2007; 62: 1363–70.
17. Canuso CM, Dirks B, Carothers J, et al. Randomized, double-blind, placebo-controlled study of paliperidone extended-release and quetiapine in inpatients with recently exacerbated schizophrenia. Am J Psychiatry 2009; 166: 691–701.
18. Kramer M, Simpson G, Maciulis V, et al. Paliperidone extended-release tablets for prevention of symptom recurrence in patients with schizophrenia: a randomized, double-blind, placebo-controlled study. J Clin Psychopharmacol 2007; 27: 6–14.
19. Emsley R, Berwaerts J, Eerdekens M, et al. Efficacy and safety of oral paliperidone extended-release tablets in the treatment of acute schizophrenia: pooled data from three 52-week open-label studies. Int Clin Psychopharmacol 2008; 23: 343–56.
20. Kramer M, Simpson G, Maciulis V, et al. One-year open-label safety and efficacy study of paliperidone extended-release tablets in patients with schizophrenia. CNS Spectr 2010; 15: 506–14.
21. Citrome L. Iloperidone for schizophrenia: a review of the efficacy and safety profile for this newly commercialised second-generation antipsychotic. Int J Clin Pract 2009; 63: 1237–48.
22. Citrome L. Iloperidone: chemistry, pharmacodynamics, pharmacokinetics and metabolism, clinical efficacy, safety and tolerability, regulatory affairs, and an opinion. Expert Opin Drug Metab Toxicol 2010; 6: 12.
23. Kane JM, Lauriello J, Laska E, Di Marino M, Wolfgang CD. Long-term efficacy and safety of iloperidone: results from 3 clinical trials for the treatment of schizophrenia. J Clin Psychopharmacol 2008; 28: S29–35.
24. Cutler AJ, Kalali AH, Weiden JP, et al. Four week, double-blind, placebo- and ziprasidone-controlled trial of iloperidone in patients with acute exacerbation of schizophrenia. J Clin Psychopharmacol 2008; 28(2 Suppl 1): S20–S8.
25. Potkin SG, Cohen M, Panagides J. Efficacy and tolerability of asenapine in acute schizophrenia: a placebo- and risperidone-controlled trial. J Clin Psychiatry 2007; 68: 1492–500.
26. Kane JM, Mackle M, Snow-Adami L, et al. A randomized placebo-controlled trial of Asenapine for the prevention of relapse of schizophrenia after long-term treatment. J Clin Psychiatry 2011; 72: 349–55.
27. Kane JM, Cohen M, Zhao J, Alphs L, Panagides J. Efficacy and safety of Asenapine in a placebo- and Haloperidol-controlled trial in patients with acute exacerbation of schizophrenia. J Clin Psychopharmacol 2010; 30: 106–15.
28. Schoemaker J, Naber D, Vrijland P, Emsley R. Long-term assessment of Asenapine vs. Olanzapine in patients with schizophrenia or schizoaffective disorder. Pharmacopsychiatry 2010; 43: 138–46.
29. Schering-Plough. Full prescribing information: Saphris (asenapine), 2009.
30. Citrome L. Lurasidone for schizophrenia: a brief review of a new second-generation antipsychotic. Clin Schizophr Relat Psychoses 2011; 4: 251–7.
31. Meyer JM, Loebel AD, Schweizer E. Lurasidone: a new drug in development for schizophrenia. Expert Opin Investig Drugs 2009; 18: 1715–26.
32. Cruz MP. Lurasidone HCl (Latuda), an oral, once-daily atypical antipsychotic agent for the treatment of patients with schizophrenia. P T 2011; 36: 489–92.
33. Buchanan RW, Kreyenbuhl J, Kelly DL, et al. The 2009 Schizophrenia PORT Psychopharmacological treatment recommendations and summary statements. Schizophr Bull 2010; 36: 71–93.
34. Lieberman JA, Phillips M, Gu H, et al. Atypical and conventional antipsychotic drugs in treatment-naive first episodes schizophrenia: a 52 week randomized-trial of clozapine vs chlorpromazine. Neuropsychopharmacology 2003; 28: 995–1003.

35. Remington G. Rational pharmacotherapy in early psychosis. Br J Psychiatry 2005; 187: 77–84.

36. Leucht S, Barnes T, Kissling W, et al. Relapse prevention in schizophrenia with new generation Antipsychotics: a systematic review and exploratory meta-analysis of randomized, controlled trials. Am J Psychiatry 2003; 160: 1209–22.

37. Jones S, Castle DJ. Management of treatment resistant schizophrenia. S Afr Psychiatry Rev 2006; 9: 17–23.

38. Kane J, Honigfeld G, Singer J, Meltzer H. Clozapine for the treatment-resistant schizophrenic. A double-blind comparison with chlorpromazine. Arch Gen Psychiatry 1988; 45: 789–96.

39. Lewis SW, Barnes TR, Davies L, et al. Randomized controlled trial of effect of prescription of clozapine versus other second-generation antipsychotic drugs in resistant schizophrenia. Schizophr Bull 2006; 32: 715–23.

40. Tandon R, Belmaker RH, Gattaz WF, et al. World Psychiatric Association Pharmacopsychiatry Section statement on comparative effectiveness of antipsychotics in the treatment of schizophrenia. Schizophr Res 2008; 100: 20–38.

41. McEvoy JP, Lieberman JA, Stroup TS, et al. Effectiveness of clozapine versus olanzapine, quetiapine, and risperidone in patients with chronic schizophrenia who did not respond to prior atypical antipsychotic treatment. Am J Psychiatry 2006; 163: 600–10.

42. Meltzer HY, Alphs L, Green AI, et al. Clozapine treatment for suicidality in schizophrenia: International Suicide Prevention Trial (InterSePT). Arch Gen Psychiatry 2003; 60: 82–91.

43. Hennen J, Baldessarini RJ. Suicidal risk during treatment with clozapine: a meta-analysis. Schizophr Res 2005; 73: 139–45.

44. Castle DJ, Lambert T, Melbourne S, et al. A clinical monitoring system for clozapine. Australas Psychiatry 2006; 14: 156–68.

45. Ronaldson KJ, Taylor AJ, Fitzgerald PB, et al. Diagnostic characteristics of clozapine-induced myocarditis identified by an analysis of 38 cases and 47 controls. J Clin Psychiatry 2010; 71: 976–81.

46. Kilian JG, Kerr K, Lawrence C, Celermajer DS. Myocarditis and cardiomyopathy associated with clozapine. Lancet 1999; 354: 1841–5.

47. Berk M, Fitzsimons J, Lambert T, et al. Monitoring the safe use of clozapine: a consensus view from Victoria, Australia. CNS Drugs 2007; 21: 117–27.

48. Ronaldson KJ, Fitzgerald PB, Taylor AJ, Topliss DJ, McNeil JJ. A new monitoring protocol for clozapine-induced myocarditis based on an analysis of 75 cases and 94 controls. Aust NZ J Psychiatry 2011; 45: 458–65.

49. Wagstaff AJ, Bryson HM. Clozapine: a review of its pharmacological properties and therapeutic use in patients with schizophrenia who are unresponsive to or intolerant of classical antipsychotics. CNS Drugs 1995; 4: 37–400.

50. Seeman P, Tallerico T. Rapid release of antipsychotic drugs from dopamine D2 receptors: an explanation for low receptor occupancy and early clinical relapse upon withdrawal of clozapine or quetiapine. Am J Psychiatry 1999; 156: 876–84.

51. Josiassen RC, Joseph A, Kohegyi E, et al. Clozapine augmented with risperidone in the treatment of schizophrenia: a randomized, double-blind, placebo-controlled trial. Am J Psychiatry 2005; 162: 130–6.

52. Anil Yagcioglu AE, Kivircik Akdede BB, Turgut TI, et al. A double-blind controlled study of adjunctive treatment with risperidone in schizophrenic patients partially responsive to clozapine: efficacy and safety. J Clin Psychiatry 2005; 66: 63–72.

53. Weiner E, Conley RR, Ball MP, et al. Adjunctive risperidone for partially responsive people with schizophrenia treated with clozapine. Neuropsychopharmacology 2010; 35: 2274–83.

54. Honer WG, Thornton AE, Chen EY, et al. Clozapine alone versus clozapine and risperidone with refractory schizophrenia. N Engl J Med 2006; 354: 472–82.
55. Wang J, Omori Ichiro M, Fenton M, Soares B. Sulpiride augmentation for schizophrenia. Cochrane Database Syst Rev 2010:[Available from: http://www.mrw.interscience.wiley.com/cochrane/clsysrev/articles/CD008125/frame.html].
56. Agelink MW, Kavuk I, Ak I. Clozapine with amisulpride for refractory schizophrenia. Am J Psychiatry 2004; 161: 924–5.
57. Assion HJ, Reinbold H, Lemanski S, Basilowski M, Juckel G. Amisulpride augmentation in patients with schizophrenia partially responsive or unresponsive to clozapine. A randomized, double-blind, placebo-controlled trial. Pharmacopsychiatry 2008; 41: 24–8.
58. Goff DC, Freudenreich O, Evins AE. Augmentation strategies in the treatment of schizophrenia. CNS Spectr 2001; 6: 904; 7–11.
59. Cipriani A, Boso M, Barbui C. Clozapine combined with different antipsychotic drugs for treatment resistant schizophrenia. Cochrane Database Syst Rev 2009: [Available from: http://www.mrw.interscience.wiley.com/cochrane/clsysrev/articles/CD006324/frame.html].
60. Chang JS, Ahn YM, Park HJ, et al. Aripiprazole augmentation in clozapine-treated patients with refractory schizophrenia: an 8-week, randomized, double-blind, placebo-controlled trial. J Clin Psychiatry 2008; 69: 720–31.
61. Fleischhacker WW, Heikkinen ME, Olie JP, et al. Effects of adjunctive treatment with aripiprazole on body weight and clinical efficacy in schizophrenia patients treated with clozapine: a randomized, double-blind, placebo-controlled trial. Int J Neuropsychopharmacol 2010; 13: 1115–25.
62. Sommer IE, Begemann MJ, Temmerman A, Leucht S. Pharmacological augmentation strategies for schizophrenia patients with insufficient response to clozapine: a quantitative literature review. Schizophr Bull 2011; doi: 10.1093/schbul/sbr004.
63. Barbui C, Signoretti A, Mule S, Boso M, Cipriani A. Does the addition of a second antipsychotic drug improve clozapine treatment? Schizophr Bull 2009; 35: 458–68.
64. Leucht S, Kissling W, McGrath J. Lithium for schizophrenia. Cochrane Database Syst Rev 2007:[Available from: http://www.mrw.interscience.wiley.com/cochrane/clsysrev/articles/CD003834/frame.html].
65. Schwarz C, Volz A, Li C, Leucht S. Valproate for schizophrenia. Cochrane Database Syst Rev 2008:[Available from: http://www.mrw.interscience.wiley.com/cochrane/clsysrev/articles/CD004028/frame.html].
66. Leucht S, Kissling W, McGrath J, White P. Carbamazepine for schizophrenia. Cochrane Database Syst Rev 2007:[Available from: http://www.mrw.interscience.wiley.com/cochrane/clsysrev/articles/CD001258/frame.html].
67. Tiihonen J, Wahlbeck K, Kiviniemi V. The efficacy of lamotrigine in clozapine-resistant schizophrenia: a systematic review and meta-analysis. Schizophr Res 2009; 109: 10–4.
68. Premkumar Titus S, Pick J. Lamotrigine for schizophrenia. Cochrane Database Syst Rev 2006: [Available from: http://www.mrw.interscience.wiley.com/cochrane/clsysrev/articles/CD005962/frame.html].
69. Lan XG, Li ZC, Li L. A randomized, placebo-controlled clinical trial of combined citalopram and clozapine in the treatment of negative symptoms of schizophrenia. Chin Ment Health J 2006; 20: 696–8.
70. Silver H, Kushnir M, Kaplan A. Fluvoxamine augmentation in clozapine-resistant schizophrenia: an open pilot study. Biol Psychiatry 1996; 40: 671–4.
71. Buchanan RW, Kirkpatrick B, Bryant N, Ball P, Breier A. Fluoxetine augmentation of clozapine in patients with schizophrenia. Am J Psychiatry 1996; 153: 1625–7.

72. Berk M, Ichim C, Brook S. Efficacy of mirtazapine add on therapy to haloperidol in the treatment of the negative symptoms of schizophrenia: a double-blind randomized placebo-controlled study. Int Clin Psychopharmacol 2001; 16: 87–92.

73. Berk M, Gama CS, Sundram S, et al. Mirtazapine add-on therapy in the treatment of schizophrenia with atypical antipsychotics: a double-blind, randomised, placebo-controlled clinical trial. Hum Psychopharmacol 2009; 24: 233–8.

74. Rasmussen KG. When is ECT indicated in psychiatric disorders. Curr Psychiatry 2002; 1: 21–6.

75. Keuneman R, Weerasundera R, Castle D. The role of ECT in schizophrenia. Australas Psychiatry 2002; 10: 385–8.

76. Levy-Rueff M, Gourevitch R, Loo H, Olie JP, Amado I. Maintenance electroconvulsive therapy: an alternative treatment for refractory schizophrenia and schizoaffective disorders. Psychiatry Res 2010; 175: 280–3.

77. Adams CE, Fenton MKP, Quraishi S, David AS. Systematic meta-review of depot antipsychotic drugs for people with schizophrenia. Br J Psychiatry 2001; 179: 290–9.

78. Kane JM, Eerdekens M, Lindenmayer J-P, et al. Long-acting injectable risperidone: efficacy and safety of the first long-acting atypical antipsychotic. Am J Psychiatry 2003; 160: 1125–32.

79. Simpson GM, Mahmoud RA, Lasser RA, et al. A 1-year Double-blind study of 2 doses of long-acting Risperidone in stable patients with schizophrenia or schizoaffective disorder. J Clin Psychiatry 2006; 67: 1194–203.

80. Kane JM, Detke HC, Naber D, et al. Olanzapine long-acting injection: a 24-week, randomized, double-blind trial of maintenance treatment in patients with schizophrenia. Am J Psychiatry 2010; 167: 181–9.

81. Citrome L. Olanzapine pamoate: a stick in time? A review of the efficacy and safety profile of a new depot formulation of a second-generation antipsychotic. Int J Clin Pract 2009; 63: 140–50.

82. Detke HC, McDonnell DP, Brunner E, et al. Post-injection delirium/sedation syndrome in patients with schizophrenia treated with olanzapine long-acting injection, I: analysis of cases. BMC Psychiatry 2010; 10: 43.

83. McDonnell DP, Detke HC, Bergstrom RF, et al. Post-injection delirium/sedation syndrome in patients with schizophrenia treated with olanzapine long-acting injection, II: investigations of mechanism. BMC Psychiatry 2010; 10: 45.

84. Gopal S, Gassmann-Mayer C, Palumbo J, et al. Practical guidance for dosing and switching paliperidone palmitate treatment in patients with schizophrenia. Curr Med Res Opin 2010; 26: 377–87.

85. Citrome L. Paliperidone palmitate - review of the efficacy, safety and cost of a new second-generation depot antipsychotic medication. Int J Clin Pract 2010; 64: 216–39.

86. Samtani MN, Gopal S, Gassmann-Mayer C, Alphs L, Palumbo JM. Dosing and switching strategies for paliperidone palmitate: based on population pharmacokinetic modelling and clinical trial data. CNS Drugs 2011; 25: 829–45.

87. Kramer M, Litman R, Hough D, et al. Paliperidone palmitate, a potential long-acting treatment for patients with schizophrenia. Results of a randomized, double-blind, placebo-controlled efficacy and safety study. Int J Neuropsychopharmacol 2010; 13: 635–47.

88. Nasrallah HA, Gopal S, Gassmann-Mayer C, et al. A controlled, evidence-based trial of paliperidone palmitate, a long-acting injectable antipsychotic, in schizophrenia. Neuropsychopharmacology 2010; 35: 2072–82.

89. Pandina GJ, Lindenmayer JP, Lull J, et al. A randomized, placebo-controlled study to assess the efficacy and safety of 3 doses of paliperidone palmitate in adults with acutely exacerbated schizophrenia. J Clin Psychopharmacol 2010; 30: 235–44.

90. Gopal S, Hough DW, Xu H, et al. Efficacy and safety of paliperidone palmitate in adult patients with acutely symptomatic schizophrenia: a randomized, double-blind, placebo-controlled, dose-response study. Int Clin Psychopharmacol 2010; 25: 247–56.

91. Hough D, Gopal S, Vijapurkar U, et al. Paliperidone palmitate maintenance treatment in delaying the time-to-relapse in patients with schizophrenia: a randomized, double-blind, placebo-controlled study. Schizophr Res 2010; 116: 107–17.

92. Gopal S, Vijapurkar U, Lim P, et al. A 52-week open-label study of the safety and tolerability of paliperidone palmitate in patients with schizophrenia. J Psychopharmacol 2011; 25: 685–97.

93. Ereshefsky L, Saklad SR, Tran-Johnson T, et al. Kinetics and clinical evaluation of haloperidol decanoate loading dose regimen. Psychopharmacol Bull 1990; 26: 108–14.

94. Knox ED, Stimmel GL. Clinical review of a long-acting, injectable formulation of Risperidone. Clin Ther 2004; 26: 1994–2002.

95. Newcomer JW. Second-generation (atypical) antipsychotics and metabolic effects: a comprehensive literature review. CNS Drugs 2005; 19(Suppl 1): 1–93.

96. De Hert M, Dekker JM, Wood D, et al. Cardiovascular disease and diabetes in people with severe mental illness position statement from the European Psychiatric Association (EPA), supported by the European Association for the Study of Diabetes (EASD) and the European Society of Cardiology (ESC). Eur Psychiatry 2009; 24: 412–24.

97. McEvoy JP, Meyer JM, Goff DC, et al. Prevalence of the metabolic syndrome in patients with schizophrenia: baseline results from the Clinical Antipsychotic Trials of Intervention Effectiveness (CATIE) schizophrenia trial and comparison with national estimates from NHANES III. Schizophr Res 2005; 80: 19–32.

98. Nasrallah HA. Metabolic findings from the CATIE trial annd their relation to tolerability. CNS Spectr 2006; 11: 32–9.

99. Kroeze WK, Hufeisen SJ, Popadak BA, et al. H1-histamine receptor affinity predicts short-term weight gain for typical and atypical antipsychotic drugs. Neuropsychopharmacology 2003; 28: 519–26.

100. Matsui-Sakata A, Ohtani H, Sawada Y. Receptor occupancy-based analysis of the contributions of various receptors to antipsychotics-induced weight gain and diabetes mellitus. Drug Metab Pharmacokinet 2005; 20: 368–78.

101. Meyer JM, Davis VG, Goff DC, et al. Change in metabolic syndrome parameters with antipsychotic treatment in the CATIE Schizophrenia Trial: prospective data from phase 1. Schizophr Res 2008; 101: 273–86.

102. L'Italien GJ, Casey DE, Kan HJ, Carson WH, Marcus RN. Comparison of metabolic syndrome incidence among schizophrenia patients treated with aripiprazole versus olanzapine or placebo. J Clin Psychiatry 2007; 68: 1510–6.

103. Allison DB, Mentore JL, Heo M, et al. Antipsychotic-induced weight gain: a comprehensive research synthesis. Am J Psychiatry 1999; 156: 1686–96.

104. Meyer JM. Effects of atypical antipsychotics on weight and serum lipid levels. J Clin Psychiatry 2001; 62: 27–34.

105. Rapaport M, Barbato LM, Heisterberg J, Yeung PP, Shapira NA. Efficacy and safety of bifeprunox versus placebo in the treatment of patients with acute exacerbations of schizophrenia (abstract 22). Neuropsychopharmacology 2006; 31: S184.

106. Bourin M, Debelle M, Heisterberg J, et al. Long-term efficacy and safety of bifeprunox in patients with schizophrenia: a 6-month, placebo-controlled study (abstract 31). Neuropsychopharmacology 2006; 31: S187.

107. Ellinger LK, Ipema HJ, Stachnik JM. Efficacy of metformin and topiramate in prevention and treatment of second-generation antipsychotic-induced weight gain. Ann Pharmacother 2010; 44: 668–79.

108. Miller LJ. Management of atypical antipsychotic drug-induced weight gain: focus on metformin. Pharmacotherapy 2009; 29: 725–35.
109. Wu RR, Zhao JP, Jin H, et al. Lifestyle intervention and metformin for treatment of antipsychotic-induced weight gain: a randomized controlled trial. JAMA 2008; 299: 185–93.
110. Ehret M, Goethe J, Lanosa M, Coleman CI. The effect of metformin on anthropometrics and insulin resistance in patients receiving atypical antipsychotic agents: a meta-analysis. J Clin Psychiatry 2010; 71: 1286–92.
111. De Leon J, Diaz FJ. A meta-analysis of worldwide studies demonstrates an association between schizophrenia and tobacco smoking behaviors. Schizophr Res 2005; 76: 135–57.
112. Kao Yc Fau - Liu Y-P, Liu Yp Fau - Cheng T-H, Cheng Th Fau - Chou M-K, Chou MK. Cigarette smoking in outpatients with chronic schizophrenia in Taiwan: relationships to socio-demographic and clinical characteristics. Psychiatry Res 2011; 190: 193–9.
113. George TP, Vessicchio JC, Termine A, et al. A palcebo controlled-trial of bupropion sustained-release for smoking cessation in schizophrenia. Biol Psychiatry 2002; 52: 53–61.
114. George TP, Vessicchio JC, Sacco KA, et al. A placebo-controlled trial of bupropion combined with nicotine patch for smoking cessation in schizophrenia. Biol Psychiatry 2008; 63: 1092–6.
115. Evins AE, Mays VK, Rigotti NA, et al. A pilot trial of bupropion added to cognitive behavioral therapy for smoking cessation in schizophrenia. Nicotine Tob Res 2001; 3: 397–403.
116. Evins AE, Cather C, Deckersbach T, et al. A double-blind placebo-controlled trial of bupropion sustained-release for smoking cessation in schizophrenia. J Clin Psychopharmacol 2005; 25: 218–25.
117. Evins AE, Cather C, Culhane MA, et al. A 12-week double-blind, placebo-controlled study of bupropion sr added to high-dose dual nicotine replacement therapy for smoking cessation or reduction in schizophrenia. J Clin Psychopharmacol 2007; 27: 380–6.
118. Fatemi SH, Stary JM, Hatsukami DK, Murphy SE. A double-blind placebo-controlled cross over trial of bupropion in smoking reduction in schizophrenia. Schizophr Res 2005; 76: 353–6.
119. Coe JW, Brooks PR, Vetelino MG, et al. Varenicline: an a4b2 nicotinic receptor partial agonist for smoking cessation. J Med Chem 2005; 48: 3474–7.
120. Cahill K, Stead Lindsay F, Lancaster T. Nicotine receptor partial agonists for smoking cessation. Cochrane Database Syst Rev 2011: [Available from: http://www.mrw.interscience.wiley.com/cochrane/clsysrev/articles/CD006103/frame.html].
121. Rollema H, Chambers LK, Coe JW, et al. Pharmacological profile of the alpha-4beta2 nicotinic acetylcholine receptor partial agonist varenicline, an effective smoking cessation aid. Neuropharmacology 2007; 52: 985–94.
122. Singh S, Loke YK, Spangler JG, Furberg CD. Risk of serious adverse cardiovascular events associated with varenicline: a systematic review and meta-analysis. CMAJ 2011; 183: 1359–66.
123. Inder WJ, Castle D. Antipsychotic-induced hyperprolactinaemia. Aust NZ J Psychiatry 2011; 45: 830–7.
124. Farver DK. Neuroleptic malignant syndrome induced by atypical antipsychotics. Expert Opin Drug Saf 2003; 2: 21–35.
125. Bazire S. Psychotropic Drug Directory 2010. Dorsington, Warwickshire, UK: Lloyd-Reinhold Communications LLP, 2011: 195.

chapter 2

Psychological approaches to the management of persistent delusions and hallucinations

Craig Steel, Rumina Taylor, and Til Wykes

As more effective treatments for schizophrenia have evolved, emphasis has been placed on defining treatments for the individual symptoms rather than on the whole schizophrenia syndrome. The hallmark positive symptoms, that is, hallucinations and delusions, are a case in point. Although the severity of these symptoms may be controlled by medication, it is not uncommon for them to persist, or at least to reappear in subsequent relapses, despite adequate doses of medication. For some patients the effects of medication on positive symptoms include making them less anxious about the symptoms (this is particularly so for delusions), and allowing them to "ignore" the symptoms so they can concentrate on their domestic and social lives. Others describe their "voices" as getting quieter and less frequent with medication. But for about one-third of patients, the positive symptoms continue despite adequate levels of antipsychotic drugs. These symptoms are distressing, and can have dramatic effects on the person's quality of life and their dependence on psychiatric care.

Symptomatic control by medication also has its costs, expressly at high doses (i.e., side effects), as well as benefits (chap. 1). Limited effectiveness and significant side effects contribute to the recent finding that half of those prescribed antipsychotic medication will discontinue within 6 months (1). Thus, alternative forms of therapy have been investigated as adjuncts to antipsychotic medication for the control of hallucinations and delusions. The recent growth in the evidence base for the effectiveness of psychological therapies in this area has led to the recommendation that they be included as part of routine clinical practice within both the United States (2) and the United Kingdom (3).

The development of psychological therapies for schizophrenia has been driven by the evolution of psychological models of the individual symptoms. Such models have enabled psychologists to establish theories of the mechanisms of the development and maintenance of these symptoms. Together with consideration of the characteristics of these symptoms, such as the levels of conviction for delusions and the physical attributes of the voices, this has led to specific treatment approaches (4–6).

Psychological approaches to the reduction of hallucinations

Even though various types of hallucination are experienced by people with schizophrenia, auditory hallucinations are the most prevalent with 60% of people with a diagnosis of schizophrenia experiencing them at some stage of their illness (7). The majority of treatment approaches for hallucinations have, therefore, been aimed at the reduction of this most prevalent category of abnormal experience: various factors affect the experience of the voice, as shown in Box 2.1. Both cognitive and behavioral approaches have been applied, and more recently there have been attempts to meld the two techniques together.

Early iterations of psychological therapies for hallucinations were largely behavioral in their approach and concentrated on providing competing stimuli, which would then divert attention away from the experience of hallucinations. Even though these interventions can reduce the experience of voices, the effect is usually only temporary. In fact, the simple task of keeping a diary of the experiences of hallucinations will, for some people, provide some temporary reduction in the frequency of the hallucinations.

Many psychological approaches to the amelioration of voices also aim to reduce the anxiety associated with them. Slade (10,11) showed that not only did the voices themselves produce anxiety, but the anxiety was then often a trigger for the experience of hallucinations. Social anxiety in particular was associated with increases in the frequency of hallucinations and controlling the anxiety in these social situations was associated with a reduction in the experience of voices. In a series of case studies these anxiety management

---

Box 2.1   Factors affecting the experience of a hallucinated voice.

- Underlying dysfunction in the perception of inner speech (8)
- Arousal (induced by social situations or particular stressors)
- Beliefs about the voices (9)

techniques were successful in reducing anxiety and subsequently the experience of hallucinations.

Later interventions were developed in line with an increased interest in cognition and brain sciences, and the associated theories about the relationship between brain functioning and the experience of voices. For instance, one theory suggested that hallucinations were the result of poor transfer of information across the corpus callosum that resulted in a mismatch between the auditory experiences in each ear. It was thought that an ear plug in the left ear would even up this information transfer and, in fact, those patients who wore an ear plug did report a significant reduction in voices. However, it was also noticed that some people returned to the clinic with two ear plugs, having invested in a further one themselves. Others returned with the ear plug in the right ear and also reported reductions in the severity of the hallucinations. It is not clear what was responsible for these reductions but on stopping the use of the earplugs the voices returned to their usual level (12).

Although there is no generally accepted psychological model of auditory hallucinations, there is an assumption that there is an underlying dysfunction in inner speech. In particular, there is thought to be a problem in the ability to monitor the source (e.g., real or imagined, internal or external) of inner speech, which leaves people vulnerable to making errors. Jones and Fernyhough (13) in their review suggest that those who experience auditory hallucinations have particular problems in tasks which demand high levels of source monitoring, such as imagining people speaking or imagining sounds. A deficit in source monitoring becomes relevant when low-level non-verbal thought is transformed into verbal thought and the subsequent dialogue within the verbal thought is not attributed to oneself and they are experienced as the voices of other people (14). The phenomenology of the majority of auditory hallucinations involves voices which appear to be attempting to regulate the ongoing actions of the voice hearer and it is argued that these voices are consistent with inner speech–based models (15).

There has been much research and speculation on a possible relationship between childhood sexual abuse (CSA) and experiencing auditory hallucinations. Several studies highlight the increased prevalence of voice hearing in people who have suffered CSA, and some studies identify links to that experience in the content of voices and earlier traumatic experiences (see Ref. (16) for a review). However, while there are some theoretical accounts that link past traumatic experiences with the content of the symptoms of psychosis (17), these processes are still poorly understood. Further, the relationship between trauma and psychotic symptoms has yet to evolve into an evidence-based psychological intervention.

As discussed above, anxiety-provoking situations appear to increase the frequency of voices. In addition, the patient's level of self-esteem is thought to affect the negative content of the voice. However, there is also a third factor which affects the experience of voices—the beliefs about the origin and potency of the voices. Birchwood and Chadwick (9) have shown that the interpretation of the voices, in particular the perceived powerfulness of the voice, affects the severity of the distress experienced. Changing the beliefs about the powerfulness of the voice has, therefore, become a further focus of interventions. The therapy of changing beliefs about voices has developed into a more comprehensive treatment intervention called cognitive–behavioral therapy (CBT) for hallucinations (Table 2.1 for a review of associated psychological interventions). The role of beliefs about voices has been incorporated into a cognitive–behavioral framework (18,19) which considers how an individual responds (behaves) to a voice-hearing experience in relation to how they make sense of the voice (e.g., patients hiding in their room due to the perception of a threat). The role of behavior is considered central to the maintenance of distress, and is therefore a target within the intervention.

Another important development within the psychological management of voices is based on the concept of "normalization." Marius Romme and Sandra Escher (20) publicised the fact that there are a large number of people who hear voices who have never been involved with the psychiatric system. Some of these people learn to cope with their voices, while others find them to be a positive part of their life. An increased awareness of this previously ignored group has led to a research which has focused on how the coping strategies of the nonpsychiatric group compare to those of people who have been diagnosed with schizophrenia. The nonpsychiatric group tend to describe a "relationship" with their voices, in which they are more able to choose when they occur, and are more in control of their own responses. The fact that many non-patients experience hearing voices enables a process of normalization and a reduction of stigma for those who do have a diagnosis. This research provided the basis for the view that the target of an intervention should be the distress associated with voices (as a result of how they are appraised) and not the voices themselves. This process is now incorporated into most modern psychological approaches, and is a fundamental aspect of group work with voice hearers (21). The role of normalization and having a safe place to discuss the experience of voices are highlighted within a recent review of the mechanisms of change within hearing voices groups (22). A voice hearer's movement, called the Hearing Voices Network, has grown in the United Kingdom (www.hearing-voices.org) and publishes a variety of useful resources. An international organization called Intervoice (www.intervoiceonline.org) serves to link hearing voices groups from around the world.

Psychological interventions for delusions

For a long time it was thought that talking to patients about abnormal beliefs (delusions) was not only unhelpful but could be potentially damaging. Hence, many early therapeutic techniques for delusions entailed trying to distract the

Table 2.1 Psychological interventions for hallucinations

Type of intervention	Therapy	Description
Competing information	Thought stopping	The person has an elastic band around their wrist and is told to snap the elastic band whenever he/she hears a voice; or the person shouts "stop it" either overtly or covertly on occurrence of the hallucination
	Competing auditory stimuli	Wearing a personal stereo, humming, singing, and speaking out loud. Using the muscles involved in vocalization seems to be the most efficacious
	Self-monitoring	Keeping a diary where information is recorded concurrently with the experience. The information includes the thoughts and feelings associated with the experience of the voices
Anxiety reduction	Anxiety management	Carrying out a functional analysis of times of high anxiety then using breathing techniques and relaxation exercises to reduce these experiences. Also use of systematic desensitization to reduce the impact of specific cues for anxiety
Cognitive	Belief modification	Investigating the events which activate the voice and the consequences. Exploring the content of the voice and providing alternative hypotheses to test with exploration of the evidence for the belief
	Focusing	Asking the person to concentrate on the physical attributes of the voices and then gradually encouraging him/her to identify the contents of the voice as internally generated
	Coping skills enhancement	Using a case formulation, the person identifies the antecedents, behaviors, and consequences as well as his/her own coping strategies for dealing with the voices

person and/or deny them attention whenever they talked about delusional beliefs. These techniques did have an effect on reducing delusional speech, but it has never been clear that there was any accompanying reduction of the ideas themselves rather than patients merely learning to talk about other things, or simply reduce their amount of speech (23).

Some early attempts to try to change patients' beliefs, by discussing them and trying to generate alternative hypotheses about the delusions in collaboration with the patient, proved more successful than challenging the beliefs directly (24). This finding led to the development of methods for changing beliefs themselves. As with the development of psychological interventions for hallucinations, these innovations have been fuelled by an enhanced understanding of the dimensions of delusions; that is, conviction, preoccupation, interference with everyday life and distres. In fact one commonly proposed route to delusional beliefs (25) is of an individual using normal reasoning processes to make sense of highly unusual perceptual experiences (such as auditory hallucinations). Recently, other psychological factors, such as an underlying problems with the recognition of the mental states of others (Theory of Mind), abnormal reasoning biases (particularly jumping to conclusions on little evidence (26)) and the effects of poor self-esteem have been integrated into the development of more sophisticated therapies.

Given that psychological therapies concentrate on the reduction of distress, there has been a particular focus on the development of understanding paranoid delusions (27,28). Attribution theory has been used in an attempt to understand paranoid delusions (29). Studies have shown that the normal "self-serving bias" in which nonclinical individuals attribute blame for negative events to an outside source, is exaggerated within those suffering from persecutory delusions. Freeman et al. (28) argue that paranoia can be understood as a "threat belief" and as such inherently contains many of the psychological processes that are associated with a state of anxiety. Therefore, a psychological approach to paranoia will need to tackle behaviors such as avoidance and safety seeking. These theories have contributed to more generic cognitive models of psychosis and their associated interventions (see below).

After a therapist has established a shared understanding of the development of a delusional belief with the patient, there are three commonly used cognitive interventions:

- *Belief modification*: Here beliefs are ordered into levels of conviction, with the least well-held belief being tackled first, by trying to disentangle the types of evidence used to support the belief and generating alternative explanations.
- *Behavioral experiments*: These test the veracity of the delusional belief and the supporting evidence.

- *Reattribution*: This is a therapy which is particularly used with paranoid ideation, where patients are encouraged to attribute negative events not to people but to situations, with an emphasis on the personal benefits (reduced distress) that these new explanations will bring.

Whilst most of the current evidence base for the psychological treatment of schizophrenia is based on clinical trials which have been aimed at a broad range of symptoms, there has been some recent success with approaches which specifically target persecutory delusions. Freeman (30) has reviewed a number of recent and ongoing studies which target specific processes that are proposed to maintain the distress associated with this symptom, including sleep deprivation and reasoning processes.

It must be emphasized that the goal of all of these approaches is to reduce the negative effects of abnormal beliefs on the lives of people with schizophrenia, and not specifically to target the content of the belief alone. Thus, change in either preoccupation or distress associated with the belief will be considered a good outcome. The reason for this is that many people who have not been diagnosed with schizophrenia hold unusual or abnormal beliefs, (i.e., those not considered normal outside the beliefs of a particular culture) but are not distressed by them and have a good quality of life (31).

Cognitive–behavioral therapy

The main developmental roots for CBT have been in understanding and treating depression and anxiety. Two early case studies reported the application of such techniques to schizophrenia (32,33), but CBT has only relatively recently been applied more rigorously, through manualized therapies, directly to psychotic symptoms. This development involved changes in the presentation of the intervention, although the underlying model of change may be similar to that adopted for mood and anxiety symptoms. The main aims of CBT are to ameliorate distress, disability and emotional disturbance as well as reduce the chance of relapse of the acute symptoms (34). CBT-based therapies are active and structured therapeutic methods and should be distinguished from psychoeducation, which tends to be simple, didactic, and educational. A recent Cochrane review (35) found psychoeducation to reduce relapse and readmission and improve medication compliance more than "treatment as usual" for people with schizophrenia. There was also some evidence that participants receiving psychoeducation were more likely to be satisfied with mental health services and have improved quality of life.

Although there are specific components of CBT that would be accepted by all its proponents, these ingredients may be given in different proportions by different groups of professionals and for different patients. Those elements accepted by most therapists are shown in Box 2.2.

Box 2.2   Elements of CBT

- Engagement with the client
- Problem identification
- Agreeing on a collaborative formulation of the problems to be assessed
- Use of alternative explanations to challenge delusional and dysfunctional thoughts
- Establishing the link between thoughts and emotions
- Encouraging the patient to examine alternative views of events
- Encouraging the patient to examine the link between thoughts and behavior
- Use of behavioral experiments to reality test
- Setting of behavioral goals and targets
- Developing coping strategies to reduce psychotic symptoms
- Development and acquisition of relapse prevention strategies

---

Further elements incorporated by some therapists include:

- improvement in self-esteem;
- increasing social support and social networks;
- schema-focused therapy.

A number of cognitive models of schizophrenia have been developed (36,37) which have attempted to integrate our current understanding of a number of psychological processes, such as those discussed in relation to hallucinations and delusions, above. These models establish the basis of a formulation-based approach which has resulted in a number of clinical casebooks (38,39).

The first clinical trials of CBT for schizophrenia were conducted in the United Kingdom in the mid-1990s and were targeted at those considered to suffer from "medication-resistant" symptoms. There have now been over 30 randomized controlled trials (RCTs) within the United Kingdom, Europe, Australia, and the United States, with the targets for interventions including command hallucinations, relapse, self-esteem, enhanced coping strategies, negative symptoms, social recovery, and comorbid substance misuse.

What are the outcomes from CBT?

Meta-analyses have all suggested that CBT for psychosis (CBTp) does have an effect on the symptoms, which is durable after treatment has been discontinued (40–43). Average effect sizes (the amount of change you can expect following treatment) found in these meta-analyses ranged from 0.3 to 0.57.

Many of these studies, however, had methodological problems such as non-blind rating of symptoms which is known to inflate the effectiveness (43). The studies have also adopted disparate methods for evaluating the efficacy of the therapy; used different rating scales; and sometimes applied idiosyncratic methods which would be difficult to replicate (see Ref. (44) for a review of methodological problems in 22 RCTs).

The most recent and comprehensive review incorporated 34 trials, with 22 of these being individual CBTp aimed at the positive symptoms of psychosis. The overall effect size for CBTp was moderate, and was broadly similar (around 0.4) whether the analysis was based on outcome in relation to positive symptoms, negative symptoms, mood, or social functioning (43).

The evidence to date predominantly provides support for CBTp as an intervention for individuals suffering from "treatment-resistant" psychosis in a chronic, but stable phase. However, most trials have adopted a generic approach to CBTp and despite these being aimed at the positive symptoms of psychosis, there has been little differential impact between psychotic and nonpsychotic symptoms. Consequently, relatively little is known about the effectiveness of CBTp for other phases of the disorder. The evidence appears to be strongest when the group to receive treatment are more specifically defined, such as Trower et al.'s study (45) which focused specifically on those individuals who heard command hallucinations. However, little is known as to which elements of CBTp are the most important in producing change, and there are few markers as to who would benefit most from this intervention.

One of most methodologically rigorous RCTs reviewed, a study of first- and second-episode patients carried out at the University of Manchester (SoCRATES), evaluated the effect of CBT for patients in the acute phase of their illness. There were small but measurable effects in the first few weeks of admission in the reduction of acute symptoms, particularly hallucinations. However, these short-term effects disappeared as the control conditions caught up with CBT group (46). Over an 18-month period following cessation of treatment, improvements in symptom scores were evident for both the CBT and supportive counseling groups compared with treatment as usual, but overall relapse rates were not diminished (47). Valmaggia et al. (48) found improvements in psychotic symptoms post treatment although these were not maintained at follow-up. It should be stressed that the fact improvements are not maintained after cessation of treatment is not grounds to conclude that the treatment does not work. Several other randomized controlled trials have also demonstrated overall symptom improvement (49–53), although typically there is a larger decrease is delusions than hallucinations.

Whilst U.K. trials have focussed on symptoms, the trials conducted in the United States more often focus on negative symptoms and social recovery. A recent trial (54) was effective in increasing functioning and reducing negative symptoms within patients diagnosed with schizophrenia and suffering from neuropsychological impairment.

Can we improve the outcome of CBT?

A methodologically rigorous trial (55) involving both CBT and family interventions showed no overall effect on relapse rates for either intervention. But a recent sophisticated analyses of these data found that those who received a significant "dose" of CBT did benefit on a wide range of outcomes (56).

Most published studies suggest improvements in positive symptoms for CBT interventions which last at least 20 sessions and are provided by highly trained and supervised therapists. However, there have been studies investigating whether mental health professionals can be trained to deliver briefer CBT interventions, thus making the therapy available to more patients. While there is evidence that training mental health nurses to deliver brief CBT leads to a durable improvement in negative symptoms, insight, depression, and readmissions, psychotic symptoms showed no improvement (57,58). Similarly, an RCT investigating group CBT for voices found that only therapy provided by highly experienced therapists who received expert supervision reduced auditory hallucinations, although an improvement in social functioning was found from therapy delivered by both highly experienced and less experienced therapists (21). Steel et al. (59) highlight that an improved outcome within CBTp is associated with therapists who receive a greater quantity of supervision, and who deliver therapy to a higher number of patients.

Another strategy that has been investigated to try to increase the number of people with access to treatment is to deliver CBT in a group format. As mentioned above, Wykes et al. (21) found an improvement in voices when group CBT was delivered by highly experienced therapists. In an RCT between group CBT and treatment as usual in which more global positive symptoms were targeted, no significant differences were found, although group CBT did reduce feelings of hopelessness and low self-esteem (60).

Despite the lack of support for cheaper alternatives to individual CBT interventions delivered by highly trained therapists, CBT has been shown to be an economical treatment for psychotic symptoms of schizophrenia. Studies that have evaluated the cost-effectiveness or cost-utility of psychological interventions for the symptoms of schizophrenia have shown that providing CBT as an adjunct to standard care is not expensive, and may even be cost effective (50,61).

The application of other forms of psychological intervention for people with persistent symptoms is still in its infancy. A recent trial of acceptance commitment therapy for command hallucinations has been reported (62) and other trials are in progress. The scope, applicability, and efficacy of such techniques remain to be established.

A note about psychological treatments

The success of medication treatments for chronic disorders such as schizophrenia is based on an acute treatment and prevention model, in the same way that diabetes and asthma treatments are evaluated. So, it would be expected that withdrawal of a drug that reduces symptoms would be followed by the return of the symptoms. However, psychological treatment is often evaluated as if it were an antibiotic, with success implying improvements in symptoms and then durability of these changes when the treatment is withdrawn. This leads to the conclusion that if symptoms return following psychological treatment then the treatment has failed. This clearly is not the case; the treatment did affect the symptoms, despite the lack of durability. However, this argument does suggest an alternative regime, that is, psychological treatments should also be provided as maintenance therapy given in a depot every few months. These assumptions about treatment mechanisms have seriously hindered the adoption of psychological treatments into health services, because although the maintenance component of the therapy will increase costs, there are likely to be further benefits in terms of quality of life for the patients.

Resources

Manuals outlining CBT for psychosis

Chadwick P, Birchwood M, Trower P. Cognitive Therapy for Delusions, Voices and Paranoia. Chichester: Wiley, 1996.

Fowler D, Garety PA, Kuipers E. Cognitive Behaviour Therapy for Psychosis: Theory and Practice. Chichester: Wiley, 1995.

Kingdon D, Turkington D. Cognitive Therapy of Schizophrenia. New York: Guilford Press, 2005.

Nelson H. Cognitive Behaviour Therapy with Schizophrenia. A Practice Manual. Cheltenham: Stanley Thornes, 1997.

Clinical casebooks of CBT for psychosis

Kingdon D, Turkington D. The Case Study Guide to Cognitive Behaviour Therapy of Psychosis. Chichester: Wiley, 2002.

Morrison AP. A Casebook of Cognitive Therapy for Psychosis. Hove: Brunner-Routledge, 2002.

Self-Help resources

Baker P. The Voice Inside. A Practical Guide to Coping with Hearing Voices. London: Mind Publications, 2003.

Freeman D, Freeman J, Garety P. Overcoming Paranoid and Suspicious thoughts. London: Constable and Robinson, 2006.

Romme M, Escher S. Making Sense of Voices. London: Mind Publications, 2000.

Romme M, Escher S, Dillon J, Corstens D, Morris M. Living with Voices: 50 Stories of Recovery. Herefordshire: PCCS Books Ltd, 2009.

Jones S, Hayward P. Coping with Schizophrenia: A Guide for Patients, Families and Caregivers. Oxford: Oneworld publications, 2004.

Steele K, Berman C. The Day the Voices Stopped: a Schizophrenic's Journey from Madness to Hope. New York: Basic books, 2002.

Watkins J. Hearing Voices: a Common Human Experience. Melbourne, Victoria: Michelle Anderson Publishing, 2008.

Useful websites

www.hearing-voices.org

www.intervoiceonline.org

www.understandingpsychosis.com

www.asylumonline.net

www.nationalparanoianetwork.org

www.mind.org.uk

References

1. Lewis S, Lieberman J. CATIE and CUtLASS: can we handle the truth? Br J Psychiatry 2008; 192: 161–3.
2. Dixon LB, Dickerson F, Bellack AS, et al. The 2009 PORT psychosocial treatment recommendations and summary statements. Schizophr Bull 2010; 36: 48–70.
3. National Institute of Clinical Excellence (NICE). Schizophrenia: core interventions in the treatment and management of schizophrenia in primary and secondary care (update). London: NICE, 2009.
4. Hemsley DR, Garety PA. The formation of maintenance of delusions: a Bayesian analysis. Br J Psychiatry 1986; 149: 51–6.
5. Frith C, Done J. Positive symptoms of schizophrenia. Br J Psychiatry 1989; 154: 569–70.
6. Chadwick P, Birchwood M. The omnipotence of voices: a cognitive approach to auditory hallucinations. Br J Psychiatry 1994; 164: 190–201.
7. Shergill SS, Murray RM, McGuire PK. Auditory hallucinations: a review of psychological treatments. Schizophr Res 1998; 32: 137–50.
8. Frith CD. The Cognitive Neuropsychology of Schizophrenia. Hillside, NJ: Lawrence Erlbaum Associates, 1992.
9. Birchwood M, Chadwick P. The omnipotence of voices: testing the validity of a cognitive model. Psychol Med 1997; 27: 1345–53.
10. Slade PD. The effects of systemic desensitization on auditory hallucinations. Behav Res Ther 1972; 10: 85–91.
11. Slade PD. The psychological investigation and treatment of auditory hallucinations: a second case report. Br J Med Psychol 1973; 46: 293–6.
12. Done D, Frith C, Owens DC. Reducing persistent auditory hallucinations through occlusion of monaural input. Br J Clin Psychol 1986; 25: 151–2.
13. Jones SR, Fernyhough C. Neural correlates of inner speech and auditory verbal hallucinations: a critical review and theoretical integration. Clin Psychol Rev 2007; 27: 140–54.
14. Fernyhough C. Alien voices and inner dialogue: towards a developmental account of auditory verbal hallucinations. New Ideas Psychol 2004; 22: 29–68.
15. Jones SR. Do we need multiple models of auditory verbal hallucinations? Examining the phenomenological fit of cognitive and neurological models. Schizophr Bull 2010; 36: 565–75.
16. McCarthy-Jones S. Voices from the storm: a critical review of quantitative studies of auditory verbal hallucinations and childhood sexual abuse. Clin Psychol Rev 2011; 31: 983–92.

17. Steel C, Fowler D, Holmes EA. Traumatic intrusions in psychosis: an information processing account. Behav Cog Psychother 2005; 33: 139–52.
18. Morrison AP. A cognitive analysis of the maintenance of auditory hallucinations: are voices to schizophrenia what bodily sensations are to panic?. Behav Cog Psychother 1998; 26: 289–302.
19. Beck AT, Rector NA. A cognitive model of hallucinations. Cog Ther Res 2003; 27: 19–52.
20. Romme M, Escher S. Accepting Voices. London: Mind, 1993.
21. Wykes T, Hayward P, Thomas N, et al. What are the effects of group cognitive behaviour therapy for voices? A randomized control trial. Schizophr Res 2005; 77: 201–10.
22. Ruddle A, Mason O, Wykes T. A review of hearing voices groups: evidence and mechanisms of change. Clin Psychol Rev 2011; 31: 757–66.
23. Liberman R, Telegan J, Patterson R, Baker V. Reducing delusional speech in chronic paranoid schizophrenics. J Appl Behav Anal 1973; 6: 57–64.
24. Watts FN, Powell GE, Austin SV. The modification of abnormal beliefs. Br J Med Psychol 1973; 46: 359–63.
25. Maher B. Delusions. In: Sutker PB, Adams HE. eds. Comprehensive Handbook of Psychopathology, 3rd edn. New York: Springer Science, Business Media LLC, 2004: 309–40.
26. Peters ER, Garety P. Cognitive functioning in delusions: a longitudinal analysis. Behav Res Ther 2006; 44: 481–514.
27. Bentall RP, Kinderman P, Kaney S. The self, attributional processes and abnormal beliefs: towards a model of persecutory delusions. Behav Res Ther 1994; 33: 331–41.
28. Freeman D, Garety PA, Kuipers E, Fowler D, Bebbington PE. A cognitive model of persecutory delusions. Br J Clin Psychol 2002; 41: 331–47.
29. Bentall RP, Corcoran R, Howard R, Blackwood N, Kinderman P. Persecutory delusions: a review and theoretical integration. Clin Psychol Rev 2001; 21: 1143–92.
30. Freeman D. Improving cognitive treatments for delusions. Schizophr Res 2011; 132: 135–9.
31. Peters ER, Day S, Mckenna J, Orbach G. The incidence of delusional ideation in religious and psychotic populations. Br J Clin Psychol 1999; 38: 83–96.
32. Beck AT. Successful outpatient psychotherapy of a chronic schizophrenic with a delusion based on borrowed guilt. Psychiatry 1952; 15: 305–12.
33. Shapiro MB, Ravenette AT. A preliminary experiment on paranoid delusions. J Ment Sci 1959; 105: 295–312.
34. Fowler D, Garety P, Kuipers E. Cognitive therapy for psychosis: formulation, treatment, effects and service implications. J Ment Health 1998; 7: 123–33.
35. Xia J, Merinder LB, Belgamwar MR. Psychoeduction for schizoprehnia. Cochrane Database Syst Rev 2011: CD002831.
36. Garety P, Kuipers E, Fowler D, Freeman D, Bebbington P. A cognitive model of the positive symptoms of psychosis. Psychol Med 2001; 31: 189–95.
37. Morrison AP. The interpretation of intrusions in psychosis: an integrative cognitive approach to psychotic symptoms. Behav Cog Psych 2001; 29: 257–76.
38. Morrison AP. A Casebook of Cognitive Therapy for Psychosis. East Sussex: Brunner-Routledge, 2002.
39. Kingdon D, Turkington D. Cognitive Therapy for Schizophrenia. New York: Guilford Press, 2005.
40. Pilling S, Bebbington P, Kuipers E, et al. Psychological treatments in schizophrenia: I. Meta-analysis of family intervention and cognitive behaviour therapy. Psychol Med 2002; 32: 763–82.
41. Zimmermann G, Favrod J, Trieu VH, Ponini V. The effect of cognitive behavioural treatment on the positive symptoms of schizophrenia spectrum disorders: a meta-analysis. Schizophr Res 2005; 77: 1–9.

42. Pfammatter M, Junghan U, Brenner H. Efficacy of psychological therapy in schizophrenia: conclusions from meta-analyses. Schizophr Bull 2006; 32(Suppl 1): 64–80.
43. Wykes T, Steel C, Everitt B, Tarrier N. Cognitive behaviour therapy for Schizophrenia: effect sizes, clinical models and methodological rigor. Schizophr Bull 2008; 34: 523–37.
44. Tarrier N, Wykes T. Is there evidence that cognitive behaviour therapy is an effective treatment for schizophrenia? A cautious or cautionary tale? Behav Res Ther 2004; 42: 1377–401.
45. Trower P, Birchwood M, Meaden A, et al. Cognitive therapy for command hallucinations: randomised controlled trial. Br J Psychiatry 2004; 184: 312–20.
46. Lewis S, Tarrier N, Haddock G, et al. Randomised controlled trial of cognitive-behavioural therapy in early schizophrenia: acute-phase outcomes. Br J Psychiatry 2002; 181(Suppl 43): 91–7.
47. Tarrier N, Lewis S, Haddock G, et al. Cognitive-behavioural therapy in first-episode and early schizophrenia. Br J Psychiatry 2004; 184: 231–9.
48. Valmaggia LR, van der Gaag M, Tarrier N, et al. Cognitive-behavioural therapy for refractory psychotic symptoms of schizophrenia resistant to atypical antipsychotic medication. Randomised controlled trial. Br J Psychiatry 2005; 186: 324–30.
49. Kuipers E, Garety P, Fowler D, et al. London-East Anglia randomised controlled trial of cognitive-behavioural therapy for psychosis: I. Effects of the treatment phase. Br J Psychiatry 1997; 171: 319–27.
50. Kuipers E, Fowler D, Garety P, et al. London-East Anglia randomised controlled trial of cognitive-behavioural therapy for psychosis: III. Follow-up and economic evaluation at 18 months. Br J Psychiatry 1998; 173: 61–8.
51. Tarrier N, Yusupoff L, Kinney C, et al. A randomised controlled trial of intensive cognitive behaviour therapy for patients with chronic schizophrenia. Br Med J 1998; 317: 303–7.
52. Tarrier N, Wittkowski A, Kinney C, et al. The durability of the effects of cognitive behaviour therapy in the treatment of chronic schizophrenia: twelve months follow up. Br J Psychiatry 1999; 174: 500–4.
53. Sensky T, Turkington D, Kingdon D, et al. A randomised controlled trial of cognitive-behavioural therapy for persistent symptoms in schizophrenia resistant to medication. Arch Gen Psychiatry 2000; 57: 165–72.
54. Grant PM, Huh GA, Perivoliotis D, Stolar NM, Beck AT. Randomised trial to evaluate the efficacy of cognitive therapy for low-functioning patients with schizophrenia. Arch Gen Psychiatry 2011; 69: 121–7.
55. Garety PA, Fowler DG, Freeman D, et al. Cognitive-behavioural therapy and family intervention for relapse prevention and symptom reduction in psychosis: randomised controlled trial. Br J Psychiatry 2008; 192: 412–23.
56. Dunn G, Fowler D, Rollinson R, et al. Effective elements of cognitive behaviour therapy for psychosis: results of a novel type of subgroup analysis based on principal stratification. Psychol Med 2011.
57. Turkington D, Kingdon D, Turner T, the Insight Group. Effectiveness of a brief cognitive behavioural therapy intervention in the treatment of schizophrenia. Br J Psychiatry 2002; 180: 523–8.
58. Turkington D, Kingdon D, Rathod S, et al. Outcomes of an effectiveness trial of cognitive-behavioural intervention by mental health nurses in schizophrenia. Br J Psychiatry 2006; 189: 36–40.
59. Steel C, Tarrier N, Stahl D, Wykes T. Cognitive behaviour therapy for psychosis: the impact of therapist training and supervision. Psychother Psychosom 2012; In press.
60. Barrowclough C, Haddock G, Lobban F, et al. Group cognitive-behavioural therapy for schizophrenia: randomi sed controlled trial. Br J Psychiatry 2006; 189: 527–32.

61. Startup M, Jackson MC, Evans KE, Bendix S. North Wales randomized controlled trial of cognitive behaviour therapy for acute schizophrenia spectrum disorders: two-year follow-up and economic evaluation. Psychol Med 2005; 35: 1307–16.
62. Shawyer F, Farhall J, Mackinnon A, et al. A randomised controlled trial of acceptance-based cognitive behaviour therapy for command hallucinations in psychotic disorders. Behav Res Ther 2012; 50: 110–21.

chapter 3

The management of negative symptoms

David L. Copolov and David J. Castle

As a common source of chronic disability, negative symptoms serve to remind clinicians of the imperfections of psychiatric therapeutics in schizophrenia. Negative symptoms are conceptualized as those occurring as a result of a loss of function (1). They can be grouped into two domains: *avolition* which includes diminished drive (amotivation), loss of pleasure (anhedonia) and lack of involvement in social relationships (asociality); *expressive deficits* which include affective flattening and poverty of speech (alogia) (2,3). They are present to varying degrees in patients with schizophrenia with estimates being that 15–25% of people with the disorder experience negative symptoms of sufficient severity to warrant symptom-targeted therapeutic intervention (4). When present to such a degree, these symptoms often contribute to social dislocation and isolation and greatly reduced activities of daily living.

Just as there is a clear overlap between the positive and negative symptoms of schizophrenia in individual patients, so too the treatment for these two classes of symptoms overlap: both involve pharmacotherapy, supportive psychotherapy and attention to broader psychosocial issues such as employment, accommodation, and interactions with others (chap. 11 and chap.12). But in dealing with negative symptoms, special emphasis is placed on the consideration of differential diagnosis and the use of psychosocial rehabilitation strategies.

Negative symptoms are often present from the onset of schizophrenia (5) but are approximately half as common as in early phase patients in comparison to more chronic ones (6,7). These symptoms respond to an extent to treatment, but less definitively than positive symptoms (8). It is instructive to subcategorize negative symptoms into *phasic* symptoms that improve in tandem with positive symptoms and *enduring* symptoms (9). The latter appear to correlate with poor premorbid function, more severe global psychopathology, and impaired neuropsychological performance (9). Such enduring negative symptoms are evident even in first-episode psychosis (10,11).

Diagnosis before treatment

There are several important causes of emotional withdrawal, avolition, reduced spontaneity, and reduced affective range in patients with schizophrenia other than the underlying disease processes (Box 3.1) (5,12–14).

One such secondary cause is that of *negative symptoms secondary to positive psychotic symptoms*. Hallucinations and delusions may lead to emotional and social withdrawal both as a response to the often threatening content of these psychotic phenomena and to the attempt to reduce external stimuli in the face of being overwhelmed by emotional experiences. During acute psychotic episodes, it may be impossible to distinguish between secondary negative symptoms originating from this cause and primary negative symptoms; such a distinction may be possible only in retrospect.

Negative symptoms due to the extrapyramidal side effects (EPSEs) of antipsychotic drugs were more common as differential diagnosis with the older generation of antipsychotics (chap. 1). But even with atypical drugs in current use, only clozapine and quetiapine carry a very low risk of EPSEs across their dose range (15), so this is still an important differential diagnosis to consider. The most obvious feature shared by primary negative symptoms and extrapyramidal syndromes is diminished spontaneous movements (bradykinesia) (12). Differentiating features, therefore, focus on the nonbradykinesic set of EPSE symptoms and signs including akathisia, tremor, and rigidity. These should be considered when assessing the likelihood that a particular antipsychotic drug might be causing EPSEs.

The features of *comorbid depression* that overlap with primary negative symptoms include a depressed affect, reduced capacity for pleasure, and decreased level of engagement with others. Clarification of the differential diagnosis is aided by a detailed consideration of the patient's mood and an inquiry into possible accompanying depressive symptoms such as recurrent suicidal ideation, persistent insomnia, significant weight loss, and intrusive feelings of worthlessness (chap. 5) (16). Although there are similarities between a flattened and a depressed affect, in terms of reduced mobility and range, several

---

Box 3.1 Differential diagnosis of negative symptoms.

1. Primary Negative Symptoms
   due to underlying disease processes
2. Secondary Negative Symptoms
   secondary to positive psychotic symptoms
   secondary to extrapyramidal side effects of antipsychotic drugs
   secondary to depression
   secondary to catatonia

studies (17,18) have shown that the distinction between these two abnormalities of affect can usually be made reliably, assisted by differentiating features such as tearfulness and observed sadness.

Although *catatonia* is relatively rare in developed countries, it still needs to be kept in mind as a cause of the type of psychomotor inhibition that can be confused with primary negative symptoms (19). Distinguishing features of catatonia include stupor, bizarre posturing, negativism, and waxy flexibility.

The management of negative symptoms

Negative symptoms warrant particular attention from clinicians because they generally fail to give rise to appropriate levels of concern from patients; instead they tend to engender an attitude of relative indifference (20). Thus, clinicians must rely on appropriate and directed history taking, discussion with family members or others who know the patient well, and on observation to diagnose and track these symptoms.

The philosophy underlying the diagnosis and treatment of negative symptoms must take into account the fact that in some circumstances it may not be possible to distinguish between primary and secondary negative symptoms. Under such circumstances it may be necessary to treat potentially reversible causes of the negative symptoms, such as depression or EPSEs if there is a reasonable level of suspicion that such causes might be relevant to the patient's presentation. When improvement occurs in the context of uncertainty about the extent to which the treatment has affected primary or secondary negative symptoms, there is a possibility that a "pseudospecific" response has been elicited (4). Although this may muddy the waters in terms of mechanisms of action, in practical terms the key issue is that the patient improves.

The prevention and management of secondary negative symptoms

The principles underlying the treatment of the *positive symptoms* of schizophrenia are outlined elsewhere in this book (chaps. 1 and 2). Treatment of these symptoms will usually result in improvements in negative symptoms either as a result of "*en bloc*" improvements in the symptoms of the disorder (with negative symptoms typically improving to a lesser extent than positive symptoms) (21) or improvements in the negative symptoms that are more directly the consequence of positive ones. One key element of such treatment is the use of antipsychotic drugs. In order to reduce the likelihood of *extrapyramidal symptoms* arising during the course of treatment with such drugs, the best approach is to choose a second-generation antipsychotic (SGA) medication such as quetiapine, olanzapine, aripiprazole, ziprasidone, asenapine, or

Box 3.2 Treatment approaches aimed at minimizing extrapyramidal side effects.

Use of newer-generation drugs if possible
The lowest effective dose of antipsychotic drugs
A judicious use of anticholinergic medications

low-dose risperidone or paliperidone (Box 3.2). It must be remembered, however, that the risk of EPSEs is not uniform across this range of drugs (15).

If financial considerations preclude the use of newer drugs, conventional antipsychotic drugs should be used at the lowest effective dose. For haloperidol this dose is likely to be in the range of 3–4 mg/day (22) or 4–6 mg/day (23); doses which are high enough to achieve the 65% or higher dopamine D2 receptor occupancy levels are required for antipsychotic efficacy (24–26).

The trend toward lower antipsychotic dosages is a welcome development but it must be recognized that increasing drug doses may need to be used in order to obtain control of positive symptoms in particular. Several groups have shown that doses in the range of 200–500 mg chlorpromazine equivalents (CPZ eq)/day result in a greater number of responders and that treatment responsiveness plateaus definitively in the 500–800 mg CPZ eq/day range (27). Doses in this latter range are, however, associated with much higher rates of EPSEs; thus, it has been estimated that to benefit one additional patient in terms of efficacy by treating with these higher doses will cause significant EPSEs in up to four patients in the first 6 months of maintenance therapy (27).

Observations such as these have two corollaries. First, there is no fixed "low dose that fits all" for each antipsychotic drug, and an individual response must be established. Second, there are doses below which a significant proportion of patients do not respond. For example, in a study of standard- versus low-dose fluphenazine decanoate (12.5–50 mg every 2 weeks vs 1.25–5 mg every 2 weeks), relapse rates over 9 months were eight times higher (56% vs 7%) in the lower-dose group (28). Similarly, studies with risperidone have shown that while there is a recommendation to start this drug at 2 mg per day, efficacy is considered to be greatest in the 4–6 mg range; below 2 mg per day, the drug is generally ineffective in non-elderly adults (29).

The fact that a substantial number of patients on conventional antipsychotic drugs (ranging from 20 to 66%) (30) experience extrapyramidal symptoms may therefore be seen as a calculated trade-off of side effects for treatment response. Nevertheless, there is also a high rate of failure to recognize EPSEs (31), so vigilance regarding these side effects should always be maintained. If EPSEs are detected, a judicious lowering of the dose to a level sufficient to maintain efficacy, or switching to a drug with a less EPSE-causing potential (32), or the addition of anticholinergic drugs such as benzotropine (33) should be considered (chap. 1). Because of side effects such as dry mouth, blurred vision, constipation, tachycardia, and urinary hesitancy, the prophylactic use of anticholinergic agents should be reserved for those being treated with conventional antipsychotic drugs with a history of EPSEs, especially those in whom EPSEs have led to the discontinuation of antipsychotic medications (34).

The third significant cause of secondary negative symptoms in schizophrenia is *depression*. The treatment of depression in schizophrenia is discussed in chapter 5.

The treatment of primary negative symptoms

There are two elements in treating primary negative symptoms: choosing the most efficacious antipsychotic drug and instigating appropriate psychosocial interventions.

Several reports have claimed efficacy for treating primary negative symptoms with atypical antipsychotic drugs including amisulpride alone (19,35–37); amisulpride as an adjunct to haloperidol (38) or clozapine (39); olanzapine (40); risperidone (41); and clozapine alone (42,43). A meta-analysis of first-generation antipsychotics (FGAs) versus SGAs showed that only amisulpiride, clozapine, olanzapine, and risperidone were superior to FGA drugs in the treatment of negative symptoms, whereas aripiprazole, quetiapine, sertindole, ziprasidone, and zotepine did not demonstrate superiority (44). There is some emergent evidence that asenapine may be particularly effective for negative symptoms in schizophrenia (45).

Despite some antipsychotics appearing to have at least a "signal" for efficacy for primary negative symptoms, it is fair to say that overall the efficacy of available antipsychotic drugs on negative symptoms is modest, inconsistent, and often of marginal clinical value (46–49). Furthermore, few studies have addressed treatment response in patients with the so-called deficit syndrome, in which negative symptoms predominate.

Alternate pharmacological approaches to negative symptoms have included the adjunctive use of antidepressants. A recent meta-analysis (50) concluded that the treatment of negative symptoms with antidepressants as adjuncts to antipsychotics is more effective than the use of antipsychotics alone, singling out fluoxetine, trazodone, and ritanserin as demonstrating adjunctive efficacy. This conclusion must be tempered by the small number of studies of each of the nine antidepressants reviewed and the small number of subjects per study.

Other pharmacotherapy trials have included N-methyl-D-aspartate agonists glycine (51) and D-cycloserine (52–54), galantamine (55), pergolide (56) modafinil (57,58), sildenafil (59), and minocycline (60). These approaches have yet to be validated.

Recently, there has been a considerable interest in the use of repetitive transcranial magnetic stimulation in the treatment of negative symptoms. Although some reports, especially those involving a frequency of stimulation of 10 Hz, have been positive, two recent meta-analyses have reported across-study efficacies that are not significant (61) or are in the small-to-medium range (62). Larger and more conclusive studies must be conducted before repetitive transcranial magnetic stimulation could be recommended for the treatment of negative symptoms on a routine basis.

Psychosocial aspects of managing negative symptoms

A subcomponent meta-analysis and review of 24 psychosocial intervention studies in which negative symptoms had been assessed, demonstrated a greater beneficial effect of such therapies on negative- than positive symptoms (63). On the basis of chronic patients responding to such treatments better than acute patients, this review also suggested that clinicians adopt a "phase of illness" orientation to treatment, with priority being given to optimizing medication in the acute phase and to optimizing psychosocial treatments in the chronic phase.

Environmental understimulation is one psychosocial factor that has been shown to exacerbate negative symptoms and is amenable to intervention. Although research in long-stay psychiatric institutions demonstrate the deleterious role of environmental understimulation in inpatient settings (64,65), it is just as important to keep track of this factor in the community settings in which patients are now usually treated. The elements comprising environmental understimulation include:

- having little contact with the outside world;
- having little or no engagement in a constructive occupation;
- spending long periods of time doing nothing.

It has been shown that the introduction of measures to address these issues can bring substantial benefits (64) in terms of reduction in negative symptoms, without a concomitant increase in positive symptoms. In a study of the postdischarge fate of patients who had been previously on long stay wards (66) it has been shown that the provision of enriched social environments is associated with a lessening of negative symptoms, but it may take a number of years for this effect to become evident. Elements that appear to be relevant to improvements in negative symptom status include increases in the number of friends, increased contact with those in the community providing services and goods (such as local shopkeepers), and the provision of less restrictive living environments.

Many of the psychosocial treatments and strategies which are valuable in the management of schizophrenia, such as case management, occupational therapy, assertive community treatment, and vocational rehabilitation (chap. 11, 12, and 16) attempt to address the negative impact of environmental understimulation on patients. Specific psychosocial interventions that have recently been shown to have some effect on negative symptoms include social skills training (67), group therapy involving multiple families (68), cognitive remediation therapy (69), vocational rehabilitation (70), and cognitive–behavioral therapy (CBT) (71–73). The CBT of negative symptoms aims to harness motivation and promote social and emotional re-engagement by techniques including behavioral self-monitoring, activity scheduling, and graded task assignments (74). It has been difficult to parse out the efficacy of CBT on overall symptoms and those relating specifically to negative symptoms, especially persistent ones. For example, only two of the 23 studies included in Wykes' meta-analysis of the efficacy of CBT in schizophrenia (75) chose negative symptoms as a primary outcome measure.

The iterative relationship between psychosocial treatments and pharmacotherapy is also of importance. Antipsychotic medications such as clozapine can facilitate patient engagement in psychosocial rehabilitation programs. In turn, these programs when used adjunctively with pharmacotherapy, but only after a period of several months, can result in additional symptom improvements and a better quality of life (76).

Negative symptoms and family members

It is imperative to recognize and help deal with the impact of schizophrenia on family members in the post-deinstitutionalization era which often sees them as the principal caregivers for adults with major psychiatric disorders (chap. 15). Family members are often more distressed by the effects of negative symptoms than are patients themselves (77,78). This is especially the case when they have inadequate knowledge about schizophrenia and perceive the symptoms to be under the patient's control (79).

Be it individually or in group settings (68), family members can be helped to cope with negative symptoms in their loved ones (77). Psychoeducation aimed at clarifying that these symptoms are not the patient's fault is important. *Blunted affect* may lead to a misreading of the patient's level of interest in activities; so relatives should be advised to ask judiciously about the patient's feelings, rather than assume that impassive facial expressions mean that interest is lacking. One strategy to deal with *poverty of speech* may be to arrange joint activities outside the home. This lessens the pressure on conversation and may provide topics for later discourse. When engaging in discussion, relatives should be encouraging but not place high expectations on what patients can contribute; they should learn to be tolerant of long pauses in conversation and to be active in filling in some of the silences with undemanding contributions. Relatives can help patients with *reduced drive* by regularly scheduling enjoyable recreational activities and making a special effort to include them in family activities.

Conclusions

Negative symptoms are a major contributor to the poor quality of life experienced by patients with schizophrenia (80). While there is a clear need to undertake more research into the pathopsychology of these symptoms in order to improve the limited therapeutic interventions currently available (46,49,81), there are practical and proven steps that clinicians can take to assist patients deal with secondary, and to a lesser extent, primary negative symptoms.

References

1. Andreasen NC, Flaum M, Swayze VW II, et al. Positive and negative symptoms in schizophrenia. A critical reappraisal. Arch Gen Psychiatry 1990; 47: 615–21.
2. Kimhy D, Yale S, Goetz RR, McFarr LM, Malaspina D. The factorial structure of the schedule for the deficit syndrome in schizophrenia. Schizophr Bull 2006; 32: 274–8.
3. Messinger JW, Trémeau F, Antonius D, et al. Avolition and expressive deficits capture negative symptom phenomenology: implications for DSM-5 and schizophrenia research. Clin Psychol Rev 2010; 31: 161–8.
4. Kirkpatrick B, Fenton WS, Carpenter WT, Marder SR. The NIMH-MATRICS consensus statement on negative symptoms. Schizophr Bull 2006; 32: 214–19.
5. Peralta V, Cuesta MJ, Martinez-Larrea A, Serrano JF. Differentiating primary from secondary negative symptoms in schizophrenia: a study of neuroleptic-naïve patients before and after treatment. Am J Psychiatry 2000; 157: 1461–6.
6. Ventura J, Nuechterlein KH, Green MF, et al. The timing of negative symptom exacerbations in relationship to positive symptom exacerbations in the early course of schizophrenia. Schizophr Res 2004; 9: 333–42.
7. Foussias G, Remington G. Negative symptoms in schizophrenia: avolition and Occam's razor. Schizophr Bull 2010; 36: 359–69.
8. Arndt S, Andreasen NC, Flaum M, et al. A longitudinal study of symptom dimensions in schizophrenia: prediction and patterns of change. J Am Med Assoc 1995; 52: 352–60.
9. Tandon R, DeQuardo JR, Taylor SF, et al. Phasic and enduring negative symptoms in schizophrenia: biological markers and relationship to outcome. Schizophr Res 2000; 45: 191–201.
10. Edwards J, McGorry PD, Waddell FM, Harrigan SM. Enduring negative symptoms in first-episode psychosis: comparison of six methods using follow-up data. Schizophr Res 1999; 40: 147–58.
11. Malla A, Norman R, Takhar J, et al. Can patients at risk for persistent negative symptoms be identified during their first episode of psychosis? J Nerv Ment Dis 2004; 192: 455–63.
12. Barnes TRE. Issues in the clinical assessment of negative symptoms. Curr Opin Psychiatry 1994; 7: 35–8.

13. Buchanan RW, Gold JM. Negative symptoms: diagnosis, treatment and prognosis. Int Clin Psychopharmacol 1996; 11(Suppl 2): 3–11.
14. Buchanan RW. Persistent negative symptoms in schizophrenia: an overview. Schizophr Bull 2007; 33: 1013–22.
15. Weiden PH. EPS Profiles: the atypical antipsychotics are not all the same. J Psychiatr Pract 2007; 13: 1.
16. Castle D, Bosanac P. Depression and schizophrenia. Adv Psychiatr Treat 2012; in press.
17. Newcomer JW, Faustman WO, Yeh W, Csernansky JG. Distinguishing depression and negative symptoms in unmedicated patients with schizophrenia. Psychiatry Res 1990; 31: 243–50.
18. Hausmann A, Fleischhacker WW. Differential diagnosis of depressed mood in patients with schizophrenia: a diagnostic algorithm based on a review. Acta Psychiatr Scand 2002; 106: 83–96.
19. Paillere-Martinot ML, Lecrubier Y, Martinot JL, Aubin F. Improvement of some schizophrenic deficit symptoms with low doses of amisulpride. Am J Psychiatry 1995; 152: 130–4.
20. Selten J-P, Wiersma D, van den Bosch RJ. Distress attributed to negative symptoms in schizophrenia. Schizophr Bull 2000; 26: 737–44.
21. Meltzer H, Kostakaglu E, Lee M. Response: negative symptoms redux. Neuropsychopharmacology 2000; 22: 642–3.
22. McEvoy JP, Hogarty GE, Steingard S. Optimal dose of neuroleptic in acute schizophrenia. Arch Gen Psychiatry 1991; 48: 739–45.
23. Nordstrom AL, Farde I, Wiesel FA, et al. Central D2-dopamine receptor occupancy in relation to antipsychotic drug effects: a double-blind PET study of schizophrenic patients. Biol Psychiatry 1993; 33: 227–35.
24. Farde L, Nordstrom AL, Wiesel FA, et al. Positron emission tomographic analysis of central D1 and D2 dopamine receptor occupancy in patients treated with classical neuroleptics and clozapine: relation to extrapyramidal side effects. Arch Gen Psychiatry 1992; 49: 538–44.
25. Kapur S, Zipursky R, Roy P, et al. The relationship between D2 receptor occupancy and plasma levels on low dose oral haloperidol: a PET study. Psychopharmacology (Berlin) 1997; 131: 148–52.
26. Kapur S, Zipursky R, Jones C, et al. Relationship between dopamine D(2) occupancy, clinical response, and side effects: a double-blind PET study of first-episode schizophrenia. Am J Psychiatry 2000; 157: 514–20.
27. Mossman D. A decision analysis approach to neuroleptic dosing: insights from a mathematical model. J Clin Psychiatry 1997; 58: 66–72.
28. Kane JM, Rifkin A, Woerner M, et al. Low-dose neuroleptic treatment of outpatient schizophrenics. I. Preliminary results for relapse rates. Arch Gen Psychiatry 1983; 40: 893–6.
29. Williams R. Optimal dosing with risperidone: updated recommendations. J Clin Psychiatry 2001; 62: 4.
30. Muscettola G, Barbato G, Pampallona S, et al. Extrapyramidal syndromes in neuroleptic-treated patients: prevalence, risk factors, and association with tardive dyskinesia. J Clin Psychopharmacol 1999; 19: 203–8.
31. Weiden PJ, Shaw E, Mann J. Causes of neuroleptic non-compliance. Psychiatr Ann 1986; 16: 571–8.
32. Weiden PJ, Aquila R, Dalheim L, Standard JM. Switching antipsychotic medications. J Clin Psychiatry 1997; 58(Suppl 10): 63–72.
33. Holloman LC, Marder SR. Management of acute extrapyramidal effects induced by antipsychotic drugs. Am J Health Syst Pharm 1997; 54: 2461–77.

34. Lehman AF, Steinwachs DM, Dixon LB, et al. At issue: translating research into practice: the Schizophrenia Patient Outcomes Research Team (PORT) treatment recommendations. Schizophr Bull 1998; 24: 1–10.
35. Boyer P, Lecrubier Y, Puech AJ, et al. Treatment of negative symptoms in schizophrenia with amisulpride. Br J Psychiatry 1995; 166: 68–72.
36. Loo H, Poirier-Littre MF, Theron M, et al. Amisulpride versus placebo in the medium-term treatment of the negative symptoms of schizophrenia. Br J Psychiatry 1997; 170: 18–22.
37. Danion JM, Rein W, Fleurol O. Improvement of schizophrenic patients with primary negative symptoms treated with amisulpride. Am J Psychiatry 1999; 156: 610–16.
38. Bogetto F, Fonzo V, Maina G, Ravizza I. Adjunctive fluoxetine or amisulpride improves schizophrenic negative symptoms. Eur J Psychiatry 1995; 9: 119–27.
39. Munro J, Matthiasson P, Osborne S, et al. Amisulpride augmentation of clozapine: an open non-randomized study in patients with schizophrenia partially responsive to clozapine. Acta Psychiatr Scand 2004; 110: 292–8.
40. Tollefson GD, Sanger TM. Negative symptoms: a path analytic approach to a double-blind, placebo- and haloperidol-controlled clinical trial with olanzapine. Am J Psychiatry 1997; 154: 466–74.
41. Moller JH, Muller H, Borison RL, et al. A path-analytical approach to differentiate between direct and indirect drug effects on negative symptoms in schizophrenic patients. A re-evaluation of the North American risperidone study. Eur Arch Psychiatry Clin Neurosci 1996; 245: 45–9.
42. Meltzer HY. Dimensions of outcome with clozapine. Br J Psychiatry 1992; 160(Suppl): 46–53.
43. Brar JS, Chengappa R, Parcpally H, et al. The effects of clozapine on negative symptoms in patients with schizophrenia with minimal positive symptoms. Ann Clin Psychiatry 1997; 9: 227–34.
44. Leucht S, Corves C, Arbter D, et al. Second-generation versus first-generation antipsychotic drugs for schizophrenia: a meta-analysis. Lancet 2009; 373: 31–41.
45. Alphs L, Panagides J, Lancaster S. Asenapine in the treatment of negative symptoms in schizophrenia: clinical trial design and rationale. Psychopharmacol Bull 2007; 40: 41–53.
46. Erhart SM, Marder SR, Carpenter WT. Treatment of schizophrenia negative symptoms: future prospects. Schizophr Bull 2006; 32: 234–7.
47. McEvoy JP, Lieberman JA, Stroup TS. Effectiveness of colzapine versus olanzapine, quetiapine, and risperidone in patients with chronic schizophrenia who did not respond to prior atypical antipsychotic treatment. Am J Psychiatry 2006; 163: 600–10.
48. Murphy BP, Chung YC, Park TW, McGorry PD. Pharmacological treatment of primary negative symptoms in schizophrenia: a systematic review. Schizophrenia Research 2006; 88: 5–25.
49. Buckley PF, Stahl SM. Pharmacological treatment of negative symptoms of schizophrenia: therapeutic opportunity or Cul-de-sac? Acta Psychatr Scand 2007; 115: 93–100.
50. Singh SP, Singh V, Kar N, Chan K. Efficacy of antidepressants in treating the negative symptoms of chronic schizophrenia: meta-analysis. Br J Psychiatry 2010; 197: 174–9.
51. Heresco-Levy U, Javitt DC, Ermilov M, et al. Efficacy of high-dose glycine in the treatment of enduring negative symptoms of schizophrenia. Arch Gen Psychiatry 1999; 56: 29–36.
52. Goff DC, Tsai G, Levitt J, et al. A placebo-controlled trial of D-cycloserine added to conventional neuroleptics in patients with schizophrenia. Arch Gen Psychiatry 1999; 56: 21–7.

53. Heresco-Levy U, Ermilov M, Shimoni J, et al. Placebo-controlled trial of D-cycloserine added to conventional neuroleptics, olanzapine, or risperidone in schizophrenia. Am J Psychiatry 2002; 159: 480–2.

54. Goff DC, Cather C, Gottlieb JD, et al. Once-weekly D-cycloserine effects on negative symptoms and cognition in schizophrenia: an exploratory study. Schizophr Res 2008; 106: 320–7.

55. Rosse RB, Deutsch SI. Adjuvant galantamine administration improves negative symptoms in a patient with treatment-refractory schizophrenia. Clin Neuropharmacol 2002; 25: 272–5.

56. Roesch-Ely D, Gohring K, Gruschka P, et al. Pergolide as adjuvant therapy to amisulpride in the treatment of negative and depressive symptoms in schizophrenia. Pharmacopsychiatry 2006; 39: 115–16.

57. Pierre JM, Peloian JH, Wirshing DA, Wirshing WC, Marder SR. A randomized, double-blind, placebo-controlled trial of modafinil for negative symptoms in schizophrenia. J Clin Psychiatry 2007; 68: 705–10.

58. Freudenreich O, Henderson DC, Macklin EA, et al. Modafinil for clozapine-treated schizophrenia patients: a double-blind, placebo-controlled pilot trial. J Clin Psych 2009; 70: 1674–80.

59. Akhondzadeh S, Ghayyoumi R, Rezaei F, et al. Sildenafil adjunctive therapy to risperidone in the treatment of the negative symptoms of schizophrenia: a double-blind randomized placebo-controlled trial. Psychopharmacology (Berl) 2011; 213: 809–15.

60. Levkovitz Y, Mendlovich S, Riwkes S. A double-blind, randomized study of minocycline for the treatment of negative and cognitive symptoms in early-phase schizophrenia. J Clin Psychiatry 2010; 71: 138–49.

61. Freitas C, Fregni F, Pascual-Leone A. Meta-analysis of the effects of repetitive transcranial magnetic stimulation (rTMS) on negative and positive symptoms in schizophrenia. Schizophr Res 2009; 108: 11–24.

62. Jozarni J, Dlabač-de Lange JJ, Knegtering R, Aleman A. Repetitive transcranial magnetic stimulation for negative symptoms of schizophrenia: review and meta-analysis. J Clin Psychiatry 2010; 71: 411–18.

63. Mojtabai R, Nicholson RA, Carpenter BN. Role of psychosocial treatments in management of schizophrenia: a meta-analytic review of controlled outcome studies. Schizophr Bull 1998; 24: 569–87.

64. Wing JK, Brown GW. Institutionalism and Schizophrenia. Cambridge, UK: Cambridge University Press, 1970.

65. Oshima I, Mino Y, Inomata Y. Effects of environmental deprivation on negative symptoms of schizophrenia: a nationwide survey in Japan's psychiatric hospitals. Psychiatry Res 2006; 136: 163–71.

66. Leff J, Thornicroft G, Coxhead N, Crawford C. The TAPS Project. 22: a five-year follow-up of long-stay psychiatric patients discharged to the community. Br J Psychiatry 1994; 165(Suppl 25): 13–17.

67. Kopelowicz A, Liberman RP, Mintz J, Zarate R. Comparison of efficacy of social skills training for deficit and nondeficit negative symptoms in schizophrenia. Am J Psychiatry 1997; 154: 424–5.

68. Dyck DG, Short RA, Hendryx MS, et al. Management of negative symptoms among patients with schizophrenia attending multiple-family groups. Psychiatr Serv 2000; 51: 513–19.

69. Wykes T, Reeder C, Corner J, et al. The effects of neurocognitive remediation on executive processing in patients with schizophrenia. Schizophr Bull 1999; 25: 291–308.

70. Bio DS, Gattaz WF. Vocational rehabilitation improves cognition and negative symptoms in schizophrenia. Schizophr Res 2011; 126: 265–9.

71. Sensky T, Turkington D, Kingdon D. A randomized controlled trial of cognitive-behavioural therapy for persistent symptoms in schizophrenia resistant to medication. Arch Gen Psychiatry 2000; 57: 165–72.
72. Rector NA, Beck AT. Cognitive behavioral therapy for schizophrenia: an empirical review. J Nerv Ment Dis 2001; 189: 278–87.
73. Rector NA, Seeman MV, Segal ZV. Sognitive therapy of schizophrenia: a preliminary randomized controlled trial. Schizophr Res 2003; 63: 1–11.
74. Rector NA, Beck AT. Cognitive behavioral therapy for schizophrenia: from conceptualization to intervention. Can J Psychiatry 2002; 47: 39–48.
75. Wykes T, Steel C, Everitt B, Tarrier N. Cognitive behavior therapy for schizophrenia: effect sizes, clinical models, and methodological rigor. Schizophr Bull 2008; 34: 523–37.
76. Rosenheck R, Tekell J, Peters. J, et al. for the Department of Veterans Affairs Cooperative Study Group on Clozapine in Refractory Schizophrenia. Does participation in psychosocial treatment augment the benefit of clozapine? Arch Gen Psychiatry 1998; 55: 618–25.
77. Mueser KT, Gingerich S. Coping with Schizophrenia A Guide for Families. Oakland, CA: New Harbinger Publications, Inc, 1994.
78. Provencher HL, Mueser KT. Positive and negative symptom behaviors and caregiver burden in the relatives of persons with schizophrenia. Schizophr Res 1997; 26: 71–80.
79. Harrison C, Dadda M, Smith G. Family caregivers' criticism of patients with schizophrenia. Psychiatr Serv 1998; 49: 918–24.
80. Mueser KT, Douglas MS, Bellack AS, Morrison RL. Assessment of enduring deficit and negative symptom subtypes in schizophrenia. Schizophr Bull 1991; 17: 565–82.
81. Carpenter WT Jr, Arango C, Buchanan RW, Kirkpatrick B. Deficit psychopathology and a paradigm shift in schizophrenia research. Soc Biol Psychiatry 1999; 46: 352–60.

chapter 4

Cognitive dysfunction in schizophrenia

Til Wykes, Evelina Medin, India Webb, and David J. Castle

Cognitive difficulties have been an integral part of the diagnosis of schizophrenia in all diagnostic systems beginning with Kraepelin and Bleuler more than 100 years ago, although they differed on the specific mechanism that was at fault; thus Bleuler stressed the loosening of the associational threads that tie thoughts together, while Kraepelin and others emphasized poor attention and memory difficulties. This chapter describes these difficulties, with particular reference to the effect they have on quality of life and life choices. Treatment options for cognitive difficulties in schizophrenia are relatively new and have not had their full potential developed. However, some detail on the most promising of the current therapeutic approaches is provided.

What cognitive systems are disturbed in schizophrenia?

Impairments are found in a wide range of cognitive systems in people with schizophrenia, but the severity of the impairment differs between systems. For instance, mild impairments are found in overall intelligence quotient (IQ), and on some perceptual tasks; moderate impairments are found on tasks that assess distractibility, delayed recall, and working memory; and severe impairments occur in the ability to manipulate information, sometimes called executive functioning (Table 4.1). People with schizophrenia are also often very slow in their responses and find it difficult to access a wide vocabulary. There is a distribution of these difficulties within the population of people with schizophrenia with the most severely disabled patients sometimes performing well below average. Of those people who continue to be involved with the psychiatric services, 85% perform below normal on one or more cognitive domains (1). In a normal population only 5% have such low levels of functioning, so cognitive deficits can be considered as a core feature of schizophrenia. However, it must be stressed here that that many people with schizophrenia fall within the normal range of cognitive functioning.

Table 4.1 A profile of cognitive deficits in schizophrenia

Mild	Moderate	Severe
Perceptual skills	Distractibility	Executive functioning
Delayed recognition memory	Memory and working memory	Verbal fluency
Verbal and full-scale IQ	Delayed recall	Motor speed

The profile of cognitive deficits found in people with schizophrenia is different from that found in patients with Alzheimer dementia (2). For example, Alzheimer's sufferers have severe impairments in recognition memory but people with schizophrenia are only mildly impaired on these tasks. However, there seems to be only quantitative differences between those with a diagnosis of schizophrenia and those with either bipolar disorder or delusional disorder, with schizophrenia patients being the most disabled.

There has been considerable debate about whether these cognitive difficulties are static or progressive. Studies of birth cohorts or population studies have produced evidence that leaves little doubt about the existence of cognitive difficulties prior to the onset of the disorder (3,4). For example (5), study in a birth cohort from Dunedin, New Zealand showed that cognitive difficulties at all developmental stages were predictive of the later development of a schizophrenia spectrum disorder (SSD) when compared with those who later developed other psychiatric disorders or none at all. Lewis et al. (6) also showed, in a cohort of Swedish military, that those who later developed schizophrenia were more likely to have low IQs than those who did not develop the disorder. Reichenberg et al. (7) replicated these results in a study of 54,000 17-year-old Israeli conscripts who were followed for up to 11 years. They also found that the risk for SSDs increased with decreasing IQ score. Only poorer nonverbal reasoning conferred a significant risk for SSD after taking into account general intellectual ability. Because these data were all collected some time before the onset of the disorder the results are unlikely to be due to the prodromal phase of the illness.

It is also clear that there is a substantial worsening of cognitive performance with the onset of the disorder. Some of the deficits seem to be related to the presence of other symptoms (such as delusions), and remit as symptoms resolve. However, mild difficulties that were evident before the first episode can worsen into a severe cognitive deficit in the months before and during the first episode, and remain relatively stable after remission (8,9).

Data from cross-sectional studies do not indicate many differences in cognitive functioning between the following:

- Young patients with a short duration of illness, old patients with a short duration of illness and old patients with a long duration of illness (3,10)
- Adolescent and chronic patients (11)
- First-episode patients and chronic patients (12)

These data suggest a relative stability of cognitive difficulties over time.

What are the effects of cognitive difficulties on symptoms, rehabilitation, and life skills?

Symptoms

It is tempting to assume that cognitive difficulties in schizophrenia are strongly correlated with positive symptoms (hallucinations and delusions), but studies tend to show that cognitive dysfunction accounts for only a small amount of variance in those symptoms (13). What is clear from high-risk and birth cohort studies is that cognitive difficulties themselves may play a causal role in the propensity for positive symptoms. However, we cannot yet distinguish within the group of people with schizophrenia, those cognitive difficulties that may underpin the severity of specific symptoms. This is in part due to the lack of subtlety in the measurement of the symptoms themselves. Furthermore, the effect of a cognitive difficulty may only manifest if the cognitive system is stressed so that subtle difficulties, which can be compensated for under normal circumstances, break down. The experiment depicted in Figure 4.1, based on the proposal by Frith (14) that difficulties in the ability to self-monitor may underlie the experience of hallucinations, demonstrates this. Thus, when asked to distinguish words spoken by themselves or others when they were fed back words with distortion of the sound, people with schizophrenia had many more problems in distinguishing their own voice and were biased to say it was some-one else's. This difficulty was measurable only when the words were distorted before feeding them back to the patient (15). It has also been suggested that a top-down bias as well as bottom-up attentional processes can account for this self-monitoring problem (16).

Rehabilitation

The presence of cognitive difficulties is related to the degree of dependence on psychiatric services, with higher levels of problems being associated with more restrictive forms of care and a lack of independence. The difficulties are also predictive of future care. In a 6-year follow-up study of people who were moved into the community following the closure of a large psychiatric hospital, cognitive difficulties were a significant predictor of how much care a person would require, such that those with the least impairment were most able to live independently (17). Cognitive difficulties also predict the amount of care people are likely to receive. In an innovative study, Patel et al. (18) showed

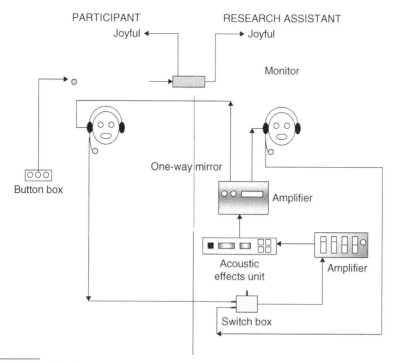

Figure 4.1 *The self-monitoring of voices: the effects of distortion. Source: Adapted from Ref. 14.*

that the overall level of cognitive difficulty led directly to the cost of care. Cognitive difficulties also predict the level of social performance. But perhaps more importantly, cognitive difficulties such as verbal memory problems appear to limit the amount that a person can learn from a traditional reha-bilitation program. Thus, those people with the worst memories achieve the least improvement, particularly in terms of social skills.

Life skills

Cognitive difficulties not only make a difference to the level of care received, but also serve to limit the vocational rehabilitation potential of patients with schizophrenia (19). Bell et al. (20) have shown that cognition rather than symptoms seems to predict improvements in work quality following a 6-month rehabilitation program. Gold et al. (21) have shown that the chance of gaining competitive paid employment following a rehabilitation program is affected by IQ, memory, and speed of processing information. But it must be emphasized that even the most severely cognitively disabled can work if they are provided with the right sort of job and effective supports (chap. 11). Several authors recently have discussed the relationship between cognition and overall functioning outcome (22) showing the difficulties in making any assessment due to overall measurement problems. However, confirmatory path analyses have revealed that neuropsychological performance predicts an intervening variable, functional capacity as measured using a controlled performance measure, and that this capacity measure then predicted the overall functioning (23).

Treatment issues

Even though the data suggest that cognitive dysfunctions in schizophrenia tend to be static over time, this does not mean that they are immutable. Indeed, there have been several recent innovative treatment approaches that have now instilled a degree of therapeutic optimism; these are outlined below. What we have also learnt is that some interaction between treatments and cognitive difficulties can make matters worse. For example, when schizophrenia patients with high levels of cognitive difficulties were moved into community placements and had to increase their decision-making capabilities, their levels of positive symptoms worsened. In contrast, those without severe cognitive difficulty both improved their social behavior and showed a reduction in symptoms (24). It is therefore essential to take into account the current cognitive state of the person when determining treatment plans.

Pharmacological approaches to improving cognition in schizophrenia

Before considering the potential role of medications in ameliorating cognitive deficits in schizophrenia, it is as well to consider whether antipsychotic medications might actually worsen cognitive ability. Rationalizing medications will avoid adding to the cognitive impairments that affect so many people with schizophrenia. However, most studies appear to show an improvement in cognition irrespective of the antipsychotic type (25).

In terms of evidence of these therapeutic effects for cognition in schizophrenia, it is the atypical antipsychotics that attracted the most recent attention. Early reports of an apparent amelioration of cognitive impairment were largely nonrandomized within-group switch studies, where patients were assessed prior to, and after, switching from a typical to an atypical agent. Such a design is flawed in that there is no control for time variables and practice effects, or for the effect of simply having withdrawn the typical agent. However, randomized control trials appear to support the notion that atypicals do exert some beneficial effect for cognition although there are also studies showing no differences (24,26). One potential confounding effect in the comparison of typicals and atypicals is the lower rate of extrapyramidal side effects (EPSEs) with the latter;

this would be most marked for tasks requiring manual dexterity. However, it seems that reduced EPSEs, even with low dosing of the typical comparator, cannot account for all of the beneficial effect of the atypicals (27,28).

What has not been established is the effect of dosage and the time required to establish a positive effect on cognition with atypical antipsychotics. It is also unclear whether particular drugs have effects on specific domains of functioning. For example, it appears that clozapine improves attention and verbal fluency, but has much more equivocal effects on working memory (29).

Furthermore, the effect size of improvement in cognition with atypicals is relatively modest, and certainly does not compensate for the deficits found in many schizophrenia patients. Put statistically, the extent of improvement in any cognitive domain with the atypical agents is less than 0.5 of a standard deviation, while the extent of abnormality (see above) is of the order of two standard deviations from the normal population mean. Thus, while of enormous potential importance, the apparent cognitive benefits of the newer atypical antipsychotics require a great deal of further careful investigation and do not obviate the need for other strategies such as psychological approaches. These partnership approaches, particularly cognitive remediation plus medication seem to produce large-effect sizes that may be clinically significant (30,31).

Other pharmacological approaches to enhancing cognition in schizophrenia include the addition of a cognitive enhancing drug such as nicotine or psychostimulant drugs. Both of these strategies have shown some promise in enhancing certain cognitive domains, notably attention (32,33). However, to date there have been only one or two studies suggesting benefits for cognitive enhancers (34) and many that show no effects. This is an exciting area of research which requires further work to validate new approaches, and establish their role, if any, in clinical practice.

Psychological approaches

Psychological approaches to dealing with cognitive dysfunction in schizophrenia can be divided into three main categories:

- Direct approaches where the cognitive difficulty is the target of the rehabilitation
- Changing the rehabilitation program so that it plays to the strengths rather than weaknesses of the patient
- Changing the environment so that it compensates for the cognitive deficits

Directly changing cognition

This approach is relatively new and various therapeutic techniques have been adopted directly to change or improve particular cognitive systems. These have shown improvements that have endured. Noneffective studies have also appeared in the literature and provide guidance on what not to do. For example, we now know that only paying people to improve their performance, simply practicing a task over and over, or merely simplifying the task is not as effective as strategy approaches (35).

The most robustly effective approach is called cognitive remediation therapy (36,37). This therapy does not simply teach tasks, but concentrates on providing strategies for dealing with problems in general. What seems to be essential is to provide tasks where patients learn to achieve goals through their own efforts; this is called "self-efficacy." This requires that the tasks are just inside the patient's level of competence so that they have to make some learning effort, but do succeed (called scaffolding). Reducing the number of errors made by the patient ("errorless learning") is also essential, as people with schizophrenia find it hard to distinguish in their memory between responses that produced errors, and responses that were correct. Thus, if they make many errors they will not be able to carry out the task correctly at a later date. The studies carried out so far have used paper and pencil tasks or computer games to teach information-processing skills and are usually supervised by clinical psychologists, but Table 4.2 shows the sort of approaches that could be provided within any psychosocial treatment program.

The most recent meta-analysis, carried out on the data from controlled and randomized controlled trials (38) demonstrates that the effect size of cognitive remediation is about 0.4. These new psychosocial techniques are more likely to have an effect of functional outcome than medication enhancement. For example, Velligan et al. (39) showed that cognition could be enhanced by quetiapine but that this had no effect on functioning. In contrast, Bell et al. (19), Spaulding et al. (40), Wykes et al. (30,41), McGurk et al. (42), and Eack et al. (43) have all shown that cognitive enhancement achieved through psychosocial means does lead to functional change. Analyses have confirmed that random changes that are apparent in the control conditions of trials do not consistently lead to functional improvement (44).

The majority of studies on the rehabilitation of cognitive deficits approached the problem in a pragmatic way with little regard to the types of techniques that may be necessary or theories about the way in which cognitive deficits impinge on daily living. Although theories are now developing, there is still plenty of room for improvement in this area (34,45). In the first book on individual cognitive enhancement, Wykes and Reeder (36) suggest three simple pathways for the impact of cognition on outcome: routine actions, routine controlled actions, and nonroutine actions. For *routine actions*, behavior is governed by a schema that requires no reflection and little cognitive control. Once the environmental trigger occurs, the behavior is automatic. These actions are unlikely to be affected by small changes in cognition functions. For *routine controlled actions*, the person has a cognitive schema to guide the action but may need to adapt it a little, for example to

Table 4.2 Cognitive enhancement strategies for people with schizophrenia

Life skill	Cognitive skills required	Useful strategies to aid relevant cognitive skills	Useful tasks to target relevant skills
Shopping for groceries	Planning Memory Sequencing	• Write a shopping list or repeat to yourself what you need to buy • Break the shopping list into categories • Order your list according to the layout of the shop(s)	• Devising a plan for how to implement a problem-solving task • Re-ordering numbers from a disorganized list • Memorizing a set of words
Reading a train timetable	Attention to detail Shifting attention Self-monitoring	• Check details frequently • Trace along lines with fingers to avoid visual neglect • Use verbal mediation to remind yourself what you are looking for	• Searching through a grid of letters for changing target letters • Line bisection tasks (estimating the midpoint of a line)
Remembering the route to the shop	Spatial memory	• Visualize the route • Generate a verbal description • Use verbal repetition • Associate landmarks with familiar objects • Make a list of landmarks • Draw yourself a map	• Memorizing sequences of squares on a grid • Memorizing designs • Generating verbal descriptions for designs or sequenced patterns
Planning your next move in a game of draughts	Spatial memory Planning Sequencing	• Visualize the moves • Find visual patterns to describe the moves • Generate a verbal description for the moves • Use verbal repetition	• Visual transformation tasks (e.g. draw what this shape would look like if it was rotated by half a turn) • Memorizing geometric patterns • Memorizing sequences of moves on a grid

Holding a conversation in a noisy room	Auditory verbal memory Comprehension Selective attention Self-monitoring	• Minimize distractions • Ask the other person to repeat what they said • Don't rush what you are saying	• Generating verbal descriptions for pictures • Listening to instructions and then carrying them out • Answering questions about a spoken passage • Counting target items whilst tapping a sequence with your hand • Comprehension tasks – learning a written passage and answering questions about it • Searching for target letters or numbers in a grid • Attentional shifting tasks: e.g. copying a design onto another sheet of paper • Sequencing tasks – describe the steps needed to carry out problem-solving tasks
Reading a magazine article	Verbal comprehension Verbal memory Attention to detail	• Use chunking • Use repetition • Follow each line with your finger to ensure nothing is missed out and reading speed is not too fast	
Baking a cake using a recipe	Sustained attention Shifting attention Sequencing Planning Memory Self-monitoring	• Take one step at a time • Organize your equipment • Use written records • Use verbal repetition • Devise a plan before you begin • Create subgoals • Check steps as you proceed	

attend to specific parts of the schema. These actions can be improved in terms of their efficiency by improvement in cognitive functions but the effects are limited. Most of our actions require flexibility and these are final-category *nonroutine controlled actions*. For these actions we must develop new cognitive schemas to guide us as to which are efficient. These actions require reflection on one's own knowledge and Wykes and Reeder (36) have termed this "metacognition." It is their contention that teaching metacognition is essential if cognitive skills are to be translated into actions. Their book provides an overview of the techniques they think should be included to enhance the transfer of cognitive improvements into everyday life. Metacognition has also recently been highlighted by Lysaker et al. (46) and Stratta et al. (47) as more likely to be a mediator of functional outcome. A recent meta-analysis on cognitive treatment in traumatic brain injury suggests that for improvements in neural plasticity in this group, and particularly for functioning, including metacognition as a target is vital (48). Others have suggested a role for brain functioning in terms of cognitive remediation reducing grey matter loss in first-episode patients (49).

Changing rehabilitation programs to fit strengths

It seems obvious that cognitive difficulties need to be taken into account in providing any psychosocial rehabilitation program. This means obtaining a profile of the cognitive difficulties of a person and then using this to guide the design of an individualized program. For example, poor verbal memory is known to limit learning in a social skills training program. The most sensible response is to change the program itself so that it does not rely too heavily on verbal memory. This sort of approach has been adopted in the learning disability literature, but has not been investigated extensively in programs for people with schizophrenia.

Changing the environment

This is the last resort for the treatment of cognitive difficulties, and is similar to the approaches made for people with dementia. Here, the environment is changed so that there is less demand on the dysfunctional cognitive systems. One randomized trial in Texas showed that by providing this sort of support, patients with cognitive difficulties improved their overall functioning (50,51). The key worker/case manager visits the person at least twice a week and provides a series of cues for carrying out particular tasks, such as alarms to remind them when to go out to the day centre. They also organize their activities minutely, for example placing all the clothes required for a single day into boxes and labeling them with the days of the week; the person then puts all the clothes on for that particular day, no more and no less. This form of therapy, known as "cognitive adaptational training" could be seen as rather intrusive, and may not be acceptable to some services and patients.

Conclusions

Cognitive impairments are common in schizophrenia, and mediate much of the disability experienced by people with the condition. The atypical antipsychotics may be associated with some degree of improvement in cognition but it is the psychosocial forms of therapy that seems to offer the most benefit. These therapies are still under development but have shown effects on a wide range of everyday behaviors such as work and social function.

References

1. Harvey P, Serper M. The nature and management of cognitive dysfunction in patients with schizophrenia. Dir Psychiatry 1999; 19: 21–35.
2. Ting C, Rajji TK, Ismail Z, et al. Differentiating the cognitive profile of schizophrenia from that of Alzheimer disease and depression in late life. PLoS One 2010; 5: e10151. doi:10.1371/journal.pone.0010151.
3. Lewandowski KE, Cohen BM, Ongur D. Evolution of neuropsychological dysfunction during the course of schizophrenia and bipolar disorder. Psychol Med 2011; 41: 225–41.
4. Reichenberg A, Caspi A, Harrington HL, et al. Static and dynamic cognitive deficits in childhood schizophrenia: a 30-year study. Am J Psychiatry 2010; 167: 160–9.
5. Cannon M, Caspi A, Moffitt TE, et al. Evidence for early-childhood pan-developmental impairment specific to schizophreniform disorder: results from a longitudinal birth cohort. Arch Gen Psychiatry 2002; 59: 449–57.
6. Lewis G, David AS, Malmberg A, Allebeck P. Non-psychotic psychiatric disorder and subsequent risk of schizophrenia: cohort study. Br J Psychiatry 2000; 177: 416–20.
7. Reichenberg A, Weiser M, Rapp MA, et al. Premorbid intra-individual variability in intellectual performance and risk for schizophrenia: a population-based study. Schizophr Res 2006; 85: 49–57.
8. Bozikas VP, Andreou C. Longitudinal studies of cognition in first episode psychosis: a systematic review of the literature. Aust NZ J Psychiatry 2011; 45: 93–108.
9. Shrivastava A, Johnston M, Shah N, Thakar M, Stitt L. Persistent cognitive dysfunction despite clinical improvement in schizophrenia: a 10-year follow-up study. J Psychiatr Pract 2011; 17: 194–9.
10. Jeste DV, Harris MJ, Krull A, et al. Clinical and neuropsychological characteristics of patients with late-onset schizophrenia. Am J Psychiatry 1995; 152: 722–30.
11. Goldberg TE, Weinberger DR. Probing prefrontal function in schizophrenia with neuropsychological paradigms. Schizophr Bull 1988; 14: 179–83.
12. Greenwood K. The Nature and Stability of Executive Impairments in Schizophrenia [PhD Thesis]. London, England: University of London, 2000.
13. Ventura J, Thames A, Wood R, Guzik L, Hellemann G. Disorganization and reality distortion in schizophrenia: a meta-analysis of the relationship between positive symptoms and neurocognitive deficits. Schizophr Res 2010; 121: 1–14.
14. Frith CD. The Cognitive Neuropsychology of Schizophrenia. Hillsdale, England: Lawrence Erlbaum Associates, Inc, England, 1992.
15. Johns LC, Rossell S, Frith C, et al. Verbal self-monitoring and auditory verbal hallucinations in patients with schizophrenia. Psychol Med 2001; 31: 705–15.
16. Ilankovic L, Allen P, Engel R, et al. Attentional modulation of external speech attribution in patients with hallucinations and delusions. Neuropsychologia 2011; 49: 805–12.

17. Wykes T, Dunn G. Cognitive deficit and the prediction of rehabilitation success in a chronic psychiatric group. Psychol Med 1992; 22: 389–98.
18. Patel A, Everitt B, Knapp M, et al. Schizophrenia patients with cognitive deficits: factors associated with costs. Schizophr Bull 2006; 32: 776–85.
19. Tsang HWH, Leung AY, Chung RCK, Bell M, Cheung W-M. Review on vocational predictors: a systematic review of predictors of vocational outcomes among individuals with schizophrenia: an update since 1998. Aust NZ J Psychiatry 2010; 44: 495–504.
20. Bell M, Bryson G, Greig T, Corcoran C, Wexler BE. Neurocognitive enhancement therapy with work therapy: effects on neurocognitive test performance. Arch Gen Psychiatry 2001; 58:763–8.
21. Gold J, Iannone V, McMahon R, Buchanon R. Cognitive correlates of competitive employment among patients with schizophrenia. Schizophr Res 2001; 49: 134.
22. Bellack AS, Green MF, Cook JA, et al. Assessment of community functioning in people with schizophrenia and other severe mental illnesses: a white paper based on an NIMH-sponsored workshop. Schizophr Bull 2007; 33: 805–22.
23. Bowie CR, Depp C, McGrath JA, et al. Prediction of real-world functional disability in chronic mental disorders: a comparison of schizophrenia and bipolar disorder. Am J Psychiatry 2010; 167: 1116–24.
24. Wykes T. Predicting symptomatic and behavioural outcomes of community care. Br J Psychiatry 1994; 165: 486–92.
25. Davidson M, Galderisi S, Weiser M, et al. Cognitive effects of antipsychotic drugs in first-episode schizophrenia and schizophreniform disorder: a randomized, open-label clinical trial (EUFEST). Am J Psychiatry 2009; 166: 675–82.
26. Keefe RSE, Silva SG, Perkins DO, Lieberman JA. The effects of atypical antipsychotic drugs on neurocognitive impairment in schizophrenia: a review and meta-analysis. Schizophr Bull 1999; 25: 201–22.
27. Green MF. Recent studies on the neurocognitive effects of second-generation antipsychotic medications. Curr Opin Psychiatry 2002; 15: 25–9.
28. Keefe RSE, Seidman LJ, Christensen BK, et al. Long-term neurocognitive effects of olanzapine or low-dose haloperidol in first-episode psychosis. Biol Psychiatry 2006; 59: 97–105.
29. Bilder RM, Goldman RS, Volavka J, et al. Neurocognitive effects of clozapine, olanzapine, risperidone, and haloperidol in patients with chronic schizophrenia or schizoaffective disorder. Am J Psychiatry 2002; 159: 1018–28.
30. Wykes T, Reeder C, Corner J, Williams C, Everitt B. The effects of neurocognitive remediation on executive processing in patients with schizophrenia. Schizophr Bull 1999; 25: 291–307.
31. Wykes T, Reeder C, Williams C. Are the effects of cognitive remediation therapy (CRT) durable? Results from an exploratory trial in schizophrenia. Schizophr Res 2003; 61: 163–74.
32. Goff D, Freudenreich O, Evins A. Augmentation strategies in the treatment of schizophrenia. CNS Spectr 2001; 6: 904–11.
33. Levin ED, Rezwani AH. Nicotinic-antipsychotic drug interactions and cognitive function in Levin ED. ESX 2006; 98: 185–205.
34. Scoriels L, Barnett JH, Soma PL, Sahakian BJ, Jones PB. Effects of modafinil on cognitive functions in first episode psychosis. Psychopharmacology 2011. DOI: 10.1007/s00213-011-2472-4. [[Available from: http://www.springerlink.com/content/m26881337u8468w0/].
35. Wykes T, Spaudling W. Thinking about the future cognitive remediation therapy – What works and could we do better? Schizophr Bull 2011; 37: 80–90.

36. Wykes T, van der Gaag M. Is it time to develop a new cognitive therapy for psychosis–cognitive remediation therapy (CRT)? Clin Psychol Rev 2001; 21: 1227–56.
37. Wykes T, Reeder C. Cognitive Remediation Therapy for Schizophrenia: Theory and Practice. London and New York: Brunner Routledge, Taylor and Francis Group, 2005.
38. Wykes T, Huddy V, Cellard C, McGurk SR, Czobor P. A meta-analysis of cognitive remediation for schizophrenia: Methodology and effect sizes. Am J Psychiatry 2011; 168: 472–85.
39. Velligan DI, Prihoda TJ, Sui D, et al. The effectiveness of quetiapine versus conventional antipsychotics in improving cognitive and functional outcomes in standard treatment settings. J Clin Psychiatry 2003; 64: 524–31.
40. Spaulding WD, Reed D, Sullivan M, Richardson C, Weiler M. Effects of cognitive treatment in psychiatric rehabilitation. Schizophr Bull 1999; 25: 657–76.
41. Wykes T, Reeder C, Landau S, et al. Cognitive remediation therapy in schizophrenia: randomised controlled trial. Br J Psychiatry 2007; 190: 421–7.
42. McGurk SR, Mueser KT, Pascaris A. Cognitive training and supported employment for persons with severe mental illness: one year results from a randomized controlled trial. Schizophr Bull 2005; 31: 898–909.
43. Eack SM, Hogarty GE, Greenwald DP, et al. Effects of cognitive enhancement therapy on employment outcomes in early schizophrenia: results from a 2-year randomized trial. Res Soc Work Pract 2011; 21: 32–42.
44. Reeder C, Smedley N, Butt K, Bogner D, Wykes T. Cognitive predictors of social functioning improvements following cognitive remediation for schizophrenia. Schizophr Bull 2006; 32(Suppl 1): S123–31.
45. Wykes T. Cognitive remediation therapy needs funding. Nature 2010; 468:165–6.
46. Lysaker PH, Shea AM, Buck KD, et al. Metacognition as a mediator of the effects of impairments in neurocognition on social function in schizophrenia spectrum disorders. Acta Psychiatr Scand 2010; 122: 405–13.
47. Stratta P, Daneluzzo E, Riccardi I, Bustini M, Rossi A. Metacognitive ability and social functioning are related in persons with schizophrenic disorder. Schizophr Res 2009; 108: 301–2.
48. Circerone K, Langenbahn D, Braden C, et al. Evidence-based cognitive rehabilitation: Updated review of the literature from 2003 through 2008. Arch Phys Med Rehabil 2011; 92: 519–30.
49. Eack SM, Hogarty GE, Cho RY, et al. Neuroprotective effects of cognitive enhancement therapy against gray matter loss in early schizophrenia: results from a 2-year randomized controlled trial. Arch Gen Psychiatry 2010; 67: 674–82.
50. Velligan D, Bow-Thomas C, Huntzinger C, et al. Randomized controlled trial of the use of compensatory strategies to enhance adaptive functioning in outpatients with schizophrenia. Am J Psychiatry 2000; 157: 1317–23.
51. Velligan D, Diamond P, Mueller J, et al. The short-term impact of generic versus individualized environmental supports on functional outcomes and target behaviours in schizophrenia. Psychiatry Res 2009; 168: 94–101.

chapter 5

Depression and anxiety in schizophrenia

David J. Castle, Til Wykes, Natalie Knoesen, and Peter Bosanac

The extent of psychiatric comorbidity in schizophrenia is often not appreciated, in part because of our heritage of an essentially hierarchical approach to psychiatric diagnosis, where schizophrenia "trumps" depression and anxiety. However, the recognition of depressive and anxiety symptoms in people with schizophrenia is important and has begun to receive increasing attention. These symptoms are common, tend to worsen the longitudinal course of illness, and can result in secondary morbidity and suicide. This chapter provides a brief overview of depression and selected anxiety disorders (social anxiety and obsessive–compulsive disorder (OCD)) in schizophrenia.

Depression and schizophrenia

The relationship between schizophrenia on the one hand, and affective disorders on the other, has dominated the nosological debate for well over a century since Kraepelin's original dichotomization of "dementia praecox" from "manic depression." Bleuler, who coined the term "schizophrenia," did include affective symptoms (anhedonia) in his definition of the disorder. But it was Kasanin, in describing patients with what he called "schizoaffective disorder," who shifted the debate to a consideration of patients with an admixture of both "schizophrenic" and "affective" symptoms; the place of such disorders in the nosology is still debated (1,2). Here we do not consider schizoaffective disorders as such, nor do we address manic psychoses, concentrating instead on depression in people with schizophrenia. For reviews of the treatment of schizoaffective disorder, see Refs. (3,1).

It is not uncommon for people with schizophrenia to manifest depressive symptoms. Indeed, the National Comorbidity Survey in the United States reported that 59% of people with schizophrenia also had a lifetime diagnosis of depression. In clinical samples of schizophrenia patients, rates of depression of anything from 7% to 65% have been reported, depending upon sample

Table 5.1   Factors that might mediate depression in schizophrenia

Social factors (unemployment, lack of social network, etc.)
Psychosocial stressors (e.g., loss of role and family stress)
Adjustment to diagnosis
Alcohol and illicit substance use
Noncompliance with antipsychotic medication
Direct dysphoric effect of antipsychotic medication
Extrapyramidal side effects of antipsychotic medication

selection and the definition of depression; Siris (4,5), who has reviewed these studies, suggests a modal figure of 25%.

The extent of this comorbidity is, in many ways, unsurprising, as many people with schizophrenia suffer from secondary social dysfunction, including the break-up of families and relationships, loss of study/work, and poverty (Table 5.1). Such factors are associated in the general population with depression. Furthermore, schizophrenia is a severe and long-term illness which carries with it a considerable stigma and which is thus difficult to adjust to for the patient.

Effect of depression on the longitudinal course of schizophrenia

Some early studies suggested that depression in schizophrenia might be a predictor of favorable outcome, but such studies were almost certainly confounded by the inclusion of people with "schizoaffective" disorders, and it is now generally accepted that depression worsens the long-term course of schizophrenia and is associated with an increased use of medications, early relapse, and increased hospital admissions (6–8). Some studies have found that patients with comorbid depressive symptoms who have a greater insight into their mental illness, its social consequences and treatment efficacy, experience a poorer overall quality of life, specifically relating to physical and psychological health, social relationships, and the environment (9–12). Such patients appear to be more at risk of depressive symptoms at the beginning of treatment, and of developing postpsychotic depression (13,14). Correlations between level of insight, distress, hopelessness, and suicidality have also been reported (11,13,15).

The rates of completed suicide are far higher in schizophrenia patients than the general population. Most recent estimates indicate that around 5% of schizophrenia patients will commit suicide, and this usually occurs near illness onset (16). In a single year, 3800 schizophrenia sufferers in the United States committed suicide (17). Given the strong correlation between depressive symptoms, notably hopelessness, and suicide in schizophrenia (7,17,18) depression is a major risk factor for suicide in patients with schizophrenia. It is thus imperative that clinicians recognize and treat depression in such individuals (5).

Recognizing depression in schizophrenia

One of the impediments to the recognition of depression in people with schizophrenia is the diagnostic hierarchy alluded to above. Thus, clinicians tend to concentrate on eliciting and monitoring psychotic symptoms, rather than depression. The problem is made worse by the fact that both psychotic symptoms and side effects of antipsychotic medication can manifest very much like those of depression, and it is difficult to make the distinction (Table 5.2).

For example, depressive lack of motivation and interest can be confused with the apathetic social withdrawal of schizophrenia, or might be considered a sign of "demoralization." It has been suggested that the eliciting of vegetative symptoms such as anorexia or insomnia, or expressions of low self-esteem and guilt, should sway the diagnosis toward one of depression (chap. 3).

Another factor to consider is that antipsychotic agents can produce side effects that can mimic depression. *Akinesia* can be missed clinically as it does not always occur in the setting of obvious parkinsonism (19). *Akathisia* is also associated with mood symptoms, notably dysphoria, and has been linked with suicide (20). It is important that such side effects are recognized and treated, as outlined in the next section.

Do antipsychotics cause depression?

There is considerable debate about whether antipsychotics actually cause depression. Siris (4) points to three sets of findings that suggest this is not a major factor:

- Depressive symptoms tend to improve as psychotic symptoms improve.
- Similar rates of depression have been reported in schizophrenia patients on and off antipsychotics.
- Studies have failed to show any consistent correlation between depressive symptoms and antipsychotic dose or plasma level.

Table 5.2 Psychotic symptoms and antipsychotic side effects presenting as depression

Positive psychotic symptoms
Negative symptoms
Akinesia
Akathisia

However, other authors refute this conclusion and have suggested a role for antipsychotic-mediated effects on dopamine-mediated reward systems in the brain as etiologically important (21).

Any dysphoric effect of antipsychotics is not likely to be prominent with the newer "atypical" agents (chap. 1). Indeed, risperidone, olanzapine, quetiapine, and ziprasidone have all been shown to have antidepressant effects in schizophrenia patients (22–26); probably the most consistent antidepressant effects are seen for quetiapine and olanzapine (27). Having said this, data from the CATIE trial involving 1460 schizophrenia patients did not show any difference of the atypical antipsychotics compared with perphenazine on depressive symptoms measured on the Calgary Depression Scale for schizophrenia (6).

It is supposed that the antidepressant effect associated with the atypical agents is dictated by the serotonergic actions of these drugs, although a number of other parameters should also be considered (Table 5.3). In an important study that controlled for the effects of lower EPS with olanzapine compared with haloperidol, Tollefson and colleagues (28) employed the path analysis to show the direct antidepressant effect of olanzapine. Similarly, Emsley et al.'s (29) path analysis study compared quetiapine with haloperidol and found a greater direct reduction in depressive symptoms, independent of positive, negative, or extrapyramidal symptoms. A randomized controlled study by Kotler et al. (30) found significant improvements in depressive symptomatology with sulpiride augmentation of olanzapine in treatment-resistant chronic schizophrenia patients.

Treating depression in schizophrenia

Table 5.4 presents some factors that should be excluded in schizophrenia patients presenting with depression. Some of these might require a therapeutic trial, for example an anticholinergic challenge if akinesia is suspected; and propranolol or benzodiazepine in patients with akathisia. It is also important

Table 5.3   Ways in which atypical antipsychotics may produce antidepressant effects

Tend not to produce extrapyramidal side effects at therapeutic doses
Tend not to produce neurolept-induced deficit symptoms (NIDS)
More efficacy against negative symptoms (notably clozapine)
Reduce illicit substance use
Enhance compliance with medication
Enable more effective psychosocial rehabilitation, including work
Direct antidepressant effect

Source: From Ref. 26.

Table 5.4 Factors to exclude in schizophrenia patients presenting with depression

Organic disorders (medical)
Alcohol abuse
Illicit substance use
"Pre-psychotic" prodromal phase of psychotic episode
Negative symptoms (e.g., anergia and apathetic social withdrawal)
Schizoaffective depression
Antipsychotic side effects (notably akinesia and akathisia)
Demoralization (diminished sense of subjective control over the illness)

Source: Adapted from Refs. 4,5,26.

to recognize that there is little evidence for the efficacy of antidepressant medication for dysphoria in patients who have prominent positive symptoms of psychosis, and the priority should be the optimal control of psychotic symptoms (4).

Psychological strategies

The treatment of depression in schizophrenia requires a multifaceted biopsychosocial approach. Life events resulting from an acute episode, the stigma attached to the illness as well as the loss of social roles are known to be associated with depression in schizophrenia (31). Psychological factors associated with psychotic symptoms are also likely to predict depression. For instance, the degree of malevolence of the content of an auditory hallucination and the powerfulness of the "voice" are predictive of depression.

Recent research suggests that greater insight into illness is associated with an increase in depression and poorer subjective quality of life in people with schizophrenia. However, insight into illness is crucial for better acceptance of illness, adherence to treatment, and rehabilitation (32). This dichotomy has important implications for treatment and suggests an emphasis on psychoeducation programs focusing on depressive symptoms and quality of life–related aspects. Recent studies have found support for such psychoeducation programs and have reported significant improvements in quality of life, competence, control, and overall well-being of the patients (33,34). This, together with an increased awareness of these issues by the clinician and a strengthening of the therapeutic alliance, may help improve insight without the risk of depressed mood and quality of life (32).

The overall psychological strategy for ameliorating depression in people with schizophrenia should be to encourage a blame-free acceptance and a mastery of the illness (31). Therefore, a cognitive approach to symptoms and the appraisal of the self should have an impact on depression. There is, however, little empirical evidence to support any specific psychological therapy in this context. Thus, interventions should be tailored to the particular needs of the individual within the overall model; for example, grief work should be provided for those experiencing loss and rehabilitation and resocialization programs for those manifesting demoralization.

Pharmacological strategies

In terms of medication, it appears clear from the earlier discussion, that atypical antipsychotics play an important role in the treatment of depression in schizophrenia. Siris (26) reviewed 13 prospective randomized controlled trials (RCTs) of atypical antipsychotics in schizophrenia, and found that 12 of these recorded antidepressant efficacy. Similarly, Tollefson's (35) review of the role of antipsychotics in the treatment of comorbid mood disorders reported more robust antidepressant treatment effects when using atypical antipsychotics. Many recent studies continue to find support for the antidepressant efficacy of atypical antipsychotics in schizophrenia (23,29,30). Thus, atypical antipsychotics seem a prudent choice in the setting of schizophrenia complicated by depression. An effect on suicidality would also be expected, and has been confirmed for clozapine (36).

The evidence regarding the efficacy of the addition of antidepressants to antipsychotics is rather mixed, and some studies have reported a worsening of psychotic symptoms with this combination. However, most studies to date are short term and limited in their generalizability (27). In their review of this literature, Siris and Bench (37) reported 13 randomized placebo controlled trials where antidepressants were added to antipsychotics, with all but two using tricyclic antidepressants; only four were positive on the primary outcome measure. The evidence regarding depressive symptoms not meeting the syndromic "caseness" is equivocal, and in this setting, strategies such as optimization of antipsychotic treatment and psychosocial interventions should be considered prior to resorting to antidepressant medication. According to Buckley (7), in acutely psychotic patients with comorbid depressive symptoms, it is best to first treat the psychosis with an atypical antipsychotic and see whether the depressive symptoms subside before adding an antidepressant or mood stabilizer. In a Cochrane review (38) of 11 RCTs, mostly with low numbers of patients, a total of 470 patients were included. The authors concluded that there was no convincing evidence either to support or refute the use of antidepressants in treating depression in people with schizophrenia. A more recent RCT found that adding citalopram to antipsychotic medication for up to 12 weeks in middle aged and older schizophrenia outpatients was associated with a reduction in suicidal ideation from baseline, particularly in those patients whose depressive symptoms were responsive (39).

Longer-term studies are few and far between. Siris (8) followed a group of patients who had been stabilized on fluphenazine decanoate and imipramine, and found that those in whom imipramine was withdrawn were more likely to experience a depressive relapse over a year follow-up. In contrast, Glick et al. (40), in a naturalistic study of schizophrenia patients with broadly defined depression, predominantly treated with atypical antipsychotics and nontricyclic antidepressants, reported most patients experienced no significant change in mood after antidepressant cessation (40). In a subsequent reflection on these and Siris' (8) data, Glick and colleagues (41) concluded that some patients with chronic schizophrenia and moderate-to-severe depressive symptoms (and/or demoralization) may benefit from antidepressant treatment, but did specify who in particular. If antidepressants are added, their effect on mood requires close monitoring of overall symptomatology, and worsening of psychotic symptoms might require their withdrawal.

Dufresne (42) has provided a useful overview of the potential problems arising from the addition of antidepressants to antipsychotic drugs in general. These include pharmacodynamic and pharmacokinetic effects that can exacerbate side effects, such as the combination of two agents with anticholinergic or cardiotoxic effects. Common sense should prevail in deciding which combination of drugs to choose, and monitoring side effects carefully, with drug levels being checked for combinations that affect each others' metabolism. In clinical practice, SSRIs are often added to atypical antipsychotics in patients with persistent depression, and this combination is usually well tolerated. Preference should be given to those SSRIs that do not perturb the metabolism of the antipsychotic. The addition of lithium to an antipsychotic, and the place of electroconvulsive therapy (ECT) in depression in schizophrenia, have not been adequately studied, although may be indicated in particular patients.

Whatever treatment is decided upon, it is best that clinicians "partner with their patients" and be guided by the patient's clinical and functional outcome to develop an appropriate and effective treatment regime (43,44).

Anxiety disorders in schizophrenia

It is often assumed that symptoms of anxiety in people with schizophrenia are secondary to positive psychotic symptoms (i.e., delusions and hallucinations). However, a number of studies have now confirmed substantial anxiety comorbidity in schizophrenia, not merely consequent upon positive symptoms. For example, Cassano et al. (45) found in their sample of 31 patients with schizophrenia spectrum disorders, 58% were comorbid for another DSM-IIIR psychiatric disorder; 19% had a lifetime diagnosis of panic disorder, 29% OCD, and 16% social phobia. In another study of patients with schizophrenia (n = 60), Cosoff and Hafner (46) found 12% were comorbid for generalized anxiety disorder, 13% for OCD, and 17% for social phobia. Similarly,

Goodwin et al. (47) reported a rate of 15% for panic attacks in their sample of 120 people with psychotic disorders; also, rates as high as 47.5% were observed for a lifetime history of panic attacks (n = 40). Similar prevalence rates have been reported in more recent studies for comorbid OCD, panic disorder, and social anxiety disorder (48–52). In fact, a comprehensive review of the literature on anxiety comorbidity in schizophrenia conducted by Pokos and Castle (53) revealed an overall average rate of anxiety comorbidity around 50% in clinical studies, significantly higher than in the general population. A meta-analysis of the prevalence of anxiety disorders in schizophrenia found pooled rates of 12.1% for OCD, 14.9% for social phobia, 10.9% for generalized anxiety disorder, 9.8% for panic disorder, and 12.4% for post-traumatic stress disorder (54). Huppert and Smith's (51) study was one of the first to examine simultaneously the interaction of specific anxiety subtypes and psychosis and found that obsessive–compulsive and social anxiety symptoms were related to increased positive symptoms (a finding also reported by Ref. (55)), bizarre behavior, and decreased quality of life, while panic and social anxiety were related to suspiciousness/paranoia.

These high comorbidity rates are not found only in clinical samples. Indeed, in the United States, the National Comorbidity Survey conducted in the general population found that 26% of individuals with schizophrenia also met criteria for panic disorder. Table 5.5 provides a summary of the average prevalence rates of specific anxiety disorders in schizophrenia and related disorders compared with those found in the general population (53).

Studies investigating the temporal relationship between schizophrenia and comorbid anxiety disorders have found that the anxiety disorders precede the onset of overt psychosis in at least 50% of patients (53). This is compatible with findings from the longitudinal Israeli High-Risk Study (57), where those who developed schizophrenia had higher anxiety ratings at the ages of 11 and 16 than those who did not. Similarly, Goodwin et al. (58) found that early neuroticism may be a precursor to the onset of psychotic symptoms, consistent with the findings of Lewis et al. (59).

A fairly uniform finding is that anxiety comorbidity in schizophrenia is associated with a relatively worse illness outcome. For example, Goodwin et al. (47) found that psychosis patients with panic comorbidity did worse on outcomes such as psychiatric symptomatology, rehabilitation outcome, and quality of life than their counterparts without panic. Similar findings were also reported by Cosoff and Hafner (46) for patients with comorbid generalized anxiety disorder. Anxiety comorbidity has also been implicated in worse quality of life in schizophrenia (60–64).

It is also the case that the anxiety comorbidity often goes unrecognized and hence not directly treated (46). It is important that all the experiences of schizophrenia patients are not dismissed as being part of their psychotic illness, as the mere acknowledgement of anxiety symptoms as "non-psychotic" can be both reassuring and empowering for the patient.

Table 5.5 Summary rates of anxiety disorders in schizophrenia spectrum disorders (SSDs)

NCS Prevalence Rates (12)		Rates in SSDs	
Any anxiety disorder	25%	Any anxiety disorder	21–85% (~50%)
Generalized anxiety disorder	5%	Generalized anxiety disorder	1–31% (10–20%)
Panic disorder	3.5%	Panic disorder	4–35% (4–20%)
Agoraphobia	5%	Agoraphobia	0–28% (5–20%)
Social phobia	13%	Social phobia	1–40% (~30%)
Specific phobia	11%	Specific phobia	0–63% (5–15%)
ECA study (56)			
OCD	2.5%	OCD	1–59% (11–15% in 1st episode vs. 22–30% in chronic patients)

Abbreviations: ECA, epidemiological catchment area; NCS, National Comorbidity Survey; OCD, obsessive–compulsive disorder.
Source: From Ref. 53.

Social anxiety disorder

Some degree of impairment of social functioning is not unusual in schizophrenia, particularly in the occupational, self-care, and independent living domains (65). Diminished social functioning might be secondary to positive symptoms, negative symptoms, or to the disruption of social maturation and adeptness that the early onset of a severe psychiatric disorder can bring. These problems are compounded by stigmatization and negative attitudes in the general population, regarding schizophrenia. Pallanti et al. (66) showed a worse outcome for schizophrenia patients with comorbid social phobia with respect to suicide attempts, substance abuse, social adjustment, and overall quality of life.

It is often assumed that social dysfunction in schizophrenia is part and parcel of the illness process, and that little can be done to ameliorate it. This is

Table 5.6   An outline of group-based program for social phobia in schizophrenia

Session 1	Overview of anxiety, social anxiety in particular; sharing of experiences/concerns by group members; setting objectives and first homework tasks (e.g., social exposure tasks, with monitoring and challenging of unhelpful automatic thoughts)
Session 2	Review of previous week and of homework; introduction to cognitive restructuring, including challenging negative automatic thoughts)
Session 3	Exposure exercise, with role play; review of cognitive restructuring
Session 4	Educational video on social phobia; further homework assignments
Sessions 5–7	Homework reviews, cognitive restructuring with increasing onus on participants to take initiative
Session 8	Social outing; closure and future individual planning

Source: Adapted from Ref. 70.

not the case. Indeed, social skills training has a track record in rehabilitation in schizophrenia, confirmed in a recent Spanish study conducted by Moriana et al. (67). However, social skills training is not effective for all patients; and when gains accrue, they often do not generalize to new situations (68). Furthermore, it is often the case that social anxiety disorder as such is not considered as a dependent variable in investigations of social skills training (69).

In terms of treatment directly for social anxiety in schizophrenia, Halperin et al. (70) piloted a group-based intervention as outlined in Table 5.6. This study reported gains in terms of social anxiety, mood, and overall quality and enjoyment of life. Similarly, Kingsep et al. (71) conducted a 12-week group CBT program consisting of psychoeducation, graded exposure simulation, cognitive restructuring and role playing, and reported significant improvements in social anxiety, general psychopathology, depression, and quality of life. Further important steps will be to determine precisely which elements of this sort of intervention (in Table 5.6) are effective, and to integrate those elements into social skills training packages.

Harvey et al. (65) investigated the benefits of a pharmacological approach to enhancing social competence in patients with schizophrenia. Short-term treatment with the atypical antipsychotics quetiapine and risperidone was associated with short-term improvements in social competence and positive correlations with cognitive ability. However, some atypical antipsychotics (notably olanzapine and clozapine) may accentuate the risk of disorders like social anxiety, necessitating careful consideration and monitoring (66). Given the lack of operational guidelines for the treatment of comorbid social anxiety disorder in schizophrenia, further research is needed to determine appropriate next-step treatments, be it psychological, pharmacological, or a combination of both.

Obsessive–compulsive disorder

The co-occurrence of obsessive-compulsive symptoms (OCSs) or full-blown OCD and schizophrenia has been recognized for decades but, until more recently, has been the principal subject of few empirical investigations (72). Indeed, Fabisch and colleagues (73) could find only nine studies between 1926 and 2001 that directly investigated the prevalence of OCS in schizophrenia. More recently, comorbid OCD has received increased attention with a number of studies investigating their co-occurrence in schizophrenia, including at different stages of the illness (49,51,55,74–76). As outlined above, reported rates vary widely (anything from 1% to 59%), depending on sample selection and diagnostic criteria employed.

Identifying OCS in patients with schizophrenia can often be a rather difficult task exacerbated by the lack of a universally accepted technique for diagnosing symptom coexpression (see Table 5.7 for diagnostic suggestions). In one of the most methodologically sound of these studies, Eisen et al. (77) found that 6 (7.7%) of 77 patients with schizophrenia or schizoaffective disorder also met DSM-IIIR criteria for OCD; this rate is two to three times that reported in general population samples. The majority of studies found that OCS tended to antedate psychotic ones (78–82).

Table 5.7 Suggestions for identifying obsessive-compulsive symptoms in psychosis

Obsessions and compulsions are phenomenologically similar to those in pure OCD, as described in the DSM-IV

A repetitious act in response to psychotic ideation, and not in response to an obsession, does not constitute a compulsion

Recurrent, intrusive, egodystonic thoughts with current delusional themes should not be regarded as an obsession. A reassessment may be necessary after acute psychotic symptoms have been treated

Thought-form disorder may confound a diagnosis of OCS. Treat the thought-form disorder first and then reassess for OCS

Primary obsessional slowness may be mistaken for prodromal schizophrenia or thought disorder, as such patients may be unable to articulate obsessions and exhibit no compulsions

In cases where it is difficult to determine real OCS in psychosis, empiric treatment with a neuroleptic and a serotonin reuptake inhibitor may be necessary

Source: From Ref. 83.

Stengel (84) and Rosen (85) believed that the occurrence of such features were to some degree protective against "personality disintegration" in schizophrenia, but more recent studies suggest that schizophrenia patients with OCSs actually have a worse longitudinal outcome and greater impairment in neuropsychological functioning (especially prefrontal dysfunction) than their counterparts without such symptoms. For example, in the Chestnut Lodge 16-year follow-up of chronic schizophrenia patients, those with OCSs had a particularly poor outcome in terms of psychopathology, social and occupational functioning, and global outcome (86). A number of studies since have confirmed higher rates of social impairment (87,88,56,89), and poorer functioning (77,90–93) in comorbid OCS patients. Lysaker et al. (75) reported greater levels of hopelessness in schizophrenia patients with significant levels of comorbid OCSs compared with those without such symptoms.

Fenton and McGlashan (86) offer the following possible explanatory hypotheses for the coaggregation of obsessive–compulsive and psychotic symptoms:

- there is a specific subtype of schizophrenia with OCSs, which has a pernicious course;
- these patients have two comorbid disorders, which additively contribute to a poor prognosis; or
- early onset of OCD impairs the individual's social development and thus contributes to social disability when schizophrenia manifests.

A more recent study conducted by Bottas et al. (83) found epidemiologic and neurobiologic evidence for a specific pattern of neurobiologic dysfunction in patients with comorbid OCD and schizophrenia, supporting the notion of a schizo-obsessive subtype of schizophrenia (hypothesis 1 of Ref. (86)). The results of their review emphasized that clinicians should distinguish between (*i*) OCSs that occur only in the context of psychosis and that may overlap with psychotic phenomenology, representing a *forme fruste* of psychosis; (*ii*) OCSs occurring only in the prodromal phase of schizophrenia; (*iii*) neuroleptic-induced OCSs or OCD and (*iv*) OCSs or OCD occurring concurrently with schizophrenia.

Treatment of OCD in schizophrenia

The treatment of OCSs or OCD in schizophrenia has not been adequately studied resulting in no standard treatment regime. However, there are some suggested therapeutic approaches to assist in the management of this often difficult-to-treat patient group. In terms of *psychological techniques*, behavioral therapy for OCS in schizophrenia can be employed effectively in some such patients, and may obviate the need for polypharmacy. A case study looking at the benefits of *exposure and response prevention (ERP)* (where OCSs were separate from the psychotic experience) reported a marked reduction in the severity, distress, and impact of long-term OCSs without leading to significant deterioration of psychotic symptoms (94). However, ERP relies on adequate perception and sustained attention, encoding and recall and executive processing, and thus neuropsychological impairment in any of these information-processing mechanisms (as often demonstrated in patients with schizophrenia and comorbid OCD) may lead to poorer outcomes with ERP treatment.

The benefits of *cognitive–behavioral therapy (CBT)* have been reported in many recent studies and have shown improvements in anxiety-related symptoms in psychosis (95,96). McKay and McKiernan (97) recommend the following stepwise procedure when using psychological techniques to treat schizophrenia with comorbid OCD: (*i*) first treat the positive symptoms with an appropriate antipsychotic; (*ii*) assess overvalued ideas; (*iii*) ERP with shorter exposure sessions; (*iv*) cognitive therapy, focusing specifically on the process of habituation and adaptive coping strategies; and (*v*) cognitive rehabilitation, focusing on memory, organization, and social skills to enhance the information-processing mechanisms.

The *pharmacological* treatment of OCSs in the setting of schizophrenia is mostly guided by the extant OCD literature. Thus, clinicians tend to rely on the compelling evidence for the efficacy of adjunctive treatment with serotonergic antidepressants (clompiramine and SSRIs) in uncomplicated OCD (98–100) and employ these in comorbid cases in addition to antipsychotic therapy (101,102). However, clompiramine's anticholinergic properties and cardiovascular and weight gain side effects may limit its use with some patients (e.g., those on clozapine), making SSRIs the favored choice in most cases.

A curious issue which has arisen with the advent of the atypical antipsychotics, notably clozapine (chap. 1) is the tendency of such agents to exacerbate, or produce *de novo*, OCSs (55,98,103–105). The putative mechanism implicates the serotonin-5HT actions of these agents, though this has not been rigorously tested. In contrast, Poyurovsky et al. (106) reported a positive therapeutic effect of olanzapine monotherapy in three schizo-obsessive patients who had otherwise been unresponsive to conventional antipsychotics in combination with anti-obsessive agents. And Reznik et al. (100) hypothesized that OCS occurring within the course of psychosis may be effectively treated with clozapine alone, while OCSs preceding psychosis may worsen with clozapine monotherapy and should rather be treated concomitantly with specific anti-obsessive agents. On the other hand, some antipsychotic medications, particularly those with sedative properties, can diminish anxiety (53).

A recent case study reported by Chaves et al. (107) found support for the benefits of ECT in treating this comorbidity. Marked reductions in aggressive, psychotic and OC symptoms were observed, indicating that ECT may be an appropriate treatment in some cases, although typically regarded as a last resort. Poyurovsky et al. (106) recommend a seven-step treatment algorithm, which is guided by patient response/lack of response, beginning with (*i*) atypical antipsychotic monotherapy, (*ii*) then adding an SSRI, (*iii*) switching to an alternative SSRI, (*iv*) trying a typical antipsychotic and SSRI combination, (*v*) a low dose of clozapine monotherapy, (*vi*) a clozapine/SSRI combination, and as a last resort (*vii*) ECT.

The treatments outlined above (i.e., serotonergic antidepressants, ERP) can be effectively employed in this clinical scenario, and discontinuation of the atypical antipsychotic is not usually necessary (10,72). However, when combining antipsychotic and anti-OC medications, it is important to be mindful of possible pharmacological interactions and thus, careful monitoring of blood levels and side effects is necessary.

Conclusions

Depression and anxiety are common in patients with schizophrenia, and are often associated with a worsening of the long-term illness outcome. Despite this clear link, the nosological implications remain unclear, necessitating more etiologically orientated classification systems. Clinically, better recognition and adequate treatment of those symptoms are required.

References

1. Levinson DF, Umapathy C, Musthaq M. Treatment of schizoaffective disorders and schizophrenia with mood symptoms. Am J Psychiatry 1999; 156: 1138–48.
2. Castle D. Schizoaffective disorder. Adv Psychiatr Treat 2012; 18: 30–3.
3. Azorin J-M, Kaladjian A, Fakra E. Current issues on schizo-affective disorder. Encephale 2005; 31: 359–65.
4. Siris SG. Diagnosis of secondary depression in schizophrenia: implications for DSM-IV. Schizophr Bull 1991; 17: 75–98.
5. Siris SG. Managing depression in schizophrenia. Psychiatr Ann 2005; 35: 60–9.
6. Addington DD, Azorin JM, Falloon IRH, et al. Clinical issues related to depression in schizophrenia: an international survey of Psychiatrists. Acta Psychiatr Scand 2002; 105: 189–95.
7. Buckley PF. Affective impairment in schizophrenia: depression/anxiety. Prim Psychiatry 2005; 12: 4–6.
8. Siris SG. Schizophrenia. In: Siris SGHirsch SR, Weinberger DR, eds. Oxford: Blackwell Science, 1995.
9. Drake RJ, Pickles A, Bentall RP, et al. The evolution of insight, paranoia and depression during early schizophrenia. Psychol Med 2004; 34: 285–92.
10. Mintz AR, Addington J, Addington D. Insight in early psychosis: a 1-year follow-up. Schizophr Res 2004; 67: 213–17.
11. Schwartz RC, Smith SD. Suicidality and psychosis: the predictive potential of symptomatology and insight into illness. J Psychiatr Res 2004; 38: 185–91.
12. Sim K, Mahendran R, Siris SG, Heckers S, Chong SA. Subjective quality of life in first episode schizophrenia spectrum disorders with comorbid depression. Psychiatry Res 2004; 129: 141–7.
13. Carroll A, Fattah S, Clyde Z, et al. Correlates of insight and insight change in schizophrenia. Schizophr Res 1999; 35: 247–53.
14. Iqbal Z, Birchwood M, Chadwick P, Trower P. Cognitive approach to depression and suicidal thinking in psychosis 2. Testing the validity of a social ranking model. Br J Psychiatry 2000; 177: 522–8.

15. Kim Y, Sakamoto K, Kamo T, Sakamura Y, Miyaoka H. Insight and clinical corre-lates in schizophrenia. Compr Psychiatry 1997; 38: 117–23.

16. Palmer BA, Pankratz VS, Bostwick JM. The lifetime risk of suicide in schizophrenia: a re-examination. Arch Gen Psychiatry 2005; 62: 247–53.

17. Jones JS, Stein DJ, Stanley B, et al. Negative and depressive symptoms in suicidal schizophrenics. Acta Psychiatr Scand 1994; 89: 81–7.

18. Siris SG. Treating depression in schizophrenia (reply to Lund et al.). Am J Psychiatry 2001; 158: 1528.

19. Van Putten T, May PRA. 'Akinetic depression' in schizophrenia. Arch Gen Psy-chiatry 1978; 35: 1101–7.

20. Drake RE, Ehrlich J. Suicide attempts associated with akathisia. Am J Psychiatry 1985; 142: 499–501.

21. Harrow M, Yonan C, Sands JR, Marengo J. Depression in schizophrenia: are neu-roleptics, akinesia, or anhedonia involved? Schizophr Bull 1994; 20: 327–38.

22. BreierA Berg PH, Thakore JH, Naber D, et al. Olanzapine versus ziprasidone: Results of a 28-week double-blind study in patients with schizophrenia. Am J Psychiatry 2005; 162: 1879–87.

23. Kinon BJ, Lipkovich I, Edwards SB, et al. A 24-week randomized study of olanzap-ine versus ziprasidone in the treatment of schizophrenia or schizoaffective disor-der in patients with prominent depressive symptoms. J Clin Psychopharmacol 2006; 26: 157–62.

24. Lieberman JA, Stroup TS, McEvoy JP, et al. Effectiveness of antipsychotic drugs in patients with chronic schizophrenia. N Engl J Med 2005; 353: 1209–23.

25. Simpson GM, Glick ID, Weiden PJ, Romano SJ, Siu CO. Randomized, controlled, double-blind multicenter comparison of the efficacy and tolerability of ziprasi-done and olanzapine in acutely ill inpatients with schizophrenia or schizoaffec-tive disorder. Am J Psychiatry 2004; 161: 1837–47.

26. Siris SG. Depression in schizophrenia: prespective in the era of 'atypical' antipsy-chotic agents. Am J Psychiatry 2000; 157: 1379–89.

27. Castle D, Bosanac P. Depression and schizophrenia. Adv Psychiatr Treat; In press.

28. Tollefson GD. Role of the novel antipsychotics in the treatment of comorbid mood disorders in schizophrenia. In: Breier A, Tran PV, Herrera JM, Tollefson GD, Bymaster FP, eds. Current Issues in the Psychopharmacology of Schizophrenia. Philadelphia, PA, US: Lippincott Williams & Wilkins Publishers, 2001: 497–512.

29. Emsley RA, Buckley P, Jones AM, Greenwood MR. Differential effect of quetiapine on depressive symptoms in patients with partially responsive schizophrenia. J Psy-chopharmacol 2003; 17: 210–15.

30. Kotler M, Strous RD, Reznik I, et al. Sulpiride augmentation of olanzapine in the management of treatment-resistant chronic schizophrenia: evidence for improve-ment of mood symptomatology. Int Clin Psychopharmacol 2004; 19: 23–6.

31. Birchwood M, Iqbal I. Depression and suicidal thinking in psychosis. In: Wykes T, Tarrier N, Lewis S, eds. Innovation and Outcome in Psychological Treatment of Schizophrenia. Wiley: Chichester, 1998: 81–118.

32. Karow A, Pajonk FG. Insight and quality of life in schizophrenia: Recent findings and treatment implications. Curr Opin Psychiatry 2006; 19: 637–41.

33. Pekkala E, Merinder L. Psychoeducation for schizophrenia. Cochrane Database Syst Rev 2002: CD002831.

34. Sibitz I, Gossler R, Katschnig H, Amering M. 'Knowing-enjoying-better living.' A seminar for persons with psychosis to improve their quality of life and reduce their vulnerability. Psychiatr Prax 2006; 33: 170–6.

35. Tollefson GD, Sanger TM, Lu Y, Thieme ME. Depressive signs and symptoms in schizophrenia: a prospective blinded trial of olanzapine and haloperidol. Arch Gen Psychiatry 1998; 55: 250–8.

36. Meltzer HY, Alphs L, Green AI, et al. International Suicide Prevention Trial Study Group. Arch Gen Psychiatry 2003; 60: 82–91.

37. Siris SG, Bench C. Depression and schizophrenia. In: Hirsch S, Weinberger D, eds. Schizophrenia, 2nd edn. Oxford: Blackwell, 2003: 142–67.

38. Furtado VA, Srihari V, Kumar A. Atypical antipsychotics for people with both schizophrenia and depression. Cochrane Database Syst Rev 2008: CD005377.

39. Zisook S, Kasckow JW, Lanouette NM, et al. Augmentation with citalopram for suicidal ideation in middle-aged or older outpatients with schizophrenia and schizoaffective disorder who have subthreshold depressive symptoms: a randomised control trial. J Clin Psychiatry 2010; 71: 915–22.

40. Glick ID, Pham D, Davis JM. Concomitant medications may not improve outcome of antipsychotic monotherapy for stabilized patients with nonacute schizophrenia. J Clin Psychiatry 2006; 67: 1261–5.

41. Glick ID, Siris SG, Davis JM. Treating schizophrenia with comorbid depressive or demoralization symptoms. J Clin Psychiatry 2008; 69: 501.

42. Dufresne RL. Issues in pharmacotherapy: focus on depression in schizophrenia. Psychopharmacol Bull 1995; 31: 789–96.

43. Ginsberg DL, Schooler NR, Buckley PF, Harvey PD, Weiden PJ. Optimizing treatment of schizophrenia. Enhancing affective/cognitive and depressive functioning. CNS Spectr 2005; 10:1–13.

44. Siris SG. Suicide and schizophrenia. J Psychopharmacol 2001; 15: 127–35.

45. Cassano GB, Pini S, Saettoni M, Rucci P, Dell'Osso L. Occurrence and clinical correlates psychiatric comorbidity in patients with psychotic disorders. J Clin Psychiatry 1998; 59: 60–8.

46. Cosoff SJ, Hafner J. The prevalence of comorbid anxiety in schizophrenia, schizoaffective disorder and bipolar disorder. Aust NZ J Psychiatry 1998; 32: 67–72.

47. Goodwin RD, Ferrgusson DM, Horwood LJ. Neuroticism in adolescence and psychotic symptoms in adulthood. Psychol Med 2003; 33: 1089–97.

48. Braga RJ, Petrides G, Figueira I. Anxiety disorders in schizophrenia. Compr Psychiatry 2004; 45: 460–8.

49. Byerly M, Goodman W, Acholonu W, Bugno R, Rush AJ. Obsessive compulsive symptoms in schizophrenia: frequency and clinical features. Schizophr Res 2005; 76: 309–16.

50. Craig T, Hwang MY, Bromet EJ. Obsessive-compulsive and panic symptoms in patients with first-admission psychosis. Am J Psychiatry 2002; 159: 592–8.

51. Huppert JD, Smith TE. Anxiety and schizophrenia: the interaction of subtypes of anxiety and psychotic symptoms. CNS Spectr 2005; 10: 721–31.

52. Muller JE, Koen L, Soraya S, Emsley RA, Stein DJ. Anxiety disorders and schizophrenia. Curr Psychiatry Rep 2004; 6: 255–61.

53. Pokos V, Castle DJ. Prevalence of comorbid anxiety disorders in schizophrenia spectrum disorders: a literature review. Curr Psychiatry Rev 2006; 2: 285–307.

54. Achim AM, Maziade M, Raymond E, et al. How prevalent are anxiety disorders in schizophrenia? A meta-analysis and critical review on a significant association. Schizophr Bull 2011; 37: 811–21.

55. Ongur D, Goff DC. Obsessive-compulsive symptoms in schizophrenia: Associated clinical features, cognitive function and medication status. Schizophr Res 2005; 75: 349–62.

56. Poyurovsky M, Hramenkov S, Isakov V, et al. Obsessive-compulsive disorder in hospitalized patients with chronic schizophrenia. Psychiatry Res 2001; 102: 49–57.

57. Kugelmass S, Faber N, Ingraham LJ, et al. Reanalysis of SCOR and anxiety measures in the Israeli High-Risk Study. Schizophr Bull 1995; 21: 205–17.

58. Goodwin R, Stayner DA, Chinman MJ, Davidson L. Impact of panic attacks on rehabilitation and quality of life among persons with severe psychotic disorders. Psychiatr Serv 2001; 52: 920–4.

59. Lewis G, David AS, Malmberg A, Allebeck P. Non-psychotic psychiatric disorder and the subsequent risk of schizophrenia: Cohort study. Br J Psychiatry 2000; 177: 416–20.

60. Braga RJ, Mendlowicz MV, Marrocos RP, Figueira IL. Anxiety disorders in outpatients with schizophrenia: Prevalence and impact on the subjective quality of life. J Psychiatr Res 2005; 39: 409–14.

61. Hofer A, Kemmler G, Eder U, et al. Quality of life in schizophrenia: the impact of psychopathology, attitude toward medication, and side effects. J Clin Psychiatry 2004; 65: 932–8.

62. Huppert JD, Weiss KA, Lim R, Pratt S, Smith TE. Quality of life in schizophrenia: contributions of anxiety and depression. Schizophr Res 2001; 51: 171–80.

63. Huppert JD, Smith TE. Longitudinal analysis of the contribution of anxiety and depression to quality of life in schizophrenia. J Nerv Ment Disord 2001; 189: 669–75.

64. Lysaker PH, Whitney KA, Davis LW. Clinical and psychosocial correlates of anxiety related symptoms in schizophrenia. In: Velotis CM, ed. Anxiety Disorder Research. Hauppauge. NY, US: Nova Science Publishers, 2005: 1–19.

65. Harvey PD, Patterson TL, Potter LS, Zhong K, Brecher M. Improvement in social competence with short-term atypical antipsychotic treatment: a randomized, double-blind comparison of quetiapine versus risperidone for social competence, social cognition and neuropsychological functioning. Am J Psychiatry 2006; 163: 1918–25.

66. Pallanti S, Quercioli L, Hollander E. Social anxiety in outpatients with schizophrenia: a relevant cause of disability. Am J Psychiatry 2004; 161: 53–8.

67. Moriana JA, Alarcon E, Herruzo J. In-home psychosocial skills training for patients with schizophrenia. Psychiatr Serv 2006; 57: 260–2.

68. Wetherell JL, Palmer BW, Thorp SR, et al. Anxiety symptoms and quality of life in middle-aged and older outpatients with schizophrenia and schizoaffective disorder. J Clin Psychiatry 2003; 64: 1476–82.

69. Penn DL, Hope DA, Spaulding W, Kucera J. Social anxiety in schizophrenia. Schizophr Res 1994; 11: 277–84.

70. Halperin S, Nathan P, Drummond P, Castle D. A cognitive-behavioural group-based treatment for social anxiety in schizophrenia. Aust NZ J Psychiatry 2000; 34: 809–13.

71. Kingsep P, Nathan P, Castle DJ. Cognitive behavioural group treatment for social anxiety in schizophrenia. Schizophr Res 2003; 63: 121–9.

72. Dowling FG, Pato MT, Pato CN. Comorbidity of obsessive-compulsive and psychotic symptoms: a review. Harv Rev Psychiatry 1995; 3: 75–83.

73. Fabisch K, Fabisch H, Langs G, Huber HP, Zapotoczky HG. Incidence of obsessive-compulsive phenomena in the course of acute schizophrenia and schizoaffective disorder. Eur Psychiatry 2001; 16: 336–41.

74. Kayahan B, Ozturk O, Veznedaroglu B, Eraslan D. Obsessive-compulsive symptoms in schizophrenia: Prevalence and clinical correlates. J Psychiatry Clin Neurosci 2005; 59: 291–5.

75. Lysaker PH, Whitney KA, Davis LW. Obsessive-compulsive and negative symptoms in schizophrenia: associations with coping preference and hope. Psychiatry Res 2006; 141: 253–9.

76. Ongur D. About 30% of men with schizophrenia or schizoaffective disorders have obsessive-compulsive symptoms. Evid Based Ment Health 2006; 9: 28.

77. Eisen JL, Beer DA, Pato MT, Venditto TA, Rasmussen STA. Obsessive compulsive disorder in patients with schizophrenia or schizoaffective disorder. Am J Psychiatry 1997; 154: 271–3.

78. Tibbo P, Kroetsch M, Chue P, Warneke L. Obsessive-compulsive disorder in schizophrenia. J Psychiatr Res 2000; 34: 139–46.
79. Krüger S, Bräunig P, Höffler J, et al. Prevalence of obsessive-compulsive disorder in schizophrenia and significance of motor symptoms. J Neuropsychiatry Clin Neurosci 2000; 12: 16–24.
80. Okasha A, Lotaief F, Ashour AM, et al. The prevalence of obsessive compulsive symptoms in a sample of Egyptian psychiatric patients. Encephale 2000; 26: 1–10.
81. Ohta M, Kokai M, Morita Y. Features of obsessive-compulsive disorder in patients primarily diagnosed with schizophrenia. Psychiatry Clin Neurosci 2003; 57: 67–74.
82. Poyurovsky M, Kriss V, Weisman G, et al. Comparison of clinical characteristics and comorbidity in schizophrenia patients with and without obsessive-compulsive disorder: Schizophrenic and OC symptoms in schizophrenia. J Clin Psychiatry 2003; 64: 1300–7.
83. Bottas A, Cooke RG, Richter MA. Comorbidity and pathophysiology of obsessive-compulsive disorder in schizophrenia: is there evidence for a schizo-obsessive subtype of schizophrenia? J Psychiatry Neurosci 2005; 30: 187–93.
84. Stengel E. A study of some clinical aspects of the relationship between obsessional neurosis and psychotic reaction types. Br J Psychiatry 1945; 91: 166–87.
85. Rosen I. The clinical significance of obsessions in schizophrenia. Br J Psychiatry 1957; 103: 778–85.
86. Fenton WS, McGlashan TH. The prognostic significance of obsessive-compulsive symptoms in schizophrenia. Am J Psychiatry 1986; 143: 437–41.
87. Berman I, Kalinowski A, Berman SM, Lengua J, Green AI. Obsessive and compulsive symptoms in chronic schizophrenia. Compr Psychiatry 1995; 36: 6–10.
88. Dominguez RA, Backman KE, Lugo SC. Demographics, prevalence and clinical features of the schizo-obsessive subtype of schizophrenia. CNS Spectr 1999; 4: 50–6.
89. Özdemir Ö, Tükel R, Turksoy N, Ücok A. Clinical characteristics in obsessive-compulsive disorder with schizophrenia. Compr Psychiatry 2003; 44: 311–16.
90. Hwang MY, Morgan JE, Losconzcy MF. Clinical and neuropsychological profiles of obsessive-compulsive schizophrenia: a pilot study. J Neuropsychiatry Clin Neurosci 2000; 12: 91–4.
91. Lysaker PH, Marks KA, Picone JB, et al. Obsessive and compulsive symptoms in schizophrenia: clinical and neurocognitive correlates. J Nerv Ment Dis 2000; 188: 78–83.
92. Lysaker PH, Bryson GJ, Marks KA, Greig TC, Bell MD. Association of obsessions and compulsions in schizophrenia with neurocognition and negative symptoms. J Neuropsychiatry Clin Neurosci 2002; 14: 449–53.
93. Nechmad A, Ratzoni GM, Poyurovsky M, et al. Obsessive-compulsive disorder in adolescent schizophrenia patients. Am J Psychiatry 2003; 160: 1002–4.
94. Ekers D, Carman S, Schlich T. Successful outcome of exposure and response prevention in the treatment of obsessive compulsive disorder in a patient with schizophrenia. Behav Cogn Psychother 2004; 32: 375–8.
95. Naeem F, Kingdon D, Turkington D. Cognitive behaviour therapy for schizophrenia: Relationship between anxiety symptoms and therapy. Psychol Psychother 2006; 79: 153–64.
96. Tarrier N. Co-morbidity and associated clinical problems in schizophrenia: Their nature and implications for comprehensive cognitive-behavioural treatment. Behav Change 2005; 22: 125–42.
97. McKay D, McKiernan K. Information processing and cognitive behaviour therapy for obsessive-compulsive disorder: comorbidity of delusions, overvalued ideas, and Schizophrenia - a response paper. Cognit Behav Pract 2005; 12: 390–4.

98. Hood S, Alderton D, Castle DJ. Obsessive-compulsive disorder: treatment and treatment resistance. Australas Psychiatry 2001; 9: 118–27.
99. Hwang MY, Yum SY, Kwon JS, Opler LA. Management of schizophrenia with obsessive-compulsive disorder. Psychiatr Ann 2005; 35: 36–43.
100. Reznik I, Yavin I, Stryjer R, et al. Clozapine in the treatment of obsessive-compulsive symptoms in schizophrenia patients: a case series study. Pharmacopsychiatry 2004; 37: 52–6.
101. Goff DC, Brotman AW, Waiters M, McCormick S. Trial of fluoxetine added to neuroleptics for treatment resistant schizophrenia. Am J Psychiatry 1990; 147: 492–4.
102. Zohar J, Kaplan Z, Benjamin J. Clomipramine treatment of obsessive-compulsive symptomatology in schizophrenic patients. J Clin Psychiatry 1993; 54: 385–8.
103. Lykouras L, Alevizos B, Michalopoulou P, Rabavilas A. Obsessive-compulsive symptoms induced by atypical antipsychotics. A review of the reported cases. Prog Neuropsychopharmacol Biol Psychiatry 2003; 27: 333–46.
104. De Haan L, Oekeneva A, van Amelsvoort T, Linszen D. Obsessive-compulsive disorder and treatment with clozapine in 200 patients with recent-onset schizophrenia or related disorders. Eur Psychiatry 2004; 19: 524.
105. Ertugrul A, Yagcioglu A, Elif A, Eni N, Yazici KM. Obsessive-compulsive symptoms in clozapine-treated schizophrenic patients. Psychiatry Clin Neurosci 2005; 59: 219–22.
106. Poyurovsky M, Weizman A, Weizman R. Obsessive-compulsive disorder in schizophrenia: clinical characteristics and treatment. CNS Drugs 2004; 18: 989–1010.
107. Chaves MPR, Crippa JAS, Morais SL, Zuardi AW. Electroconvulsive Therapy for coexistent schizophrenia and obsessive-compulsive disorder. J Clin Psychiatry 2005; 66: 542–3.

chapter 6

The general health of people with schizophrenia

Urban Ösby, Ginger E. Nicol, and John W. Newcomer

Consistent evidence spanning multiple countries and practice settings indicates that individuals with schizophrenia have a shortened life expectancy, are at a higher risk for development of medical conditions that negatively impact their health, are less likely to receive and benefit from medical treatment, are more likely to experience unfavorable clinical outcomes, and are more likely to die prematurely (1–7). These observations have led investigators to focus on risk factors that contribute to morbidity and mortality in patients with schizophrenia, and to characterize more precisely the incidence of natural and unnatural causes of death.

The average lifespan for individuals with schizophrenia is from 10 to more than 30 years shorter than that of the general population (8,9). Standardized mortality ratios (SMRs: a ratio of observed deaths to expected deaths within a given age range) are a useful way to quantify the additional mortality risk associated with schizophrenia. The "expected" mortality rate is the rate seen in the general population, whereas the "observed" mortality rate is that seen in the population in question (e.g., schizophrenia patients). SMRs are particularly useful for identifying factors that contribute to the relative risk for different causes of death for psychiatric patients in comparison to the general population. They are less useful, however, for identifying factors that contribute to the absolute risk of death, and can therefore be potentially misleading. For example, as discussed below, cardiovascular disease (CVD) is responsible for the largest number of absolute deaths in patients with schizophrenia (6). However, since rates of death from CVD are large in the general population as well, the SMR for CVD is lower than the SMR for suicide, which is responsible for a lower number of absolute deaths of schizophrenia patients, but is relatively rare in the general population.

Medical causes of excess mortality in schizophrenia

Although SMRs for death by suicide are particularly high among persons with schizophrenia, comorbid medical conditions actually confer the largest share of excess mortality in this population. Brown et al. (10) studied 370 patients with schizophrenia over 13 years and confirmed that more patients died from natural causes than unnatural causes: 73% died as a result of medical diseases. All-cause mortality SMR was 2.98 in the overall study population; disease-specific SMRs are shown in Box 6.1.

Data from public mental health systems in the United States show that the leading cause of early death among people with serious mental illness is CVD; combining heart disease and cerebrovascular disease, CVD was responsible for roughly 35% of deaths in this population. Suicide, by contrast, was responsible for fewer than 5% of deaths (5).

Cardiovascular disease

CVD accounts for over 50% of all deaths in the U.S. general population (11). Patients with schizophrenia are even more likely to have CVD, which is in fact the leading cause of mortality in schizophrenia patients (5,12–14). Goff and colleagues, comparing schizophrenia patients from the Clinical Antipsychotic Trials in Intervention Effectiveness (CATIE) to matched controls from National Health and Nutrition Examination Survey (NHANES) III, reported that schizophrenia patients had a significantly higher 10-year risk of CVD than matched controls (15). A retrospective cohort study comparing 3022 individuals with schizophrenia to a general population cohort found the prevalence of CVD was increased in schizophrenia (10.6% vs. 8.7%), along with the incidence of ventricular arrhythmia (OR = 2.3, 95% CI = 1.2 to 4.3), stroke (OR = 1.5, 95% CI = 1.2 to 2.0), diabetes (OR = 1.8, 95% CI = 1.2 to 2.6), and heart failure (OR = 1.6, 95% CI = 1.2 to 2.0) (12).

> **Box 6.1**   Disease-specific standardized mortality ratios in 370 schizophrenia patients (10).
>
> - Any cancer: 1.46
> - Lung cancer: 2.08
> - Cardiovascular disease: 1.87
> - Circulatory diseases: 2.49
> - Cerebrovascular disease: 5.34
> - Diseases of the nervous system: 6.14
> - Diabetes mellitus: 9.96
> - Endocrine diseases: 11.66
> - Respiratory diseases: 3.19
> - Epilepsy: 26.13

Diabetes Mellitus

The prevalence of type 2 diabetes mellitus is estimated to range from two to four times higher in schizophrenia patients than in the general population (15–18% vs. around 4% of the general population) (1,16–18). Furthermore, schizophrenia is associated with an increase in the incidence of diabetes in earlier adult years (19,20).

While limited data from drug-naïve schizophrenia patients suggest that the increased activation of the hypothalamic-pituitary-adrenal axis and the sympathetic nervous system may contribute to the onset or worsening of diabetes in patients with schizophrenia (21), the finding of increased adiposity or glucoregulatory impairments in unmedicated patients is not consistently observed (22). Furthermore, hypothalamic-pituitary-adrenal activation is only variably associated with schizophrenia and is largely reduced by antipsychotic treatment. Genetic and/or familial factors might play a role, as around a fifth of schizophrenia patients have a family history of type 2 diabetes mellitus (23); however, it remains to be seen to what extent the increased prevalence of diabetes in this population cannot be fully explained by increases in the prevalence of overweight and obesity as well as reductions in the level of fitness (24).

Infectious disease

In developing countries, infectious diseases remain a pressing issue for persons with schizophrenia. In industrialized nations, these are a less important cause of morbidity and mortality, though rates of infectious disease among patients with schizophrenia are higher than in the general population (1). For example, rates of HIV infection have increased eightfold in patients with a severe mental illness, and data have shown that the knowledge of exposure risks is generally low among patients (25). Rates of hepatitis C infection are also elevated among those with a severe mental illness (25).

Cancer

The association between schizophrenia and risk of cancer has been of increasing interest and debate. While some studies have emphasized an increased risk of cancer associated with schizophrenia, others have suggested that schizophrenia could provide a protective effect with respect to some cancers. While there is variability in available data and the analytic approach, schizophrenia has generally been associated with a higher risk of cancer-related morbidity and mortality (26,27). A major analytic issue for surveys in this area is that increases in premature cardiovascular mortality in persons with schizophrenia (5) may greatly reduce the probability of living long enough to develop many cancers.

Pulmonary Disease

In one sample of outpatients with severe mental illnesses, including schizophrenia, the prevalence of chronic obstructive pulmonary disease (COPD) was 22.6% (28). In addition, people with schizophrenia are more than twice as likely as the general population to develop asthma (7). Abdominal adiposity can be hypothesized to contribute to the risk of COPD; however, smoking is the strongest independent risk factor for COPD, accounting for 60% of all smoking-related deaths. People with serious mental illnesses, including individuals with schizophrenia, are more than twice as likely to smoke as the general population, and are also more likely to be exposed to the effects of secondhand smoke (29). In a sample of 200 patients with schizophrenia, 17.8% had a lifetime history of asthma, 20.1% had a lifetime history of chronic bronchitis, and 8.1% had a lifetime history of emphysema (3,28,30).

Modifiable risk factors in people with schizophrenia

An important consideration in any effort to understand and address the excess mortality observed in persons with schizophrenia is the increased prevalence of key modifiable risk factors for medical disease and low utilization of prevention approaches with established effectiveness in the general population. Key risk factors for major causes of mortality that form the basis of public health efforts in the general population are shown in Box 6.2.

Obesity

Obesity is approximately twice as prevalent in people with severe mental illnesses such as schizophrenia (24,32). In one analysis, a total of 73% of all schizophrenia patients were overweight, while 86% of the women were either overweight or obese (30). Patients with schizophrenia may be at a higher risk of becoming obese due to a constellation of clinical, physiologic, genetic, psychosocial, and environmental factors. Importantly, it is now well known that treatment with many antipsychotic medications can induce considerable increases in weight and adiposity (9,33–37). In particular, drugs with greater antagonism for histamine (H_1) receptors, and to a lesser extent 5-HT2C receptors and α_1–adrenoceptors, have been associated with greater degrees of antipsychotic-induced weight gain (38). Rates of clinically significant weight

---

Box 6.2 Key modifiable risk factors for major causes of mortality (31).

Overweight and obesity
Smoking
Hypertension
Dyslipidemia
Hyperglycemia

gain associated with the atypical antipsychotics are shown in Box 6.3 (according to pooled registration trial data reported in the U.S. package inserts (33,34).

Given the differential weight gain associated with different antipsychotic medications, reductions in weight can be hypothesized to occur with a switch from a high weight gain drug to a lower weight gain drug (34). Indeed, this effect has been observed in short-term clinical trials involving both aripiprazole and ziprasidone (33). In a longer-term study, patients were switched to ziprasidone from risperidone, olanzapine, or a first-generation antipsychotic. After 52 weeks of treatment with ziprasidone, patients switched from olanzapine had lost a mean 9.8 kg of weight, versus 6.9 kg in those switched from risperidone (41). In phase 2 of the CATIE study, patients switched to ziprasidone from other atypical antipsychotics lost a mean 1.7 lbs. per month (42).

Hypertension

Estimates of the rate of hypertension in schizophrenia patients range from 19% (1,43) to 27% (15) compared with an estimated rate of 15% in the general population (43,44). Increases in adiposity and insulin resistance are associated with increased sympathetic nervous system activity and sodium retention, and increasing risk for hypertension (45). Factors that contribute to obesity

---

Box 6.3 Weight gain associated with atypical antipsychotics.

Increase in ≥7% of body weight
- olanzapine: 29% (vs. 3% for placebo)
- quetiapine: 23% (vs. 6% for placebo)
- risperidone: 18% (vs. 9% for placebo)
- ziprasidone: 10% (vs. 4% for placebo)
- aripiprazole: 8% (vs. 3% for placebo)
- iloperidone: 18% (vs. 4% for placebo)
- asenapine: 5% (vs. 2% for placebo)
- lurasidone: 6% (vs. 4% for placebo)

Mean weight gain over 1 year of treatment
- olanzapine: 12 kg of weight gain at doses from 12.5 to 17.5 mg/day (39)
- quetiapine: 3.2 kg (40) (note: based on an "observed case" analysis, in contrast to the "last observation carried forward" method used for the other medications)
- risperidone: 2.2 kg
- ziprasidone approximately 1 kg
- aripiprazole approximately 1 kg (33)
- iloperidone: 2.1 kg
- asenapine: 1.7 kg
- lurasidone: –0.71 kg

and insulin resistance in patients, such as treatment with antipsychotic medications associated with weight gain, can therefore contribute to the risk for hypertension in this patient population (38,46).

Dyslipidemia

Dyslipidemia is a key risk factor for CVD. Increased adiposity, independent of the cause, is associated with increased prevalence of dyslipidemia. In a study of patients with schizophrenia (47), 31% had serum triglyceride levels >1.7 mmol/l. In addition, 58% of men had serum high-density lipoprotein (HDL) cholesterol levels below 1 mmol/l and 25% of women had HDL cholesterol levels below 1.2 mmol/l.

Some antipsychotic medications are associated with clinically significant increases in lipid parameters, generally in proportion to their association with weight gain (9,33–36,48). In CATIE phase 1, olanzapine was associated with the greatest increase in lipid parameters from baseline. Olanzapine-treated patients experienced a mean triglyceride increase of 42.9 ± 8.4 mg/dl and a mean increase in total cholesterol of 9.7 ± 2.1 mg/dl, versus mean decreases of 18.1 ± 9.4 mg/dl and 9.2 ± 5.2 mg/dl, respectively, in for example, ziprasidone-treated patients (37). In CATIE phase 2, patients switched to ziprasidone from other atypical antipsychotics showed mean decreases in triglycerides of 19.3 ± 10.3 mg/dl and mean decreases in total cholesterol of 9.0 ± 3.5 mg/dl (42); this is consistent with the effect of removing the prior treatments, rather than indicating any direct lipid-lowering effect of this agent.

Insulin resistance and hyperglycemia

In patients with schizophrenia, the prevalence of insulin resistance has been estimated at 1.5–2.0 times the prevalence in the general population (17). When patients with hyperglycemia progress to type 2 diabetes mellitus, they are at a greater risk for increased morbidity and mortality due to acute metabolic complications, as well as chronic vascular disease (9). Antipsychotic medications are associated with differing levels of risk for hyperglycemia, generally proportional to their association with weight gain (9,33–36,48). In CATIE phase 1, plasma glucose levels increased by a mean 15.0 ± 2.8 mg/dl in olanzapine-treated patients, versus 2.3 ± 3.9 mg/dl in ziprasidone-treated patients (37).

While antipsychotics confer most of their associated risks through weight gain, evidence from controlled studies suggests the existence of some adiposity-independent antipsychotic-related treatment effects on blood glucose and insulin resistance (35,49). While most treatment-induced insulin resistance arises from increased abdominal adiposity secondary to antipsychotic-induced weight gain, it may also be caused by direct activity of antipsychotics, for example, their effect on glucose transporter function (50).

Metabolic syndrome

The key elements that compose the metabolic syndrome are shown in Box 6.4. These are also the major risk factors for type 2 diabetes mellitus and CVD (9). The prevalence of metabolic syndrome in patients with schizophrenia ranges from 37% to 46%, versus approximately 25% in the adult U.S. population (51,52).

Antipsychotic medications are associated with the development of the metabolic syndrome to differing degrees, again in proportion to their association with weight gain (9,33,34,36,50). Pooled data from two 26-week randomized double-blind trials, one comparing aripiprazole with placebo (53) and the other comparing aripiprazole with olanzapine (54), showed an incidence of metabolic syndrome of $19.2 \pm 4.0\%$ for olanzapine, $12.8 \pm 4.5\%$ for placebo, and $7.6 \pm 2.3\%$ for aripiprazole (55).

Smoking and substance abuse

Up to 81% of people with schizophrenia are addicted to nicotine through cigarettes, compared with 28% of the general population (3,30,56,57). There are also significantly more heavy cigarette users among schizophrenia patients, with 61% of men with schizophrenia and 42% of women with schizophrenia, respectively, inhaling more than 20 cigarettes per day, compared with 15% of men and 11% of women in the general population ($P < 0.001$) (10). In the CATIE schizophrenia trial, 68% of patients were nicotine dependent (58). Among 233 dual-diagnosis individuals with serious mental disorders (including schizophrenia) and substance use, 82% were classified as alcohol abusers (59). In another analysis of dual-diagnosis patients with schizophrenia, 71% were documented as stimulant users. Patients with schizophrenia and concomitant substance use disorders have higher adjusted odds for heart disease, asthma, gastrointestinal disorders, skin infections, and respiratory disorders than patients with schizophrenia who do not abuse substances (60).

Box 6.4   Elements of the metabolic syndrome (international diabetes federation).

Waist circumference (obligatory criterion)	M ≥ 94, F ≥ 80 cm
plus at least two of the following:	
Blood pressure	≥30/85 mmHg
High-density lipoprotein	M <40, F <50 mg/dl
Triglycerides	≥150 mg/dl
Fasting glucose	≥100 mg/dl

Primary and secondary prevention

There are substantial opportunities to improve primary and secondary prevention in persons with schizophrenia. In a study by McCreadie and colleagues, 19% and 28% of the women and men, respectively, had a CHD risk that was >15%, a risk threshold at which treatment of dyslipidemia with a statin would be considered a valuable intervention (16,30). In the CATIE study, 88% of patients with dyslipidemia were receiving no lipid lowering therapy, and 62% of those with hypertension were receiving no antihypertensive agent (61). Druss and colleagues studied a national cohort of 88,241 Medicare patients 65 years of age and older, and found that patients with a mental illness were significantly less likely to receive reperfusion therapy post-myocardial infarction, or treatment with aspirin, an ACE inhibitor, or a beta-adrenergic antagonist (62). A study of approximately 300,000 persons with diabetes from the Veteran Health Authority, with about 25% of the sample having a mental health condition, indicated significantly decreased odds of appropriate monitoring and control of diabetes and dyslipidemia in patients with psychotic disorders and other mental health conditions (63).

These data indicate a pervasive underutilization of primary and secondary prevention approaches in patients with schizophrenia. Lack of timely recognition of medical conditions by physicians, combined with patient nonadherence, contributes to the higher mortality rates seen in these patients (10,64). Although there is no single optimal model for healthcare delivery to the mentally ill, one proposed model suggests creating an integrated clinic in which medical care providers are on site and continually communicating with treating

---

Box 6.5   Educational tips for patients regarding physical health (67).

People with a mental illness are at an increased risk for a number of medical conditions that can have a negative impact on quality of life and longevity. Also, some psychiatric medications have side effects that can increase the risk of certain medical conditions, notably heart disease. It is very important for people with a mental illness to be aware of these issues and to ensure that their physical health is monitored and any problems appropriately treated

Discuss these issues with your doctor and make sure you keep a record of your weight, waist measurement, and blood pressure

Your doctor should arrange regular blood tests for you, the frequency depending upon your particular risk factors as well as the medication you are on. Tests include the following:

   Fasting blood sugar (for diabetes)
   Fasting blood fats ("lipid profile")
   Liver function
   Kidney function

METABOLIC SCREENING AND MONITORING FORM

NAME: _____

There is a growing awareness that some psychiatric illnesses and atypical antipsychotics can increase metabolic risks.
Frequency of monitoring for modifiable risk factors depends on level of risk present at baseline screening.

OBESITY SCREENING [71,72]

Consider BMI (weight/height in kg/m²) at each visit.
Normal (18.5–24.9); Overweight (25–29.9); Obese (≥30)

		Baseline	Dates/values from subsequent visits				
Height	Date __/__/__	__/__/__	__/__/__	__/__/__	__/__/__	__/__/__	__/__/__
	BMI _____						
	Wt _____						

LIPID SCREENING – CHOLESTEROL, TRIGLYCERIDES (TG) [73]

	Optimal/ desirable (mg/dl)	Near/Above optimal (mg/dl)	Borderline high (mg/dl)	High/ undesirable (mg/dl)	Very high (mg/dl)	Baseline __/__/__	Dates/values from subsequent visits __/__/__	__/__/__	__/__/__	__/__/__	__/__/__
Total	<200		200–239	≥240							
LDL	<100	100–129	130–159	160–189	≥190						
HDL	≥60			<40		Enter values as indicated in the Metabolic syndrome (MS)					
TG	<150		150–199	200–499	≥500*	screening section of the form below.					

*≥500 for TG requires immediate pharmacotherapeutic intervention without waiting for therapeutic lifestyle changes.

METABOLIC SYNDROME (MS) SCREENING [73]

Risk criteria	Baseline __/__/__	Dates/values from subsequent visits __/__/__	__/__/__	__/__/__	__/__/__	__/__/__
Abdominal obesity measured in waist circumference (men >40 inches, women >35 inches)						
Triglycerides (mg/dl) (≥150; or drug treatment)						
HDL cholesterol (mg/dl) (men <40, women <50; or drug treatment)						
Blood pressure (mmHg) (≥130/≥85; or drug treatment)						
Fasting plasma glucose (≥100 mg/dl; or drug treatment) [74]						
Total criteria for each visit (≥3 = MS diagnosis*)						

*Risk for cardiovascular disease increases with each criterion present, motivating intervention for any single criterion. [75]

TYPE 2 DIABETES MELLITUS (T2DM) SCREENING [71]

Risk factors: ☐ Age (≥45) ☐ Overweight (BMI ≥25 kg/m²)† ☐ Family history
☐ Habitual physical inactivity ☐ History of GDM or delivery of baby >9 lbs ☐ Previously identified IFG or IGT
☐ Race/ethnicity* ☐ Hypertension (>140/90 mmHg in adults) ☐ HDL ≤35 mg/dl and/or triglyceride ≥250 mg/dl
☐ Polycystic ovary syndrome ☐ History of vascular disease

Diagnostic criteria for prediabetes and T2DM ‡ [71]	Baseline __/__/__	Dates/values from subsequent visits __/__/__	__/__/__	__/__/__	__/__/__	__/__/__
Fasting plasma glucose (FPG)§ Normal: <100 mg/dl; prediabetes: 100–125 mg/dl; T2DM: ≥126 mg/dl						
Two-hour postload glucose (OGTT)§ Normal: <140 mg/dl; prediabetes: 140–199 mg/dl; T2DM: ≥200 mg/dl						
Symptoms of T2DM (yes + casual (random) PG ≥200 mg/dl) ‖						
Random plasma glucose (≥100 mg/dl requires formal screening with FPG or OGTT) [76]						

* Includes African Americans, Hispanic Americans, Native Americans, Asian Americans, Pacific Islanders.
† May not be correct for all ethnic groups.
‡ Screen at 3-year intervals beginning at age 45, particularly for those with BMI of ≥25; test at <45 or more frequently when overweight and have 1+ other risk factors. [71]
§ FPG and OGTT are the **only** measures currently approved by the ADA for diabetes screening/diagnosis; ADA recommends preferential use of FPG due to ease of use/acceptance. [71]
‖ Diagnosis must be confirmed on a subsequent day with FPG, 2-h PG, or casual (random) PG if symptoms (e.g. polyuria, polydipsia) are present, unless unequivocal hyperglycemia with acute metabolic decompensation is present. [71]

ATP-III recommends therapeutic lifestyle changes (TLC) for those with prediabetes, [77] hypertension, [78] 0–1 CHD risk factor and LDL ≥160 mg/dl, [73] 2+ CHD risk factors and LDL ≥130, [73] MS, [73] and perhaps subsyndromal MS. [76] Follow-up monitoring of 6- to 12-week intervals to monitor TLC response [73] is recommended and pharmacotherapy intervention if TLC fails after 3 months – unless lipid, blood pressure, or glucose values demand immediate drug treatment. [78]

ADA/APA Consensus Statement recommends considering antipsychotic medication switch for those who gain ≥5% of baseline body weight. [79]

Authored by John W. Newcomer, MD and Dan W. Haupt, MD. Compiled primarily from ADA and ATP-III guidelines.

©2006 **Compact** Clinicals
Produced by **Compact** Clinicals Kansas City, MO

Figure 6.1 *An example of a metabolic screening form for tracking cardiometabolic risk in psychiatric patients. Abbreviations: ADA, American Diabetes Association; BMI, body mass index; CHD, coronary heart disease; HDL, high density lipoprotein; IFG, impaired fasting glucose; IGT, impaired glucose tolerance;. Source: Compact Clinicals, Kansas City, MO, USA. www.compact clinicals.com 2006 Compact Clinicals (Continued).*

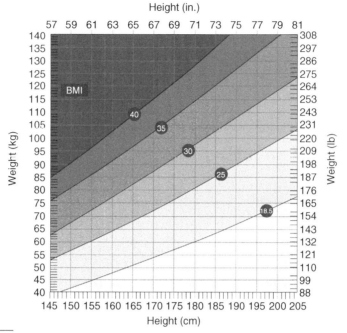

Figure 6.1 *(Continued)*

psychiatrists. This approach has been documented to improve medical outcomes without increasing the total costs. Such an approach will increase primary prevention as well as diagnostic and treatment programs that specifically target patients with major mental illnesses (65). The role of the psychiatrist may involve coordination of medical care with a patient's primary care physician (15,66). Whatever model is adopted, patient education is a key component: a suggested patient education pro forma is shown in Box 6.5.

During an initial visit between a treating psychiatrist and a patient, it is important that results of the most recent physical examination are reviewed. If such records do not exist, a medical screening should be arranged. Drug-naïve patients initiating antipsychotic therapy, as well as those changing antipsychotic treatment, should have a baseline assessment of family and personal medical history, as well as metabolic risk indicators including weight (body mass index) and/or waist circumference, blood pressure, fasting plasma glucose, and fasting lipid measurements (total, LDL and HDL cholesterol, and triglyceride), and possibly glycosylated hemoglobin (HBA$_{1C}$), with repeat measurements of weight at every visit thereafter. The overall panel of laboratory indicators should be repeated at least 3 months into initial treatment and at least annually thereafter, or more often in the setting of increased risk (17). A longitudinal tracking system is shown in Figure 6.1.

INSTRUCTIONS FOR PHYSICIANS — Metabolic Screening And Monitoring Form

Obesity screening

Overweight and obesity predispose patients to coronary heart disease (CHD), stroke, and a variety of other medical conditions, and are associated with an increase in all-cause mortality[80]. Overweight and obesity increase the risk of additional CHD risk factors, including:

- Type 2 diabetes mellitus (T2DM)
- Hypertension
- Dyslipidemia (e.g. increased low density lipoprotein (LDL) cholesterol and triglycerides (TG), and decreased high density lipoprotein (HDL) cholesterol)

Using the Body Mass Index Table on the back of the form*, determine BMI at baseline and subsequent visits to determine whether a patient's BMI falls within the 'Normal', 'Overweight', or 'Obese' range. Although some individuals with high BMIs have normal body fat and increased muscle mass, most individuals with BMIs above 25 have excess body fat.

Alternate BMI thresholds have been proposed for Asian Americans (e.g. onset of overweight/obesity at a BMI of 23/25). The BMI Table is also included on the inside of the back cover of the tear pad.

Lipid screening

The National Cholesterol Education Project (NCEP) recommendations focus on preventing CHD, metabolic syndrome (MS), and T2DM through preventive strategies that target primary prevention risk factors, including elevated LDL cholesterol[73].

CHD risk factors that guide NCEP treatment goals include:

- Cigarette smoking
- Hypertension (BP >140/90 mmHg or on antihypertensive medication)
- Low HDL cholesterol (<40 mg/dl)
- Family history of premature CHD (CHD in male first-degree relative <55 years; CHD in female first-degree relative <65 years)
- Age (men >45 years; women >55 years)

Risk assessment begins with a fasting lipoprotein profile (total cholesterol, LDL, HDL, and TG) at 5-year intervals for adults aged >20 years. More frequent monitoring and risk-reduction interventions are initiated based on risk level.

This section of the form presents the range of values by category of risk (optimal/desirable to very high) as well as space to record baseline measurements and those taken on subsequent visits. Alert values, such as TG ≥500 mg/dl, may require immediate pharmacotherapeutic intervention without a trial of therapeutic lifestyle changes (TLC) alone.

Guidelines are indicated for HDL and TG, but these values are recorded in the space provided under Metabolic Syndrome (MS) Screening.

For more information on determining risk of CHD using lipid and non-lipid risk factors, see the full NCEP report[73].

Metabolic syndrome screening

Metabolic syndrome (MS) is a constellation of lipid and non-lipid risk factors of metabolic origin, closely related to each other via insulin resistance.

Associated features of MS include:

- Abdominal obesity
- Atherogenic dyslipidemia (elevated TG, small LDL particles, low HDL cholesterol)
- Raised blood pressure
- Insulin resistance (with or without glucose intolerance)
- Prothrombotic and proinflammatory states

For this portion of the form, fill in the individual values, and total the number of out-of-range results at the bottom of each column. ATP III recommends a diagnosis of MS when three or more of the risk determinants shown are present[73]. However, it is worth noting that CHD risk can increase with one or two MS criteria[75].

Type 2 diabetes mellitus screening

The factors presented in the form reflect those that increase the risk of developing T2DM[71,73,75]. *Note:* the presence of mental disorders, including schizophrenia and depression, has been associated with increased risk[81,82].

The American Diabetes Association (ADA) recommends that screening should be considered at 3-year intervals beginning at age 45, particularly in those with BMI ≥25. Screening should be considered at an earlier age and more frequently in those who are overweight if additional diabetes risk factors are present[71,81]. Because some mental disorders and treatment have been associated with an increased risk of diabetes, clinicians should incorporate these risk factors into the determination of testing frequency[71,81].

The ADA recommends that screening for diabetes be performed using fasting plasma glucose (FPG) or an oral glucose tolerance test (OGTT). Of these recommended tests, the FPG is the easiest, fastest, and most convenient, but is less sensitive. The OGTT is more sensitive but more time consuming and costly to administer. If symptoms of T2DM are present, conduct a casual (random) glucose test to see if patient meets T2DM diagnostic criteria (casual plasma glucose ≥200 mg/dl). Note that diagnosis must be confirmed on a subsequent day with FPG, 2-h PG, or casual plasma glucose with symptoms, unless unequivocal hyperglycemia with acute metabolic decompensation is present.

Although not ADA recommended, some groups support the use of a casual (random) plasma glucose for screening, recommending that a value of >100 mg/dl be followed by formal screening with FPG or OGTT[76].

References are located on the back of the Metabolic Screening and Monitoring Form.

Figure 6.1   (*Continued*)

According to a feedback from patients with schizophrenia who were being treated for comorbid type 2 diabetes mellitus, more of these individuals were satisfied with their lives than patients with the same comorbid status who were not receiving treatment for diabetes (23). Thus, it is likely that concern for the physical health of schizophrenia patients will also increase the effects of, and compliance with, psychiatric treatment. In addition, behavioral therapy can be an effective method for overweight or obese patients with schizophrenia to manage unwanted weight gain (68).

Conclusions

Schizophrenia is frequently accompanied by medical comorbidities such as CVD, cancer, and diabetes, in addition to other prevalent complications including substance use (1–4). Therefore, addressing the risk and treatment of comorbidities is essential in improving health outcomes among patients in this population. Psychiatric and medical care systems have a particular responsibility to address those components of risk that are iatrogenic in origin, notably the contribution of medication side effects. The Institute of Medicine suggests that all psychiatric and medical systems and their associated providers involved in the care of patients with schizophrenia—including mental health, substance use, general health care, and other services—need to collaborate effectively in an effort to coordinate care of their patients (69). This cooperation should include the establishment of structured and routine comorbidity risk assessments for patients, in addition to scheduled monitoring of antipsychotic treatment for side effects and adherence issues (69). Implementation of such screening before the initiation of antipsychotic treatment and during therapy will likely improve outcomes among individuals with schizophrenia.

References

1. Dixon L, Postrado L, Delahanty J, Fischer PJ, Lehman A. The association of medical comorbidity in schizophrenia with poor physical and mental health. J Nerv Ment Dis 1999; 187: 496–502.
2. Lyketsos CG, Dunn G, Kaminsky MJ, Breakey WR. Medical comorbidity in psychiatric inpatients: relation to clinical outcomes and hospital length of stay. Psychosomatics 2002; 43: 24–30.
3. Sokal J, Messias E, Dickerson FB, et al. Comorbidity of medical illnesses among adults with serious mental illness who are receiving community psychiatric services. J Nerv Ment Dis 2004; 192: 421–7.
4. Goldman LS. Medical illness in patients with schizophrenia. J Clin Psychiatry 1999; 60(Suppl 21): 10–15.
5. Colton CW, Manderscheid RW. Congruencies in increased mortality rates, years of potential life lost, and causes of death among public mental health clients in eight states. Prev Chronic Dis 2006; 3: A42.

6. Osby U, Correia N, Brandt L, Ekbom A, Sparen P. Mortality and causes of death in schizophrenia in Stockholm county, Sweden. Schizophr Res 2000; 45: 21–8.
7. Druss BG, Rosenheck RA. Use of medical services by veterans with mental disorders. Psychosomatics 1997; 38: 451–8.
8. Jeste DV, Gladsjo JA, Lindamer LA, Lacro JP. Medical comorbidity in schizophrenia. Schizophr Bull 1996; 22: 413–30.
9. Casey DE, Haupt DW, Newcomer JW, et al. Antipsychotic-induced weight gain and metabolic abnormalities: implications for increased mortality in patients with schizophrenia. J Clin Psychiatry 2004; 65: 4–18.
10. Brown S, Inskip H, Barraclough B. Causes of the excess mortality of schizophrenia. Br J Psychiatry 2000; 177: 212–17.
11. Rosamond W, Flegal K, Friday G, et al. Heart disease and stroke statistics–2007 update: a report from the American Heart Association Statistics Committee and Stroke Statistics Subcommittee. Circulation 2007; 115: e69–171.
12. Curkendall SM, Mo J, Glasser DB, Rose Stang M, Jones JK. Cardiovascular disease in patients with schizophrenia in Saskatchewan, Canada. J Clin Psychiatry 2004; 65: 715–20.
13. Osborn DP, Levy G, Nazareth I, et al. Relative risk of cardiovascular and cancer mortality in people with severe mental illness from the United Kingdom's general practice research database. Arch Gen Psychiatry 2007; 64: 242–9.
14. Miller BJ, Paschall CB 3rd, Svendsen DP. Mortality and medical comorbidity among patients with serious mental illness. Psychiatr Serv 2006; 57: 1482–7.
15. Goff DC, Sullivan LM, Mcevoy JP, et al. A comparison of ten-year cardiac risk estimates in schizophrenia patients from the CATIE study and matched controls. Schizophr Res 2005; 80: 45–53.
16. Wood D, Durrington P, Mcinnes G, et al. Joint British recommendations on prevention of coronary heart disease in clinical practice. Heart 1998; 80: s1–s29.
17. Expert Consensus Group Schizophrenia and Diabetes 2003. Expert Consensus Meeting, Dublin, 3–4 October 2003: consensus summary. Br J Psychiatry Suppl 2004; 184(Suppl 47): S112–4.
18. Bushe C, Holt R. Prevalence of diabetes and impaired glucose tolerance in patients with schizophrenia. Br J Psychiatry Suppl 2004; 47: S67–71.
19. Harris MI. Diabetes in America: epidemiology and scope of the problem. Diabetes Care 1998; 21(Suppl 3): C11–4.
20. Mukherjee S, Decina P, Bocola V, Saraceni F, Scapicchio PL. Diabetes mellitus in schizophrenic patients. Compr Psychiatry 1996; 37: 68–73.
21. Ryan MC, Thakore JH. Physical consequences of schizophrenia and its treatment: the metabolic syndrome. Life Sci 2002; 71: 239–57.
22. Reynolds GP. Metabolic syndrome and schizophrenia. Br J Psychiatry 2006; 188: 86; author reply 86–7.
23. Dixon L, Weiden P, Delahanty J, et al. Prevalence and correlates of diabetes in national schizophrenia samples. Schizophr Bull 2000; 26: 903–12.
24. Allison DB, Fontaine KR, Heo M, et al. The distribution of body mass index among individuals with and without schizophrenia. J Clin Psychiatry 1999a; 60: 215–20.
25. Cournos F, Mckinnon K, Sullivan G. Schizophrenia and comorbid human immunodeficiency virus or hepatitis C virus. J Clin Psychiatry 2005; 66(Suppl 6): 27–33.
26. Grinshpoon A, Barchana M, Ponizovsky A, et al. Cancer in schizophrenia: is the risk higher or lower? Schizophr Res 2005; 73: 333–41.
27. Lichtermann D, Ekelund J, Pukkala E, Tanskanen A, Lonnqvist J. Incidence of cancer among persons with schizophrenia and their relatives. Arch Gen Psychiatry 2001; 58: 573–8.

28. Himelhoch S, Lehman A, Kreyenbuhl J, et al. Prevalence of chronic obstructive pulmonary disease among those with serious mental illness. Am J Psychiatry 2004; 161: 2317–19.

29. National Association of State Mental Health Program Directors (NASMHPD) Medical Directors Council Technical report on smoking policy and treatment in state operated psychiatric facilities. Twelfth in a Series of Technical Reports. In: Parks J, Jewell P, eds. Technical Writer Maile Burke, MPA [Available from: http://www.nasmhpd.org], 2006.

30. Mccreadie RG. Diet, smoking and cardiovascular risk in people with schizophrenia: descriptive study. Br J Psychiatry 2003; 183: 534–9.

31. National Cholesterol Education Program. Executive Summary of The Third Report of The National Cholesterol Education Program (NCEP) Expert Panel on Detection, Evaluation, And Treatment of High Blood Cholesterol In Adults (Adult Treatment Panel III). JAMA 2001; 285: 2486–97.

32. Susce MT, Villanueva N, Diaz FJ, De Leon J. Obesity and associated complications in patients with severe mental illnesses: a cross-sectional survey. J Clin Psychiatry 2005; 66: 167–73.

33. Newcomer JW. Second-generation (atypical) antipsychotics and metabolic effects: a comprehensive literature review. CNS Drugs 2005; 19(Suppl 1): 1–93.

34. Newcomer JW. Antipsychotic medications: metabolic and cardiovascular risk. J Clin Psychiatry 2007; 68(Suppl 4): 8–13.

35. Newcomer JW, Haupt DW, Fucetola R, et al. Abnormalities in glucose regulation during antipsychotic treatment of schizophrenia. Arch Gen Psychiatry 2002; 59: 337–45.

36. American Diabetes Association. Consensus development conference on antipsychotic drugs and obesity and diabetes. Diabetes Care 2004; 27: 596–601.

37. Lieberman JA, Stroup TS, Mcevoy JP, et al. Effectiveness of antipsychotic drugs in patients with chronic schizophrenia. N Engl J Med 2005; 353: 1209–23.

38. Kroeze WK, Hufeisen SJ, Popadak BA, et al. H1-histamine receptor affinity predicts short-term weight gain for typical and atypical antipsychotic drugs. Neuropsychopharmacology 2003; 28: 519–26.

39. Emeroff CB. Dosing the antipsychotic medication olanzapine. J Clin Psychiatry 1997; 58(Suppl 10): 45–9.

40. Brecher M, Leong RW, Stening G, Osterling-Koskinen L, Jones AM. Quetiapine and long-term weight change: a comprehensive data review of patients with schizophrenia. J Clin Psychiatry 2007; 68: 597–603.

41. Weiden PJ, Newcomer JW, Loebel AD, Yang R, Lebovitz HE. Long-term changes in weight and plasma lipids during maintenance treatment with ziprasidone. Neuropsychopharmacology 2008; 35: 985–94.

42. Stroup TS, Lieberman JA, Mcevoy JP, et al. Effectiveness of olanzapine, quetiapine, risperidone, and ziprasidone in patients with chronic schizophrenia following discontinuation of a previous atypical antipsychotic. Am J Psychiatry 2006; 163: 611–22.

43. Hennekens CH, Hennekens AR, Hollar D, Casey DE. Schizophrenia and increased risks of cardiovascular disease. Am Heart J 2005; 150: 1115–21.

44. Hennekens CH. Increasing burden of cardiovascular disease: current knowledge and future directions for research on risk factors. Circulation 1998; 97: 1095–102.

45. Reaven G. Insulin resistance, hypertension, and coronary heart disease. J Clin Hypertens (Greenwich) 2003; 5: 269–74.

46. Henderson DC, Nguyen DD, Copeland PM, et al. Clozapine, diabetes mellitus, hyperlipidemia, and cardiovascular risks and mortality: results of a 10-Year Naturalistic Study. J Clin Psychiatry 2005; 66: 1116–21.

47. Heiskanen T, Niskanen L, Lyytikainen R, Saarinen PI, Hintikka J. Metabolic syndrome in patients with schizophrenia. J Clin Psychiatry 2003; 64: 575–9.
48. Haupt DW, Fahnestock PA, Flavin KA, et al. Adiposity and insulin sensitivity derived from intravenous glucose tolerance tests in antipsychotic-treated patients. Neuropsychopharmacology 2007; 32: 2561–9.
49. Houseknecht KL, Robertson AS, Zavadoski W, et al. Acute effects of atypical antipsychotics on whole-body insulin resistance in rats: implications for adverse metabolic effects. Neuropsychopharmacology 2007; 32: 289–97.
50. Haupt DW, Newcomer JW. Hyperglycemia and antipsychotic medications. J Clin Psychiatry 2001; 62(Suppl 27): 15–26; discussion 40–1.
51. Park YW, Zhu S, Palaniappan L, et al. The metabolic syndrome: prevalence and associated risk factor findings in the US population from the Third National Health and Nutrition Examination Survey 1988–1994. Arch Intern Med 2003; 163: 427–36.
52. Ford ES, Giles WH, Mokdad AH. Increasing prevalence of the metabolic syndrome among U.S. Adults. Diabetes Care 2004; 27: 2444–9.
53. Pigott TA, Carson WH, Saha AR, et al. Aripiprazole for the prevention of relapse in stabilized patients with chronic schizophrenia: a placebo-controlled 26-week study. J Clin Psychiatry 2003; 64: 1048–56.
54. Mcquade RD, Stock E, Marcus R, et al. A comparison of weight change during treatment with olanzapine or aripiprazole: results from a randomized, double-blind study. J Clin Psychiatry 2004; 65(Suppl 18): 47–56.
55. L'italien GJ. Pharmacoeconomic impact of antipsychotic-induced metabolic events. Am J Manag Care 2003; 3: S38–42.
56. Holmberg SK, Kane C. Health and self-care practices of persons with schizophrenia. Psychiatr Serv 1999; 50: 827–9.
57. Cormac I, Ferriter M, Benning R, Saul C. Physical health and health risk factors in a population of long-stay psychiatric patients. Psychiatr Bull 2005; 29: 18–20.
58. Goff DC, Cather C, Evins AE, et al. Medical morbidity and mortality in schizophrenia: guidelines for psychiatrists. J Clin Psychiatry 2005a; 66: 183–94; quiz 147, 273–4.
59. Miles H, Johnson S, Amponsah-Afuwape S, et al. Characteristics of subgroups of individuals with psychotic illness and a comorbid substance use disorder. Psychiatr Serv 2003; 54: 554–61.
60. Dickey B, Normand SL, Weiss RD, Drake RE, Azeni H. Medical morbidity, mental illness, and substance use disorders. Psychiatr Serv 2002; 53: 861–7.
61. Nasrallah HA, Meyer JM, Goff DC, et al. Low rates of treatment for hypertension, dyslipidemia and diabetes in schizophrenia: data from the CATIE schizophrenia trial sample at baseline. Schizophr Res 2006; 86: 15–22.
62. Druss BG, Bradford WD, Rosenheck RA, Radford MJ, Krumholz HM. Quality of medical care and excess mortality in older patients with mental disorders. Arch Gen Psychiatry 2001; 58: 565–72.
63. Frayne SM, Halanych JH, Miller DR, et al. Disparities in diabetes care: impact of mental illness. Arch Intern Med 2005; 165: 2631–8.
64. Munk-Jorgensen P, Mors O, Mortensen PB, Ewald H. The schizophrenic patient in the somatic hospital. Acta Psychiatr Scand 2000; 102: 96–9.
65. Davidson M. Risk of cardiovascular disease and sudden death in schizophrenia. J Clin Psychiatry 2002; 63(Suppl 9): 5–11.
66. Daumit GL, Crum RM, Guallar E, Ford DE. Receipt of preventive medical services at psychiatric visits by patients with severe mental illness. Psychiatr Serv 2002; 53: 884–7.

67. Castle DJ, Tran N. Psychiatric Medication Information: A Guide for Patients and Carers. Melbourne: St Vincent's Mental Health, 2007.
68. Brar JS, Ganguli R, Pandina G, et al. Effects of behavioral therapy on weight loss in overweight and obese patients with schizophrenia or schizoaffective disorder. J Clin Psychiatry 2005; 66: 205–12.
69. Institute of Medicine. Improving Quality of Health Care for Mental and Substance-use Conditions. Washington, DC: The National Academies Press, 2006.

chapter 7

Substance abuse comorbidity in schizophrenia

Wynne James, Kim T. Mueser, and David J. Castle

Research over the past 35 years has explored the prevalence and possible causes of substance misuse among people with schizophrenia, as well as highlighting some of the complications that can occur as a consequence. While these studies have significantly improved our understanding of the complex interplay between drug misuse and schizophrenia, only few research studies have properly evaluated treatment interventions aimed at improving outcomes for this group.

This chapter discusses a number of important considerations essential for a clear understanding of the relationship between substance misuse and schizophrenia. These include prevalence, impact on the course of the illness, clinical implications, and reasons for use. We review studies addressing substance misuse in schizophrenia, provide a brief overview of a novel psychosocial treatment program aimed at directly addressing substance misuse in this population, and conclude by outlining medication strategies for people with schizophrenia and substance misuse.

It should be noted that cigarette smoking and caffeine abuse are also very common among people with schizophrenia (e.g., Jablensky et al. (1)), and these carry their own health risks. In this chapter, however, we concentrate on alcohol and illicit substances.

Prevalence

The prevalence of substance abuse among people with schizophrenia attracts considerable attention from service providers and researchers (2). However, studies in this area frequently suffer from a number of shortcomings, notably with respect to defining "caseness" (Box 7.1). This problem arises from the lack of standardized instruments used to determine diagnoses and for indexing

Box 7.1 Summary of weaknesses of prevalence studies of substance abuse in schizophrenia.

Lack of standardized instruments used to determine diagnosis
No consensus about "caseness"
Research sampling procedures likely to reflect bias
Berkson's Bias
Poor distinction between various degrees of substance use
Varying global patterns of drug use

degrees of substance use. Poor sampling procedures contribute by overrepresenting patients from urban areas, where substance use is often more prevalent. Berkson's bias also operates, in that the effect of coming to the attention of services consequent upon each individual disorder is additive, and results in higher rates of comorbidity than in nonclinical samples (3).

There is also considerable variability in reported prevalence rates with respect to the different groups of drugs used, a fact easily obscured by use of umbrella terms such as "drug abuse." Different drugs have different physical and psychological consequences and any evaluation regarding treatment interventions should be as specific as possible about what works best with respect to each individual drug class. Finally, any findings regarding prevalence rates are strongly influenced by local trends and the legal and social status of particular drugs in particular settings, making the generalizability of results questionable.

These issues aside, there is now a general consensus that substance abuse disorders occur more frequently among people with schizophrenia than the general population. In a review of the international literature, Cantor-Graae and colleagues (4) found 47 studies since 1990, recording prevalence of substance abuse/dependence among people with a psychotic illness. Of these, 37 were conducted in North America, eight in Europe, and one each in Australia and Africa. Rates of use varied widely, depending upon the criteria applied and the setting, but lifetime rates for substance use disorder tended to aggregate around 40–60% (5). Alcohol and cannabis were the leading drugs in all settings; other drugs of abuse varied by setting. Polydrug abuse is also a feature of this clinical group. For example, Spencer et al. (6), in an Australian sample, found that around 50% of psychosis patients regularly used more than one substance.

Community studies give a less biased assessment of rates of substance use, and allow comparison with controls who do not have a mental illness. Perhaps the most comprehensive and frequently cited community prevalence study of mental disorders, the U.S. Epidemiological Catchment Area Survey (7), estimated that 47% of people with schizophrenia also met criteria for lifetime substance abuse or dependence. Around a third of this group had a substance abuse disorder in the previous 6 months (8). The lifetime rate of substance abuse in controls was around 17%.

In the *People Living with Psychotic Illness: 2010* Australian survey (9), lifetime rates for alcohol abuse or dependence among people with psychotic disorders were 58.3% for men and 38.9.0% for women (compared with 35.3% and 14.1% respectively in the general population) and 63.2% for men and 41.7% for women (compared to 12.0% and 5.8% in the general population) for illicit substances. The most commonly abused illicit substance was cannabis, followed by amphetamines, tranquilizers, ecstasy, and heroin. These findings reflect significant increases in the proportion of men and women with psychotic illness with a lifetime history of abusing alcohol and illicit substances, compared with the previous 1997–1998 psychosis survey (10).

Impact on the course of schizophrenia

Although it has been shown in a number of studies that substance abuse often precedes the onset of psychotic symptoms in psychotic disorders (11,12), this does not imply causality; indeed, whether such substances can actually cause disorders such as schizophrenia is open to considerable conjecture (13). What is generally accepted is that use of substances such as cannabis can precipitate psychotic episodes in vulnerable individuals (14). Furthermore, most studies (but not all: see Ref. (15)) report that substance abuse is associated with a poorer illness trajectory among this group.

Substance abuse is identified as a significant factor in contributing to an increase in the number of psychotic symptoms and relapses—a finding strongly associated with patients who abuse psychotogenic drugs such as cannabis and cocaine (with a heavier use of these drugs correlating with a worse symptom profile) (16). However, it is also the case that some patients with psychotic disorders who abuse substances have a better longitudinal course than their nonusing counterparts if they stop using (17). This latter finding reinforces the need to assist people with a vulnerability to psychotic illnesses to gain control, and at least limit, their use of alcohol and illicit substances.

Clinical implications

Substance abuse is positively correlated with poor *treatment adherence* and as a result is a contributing factor to the worse outcome observed in this clinical group (18). Another major cause for concern among service providers and clinicians is *violence and crime* (chap. 9). A number of studies have identified substance abuse as a risk factor for violence in people with psychotic disorders (19), with polysubstance abuse associated with a significant increase in

> **Box 7.2** Clinical implications of substance abuse in schizophrenia.
>
> Result in increased positive symptoms
> Difficulty in maintaining stable housing
> Money management problems
> Blood-borne virus risk behavior
> Higher rates of violent behavior
> Higher rates of hospitalization

the likelihood of violent behaviors, including threats, destruction of property, assault, and suicide (20).

Prevalence rates for *blood-borne viruses* such as HIV and hepatitis C virus are high among people with psychotic disorders complicated by substance abuse (21,22). These findings underscore the requirement for ongoing health education strategies that are sensitive to the needs of specific groups. Harm reduction interventions should be a priority for patients involved in high-risk activities such as intravenous drug use, and clinicians should be proactive in delivering them.

Homelessness is another significant problem for this group (23); this in turn complicates ongoing management by treatment services. Not surprisingly, rates of psychiatric *hospitalization* are higher among people with substance abuse comorbidity (24) and while inpatient psychiatric services remain an expensive and limited resource, this is a major concern for service providers.

Thus, it is clear that the abuse of alcohol and illicit substances has a negative impact on people with psychotic disorders. Box 7.2 summarizes these parameters. It is important to develop more effective methods of engaging such individuals in treatments that address their substance use.

Motivations for use

Gaining a better understanding of motivations for substance use is an important first step in developing more effective treatments for people with psychotic disorders. This aspect of substance use is still poorly understood. The notion of "self-medication" was for many years the predominant theory used to explain the higher rates of substance abuse among people with psychotic disorders (25). This hypothesis suggests that substance abuse is an attempt by the individual to deal with symptoms of their illness, or to counteract some of the unwanted side effects attributed to psychiatric medications. While this theory cannot be discounted, recent studies report that substance use within psychiatric populations appears to be motivated by many of the same reasons as those identified within the general population (Box 7.3) (26–28).

Box 7.3   Reasons for substance abuse by people with schizophrenia.

Self-medication: the relief of distressing symptoms and/or side effects of
   medication
Enhancement: "to make you feel good"
Social motives: "it's what others do"
Coping with unpleasant affect: "to forget your worries"
Conformity: "not to be left out"
Acceptance: "to be liked"
Changing moral attitudes toward drugs use
Increased availability
Community psychiatric care

In a study investigating motivations for use in people with psychosis (mainly schizophrenia) Spencer et al. (29) found that most respondents attributed their substance use to the same motivations as those given by the general population. Thus, they reported that their substance use was driven by negative emotions such as boredom and depression; social motives such as conformity and acceptance and improving social interaction; and was seen by some as a way of enhancing mood. Another consideration lending support to these findings is that, as stated above, drug use among this group generally reflects local community drug trends, rather than there being a specific correlation between certain symptoms or side effects, and use of certain drugs of abuse (30). It is probable that a number of factors contribute to the high rates of substance abuse in people with psychotic disorders, and that many of these factors are the same as those mediating abuse in patients without such disorders. The challenge for the field is to establish treatments that are responsive to these motivations for use, such that patients can be engaged in a treatment that is relevant and responsive to their particular makeup and situation.

Treatments for substance abuse in psychosis

While substance abuse is an acknowledged problem in mental health settings, it often goes undetected, and thus untreated. Part of the reason for this is the traditional dichotomy between substance misuse and mental health services, and also the lack of acceptable and well-validated treatments (31).

Integrated treatment approaches that incorporate aspects from both mental health and substance abuse treatments, and are delivered simultaneously by the same personnel, are widely accepted as the preferred model of care for people with co-occurring problems (32,33). Within this approach treatments are nested in clinical practice settings and involve collaboration between different health professionals. Unfortunately this is often not reflected in current clinical practice, with mental health and substance abuse services more often than not polarized (or siloed), resulting in substance-using persons with a psychotic illness "falling between the cracks."

Furthermore, there remains a major deficit in terms of defining the most effective content, shape, and form of interventions, which will assist people with substance abuse comorbidity control their substance use. Cleary and colleagues (34) recently reviewed published randomized controlled studies in the area. They found 25 relevant studies containing a total of 2478 people, including patients with an array of psychiatric disorders. Studies were conducted in the United States, United Kingdom, and Australia and interventions were delivered across settings that included psychiatric hospitals, community mental health services, and jails. A mixture of psychosocial interventions were trialed: four used integrated approaches; four used nonintegrated approaches; three combined motivational interviewing (an approach that builds motivation for positive change) and cognitive–behavioral therapy (an approach that promotes adaptive behavior by improving coping strategies); four used mainly cognitive–behavioral therapy; five used mainly motivational interviewing; and two using skills training.

Significant differences were evident across these interventions in terms of intensity, duration, theoretical model used, mode and location of administration, the target group to which they had been applied, and the way that they had been evaluated. These differences hindered comparison between studies and therefore give little indication of precisely which elements of the intervention were effective (or not) (35). Many of the strategies described may not be practical to implement outside research settings and do not appear to be generalizable either across treatment settings (e.g., mental health and non-government services; early episode and chronic rehabilitation settings), or to patients at different stages of their illness (e.g., early episode, chronic). Finally, they were generally not informed by assessment of the motivations for use by the particular individual, preventing tailoring of the intervention to the individual patient.

Psychosocial treatments

Despite the flaws in the literature on treatment interventions for substance abuse in schizophrenia, there is growing consensus about what features such interventions should contain (Box 7.4) (36).

We provide here an outline of a group psychosocial treatment intervention for substance abuse in schizophrenia that incorporates many of these elements (37,38). This example illustrates many of the features currently advocated in the literature and draws from work undertaken by, among others, Marlatt and Gordon (39), Miller and Rollnick (40), Zeidonis and Fisher (41), Kavanagh (42), Graham (43), and Spencer et al. (44).

The intervention is delivered in an outpatient setting over a 6- to 8-week period and utilizes peer support, motivational enhancement strategies, relapse

Box 7.4   Content of psychosocial treatment interventions for substance abuse in schizophrenia.

Interventions congruent with readiness to change
Not abstinence focused
Psychoeducation
Harm reduction interventions
Motivation enhancement strategies
Relapse prevention strategies
Peer orientated
Offers links to other supportive agencies

Source: Based on Ref. 36.

prevention, and harm minimization approaches. It is available as an adjunct to existing multidisciplinary case management services and is for people who have a psychotic condition and also abuse drugs. The intervention was designed with the following broad aims:

1. Establish motivations for use, and tailor intervention strategies for individuals on the basis of these motivations.
2. Provide a forum for participants to discuss the pros and cons of drug use.
3. Provide up-to-date information to enable participants to make informed choices.
4. Enhance motivation to reduce drug abuse or minimize associated problems.
5. Encourage participants to develop ways of managing their symptoms, relieving boredom, or engaging in social activities without relying on drugs.

Importantly, there is the capacity to tailor the precise elements of the intervention to individuals within the group, based on and responsive to the factors that motivate their use of substances. This is accomplished through exercises and examples used in the groups themselves, as well as those being incorporated into the homework that each participant is expected to complete. The group is divided into five modules, which can be completed in one or two sessions each. A more detailed description can be found in James et al. (45).

A further influential study in this field is that of Barrowclough and colleagues (46), who employed a comprehensive package incorporating motivational interviewing, cognitive–behavioral treatment and family/care giver intervention over a 9-month period. In a randomized trial against treatment as usual, there were modest improvements in general functioning and positive symptoms, and an increase in the number of days abstinent from drugs. Importantly, significant improvements were maintained in the treatment group at 18-month follow-up (47).

Pharmacological strategies

Another element of treatment for comorbid substance use in schizophrenia is medication. Krystal and colleagues (48) have provided a useful guide to pharmacotherapy of such patients. They detail the importance of optimal treatment of symptoms and prevention of side effects, to counter the "self-medication" component of motivation for substance use. Their suggested strategies are detailed in Table 7.1.

In a review of the pharmacological management of schizophrenia with substance abuse comorbidity, Wobrock and Soyka (49) suggest that there is evidence (albeit from a limited range of largely uncontrolled studies) that atypical antipsychotics (aripiprazole, clozapine, olanzapine, quetiapine, and risperidone) are associated with lower rates of substance misuse, certainly compared with typical agents. Picking up on this theme, and concentrating on clozapine in particular, Green et al. (50) conjecture that this effect might be mediated by the particular receptor-binding profile of such agents, for example the blockade of serotonin 5HT-2 receptors (potentially decreasing impulsivity), and of alpha 1 and alpha 2 receptors; and, for clozapine at least, the relatively weak dopamine D2 blockade in association with relative tenacity for dopamine D1 and D4 receptors (perhaps diminishing novelty-seeking behaviors). Such theories are worthy of further exploration in the quest for more effective pharmacological approaches to the treatment of dual diagnosis patients.

Table 7.1 Medication strategies to reduce "self-medication" with nonprescribed substances by people with schizophrenia

Symptom/side effect	Therapeutic intervention
Extrapyramidal side effects	Lower dose of a typical antipsychotic
	Use an atypical antipsychotic
Persistent positive symptoms	Optimize control; consider clozapine
Enduring negative symptoms	Ensure not secondary to any typical antipsychotic, depression, or positive symptoms
	Consider an atypical agent, notably clozapine
"Emotional distress"	Antidepressant/benzodiazepine
	Mood stabilizer
	Atypical antipsychotic
Cognitive dysfunction	Lower dose of a typical antipsychotic
	Reduce benzodiazepines and anticholinergics
	Switch to an atypical agent

Source: Adapted from Ref. 48.

Another consideration in the pharmacological management of substance use in schizophrenia is the addition of other agents to the antipsychotic. In their review, Wobrock and Soyka (49) identified two prospective studies with desipramine and two with imipramine as adjuncts to antipsychotics, which showed reductions in cocaine craving and use in a cocaine-dependent schizophrenia patient: the effect was not seen for cannabis and was apparently not mediated by amelioration of mood symptoms. A case series of treatment-resistant schizophrenia patients with comorbid alcohol use disorder reported beneficial effects for the mood stabilizing anticonvulsant lamotrigine in terms of alcohol consumption and craving (51). Further investigation of such agents appears warranted.

A further strategy is the use of antiaddiction agents such as naltrexone and acamprosate. Wobrock and Soyka (49) identified two retrospective open studies and one prospective randomized controlled trial of naltrexone for alcohol abuse in schizophrenia, all with encouraging outcomes. We are aware of no published studies of acamprosate in schizophrenia patients. The relapse-prevention agent disulfiram may have a limited role in people with schizophrenia, but compliance is often erratic and it can exacerbate psychotic symptoms (48).

Conclusions

Substance abuse comorbidity in schizophrenia is a major problem both in terms of prevalence and of having the potential negative impact on illness course. Much needs to be done to enhance our understanding of what drives this comorbidity, and to refine therapeutic interventions.

References

1. Jablensky A, McGrath JJ, Herrman H, et al. Psychotic disorders in urban areas: an overview of the study on low prevalence disorders. Aust NZ J Psychiatry 2000; 34: 221–36.
2. Mueser K, Yarnold P, Rosenberg S, et al. Substance use disorder in hospitalised severely mentally ill psychiatric patients: prevalence, correlates and sub groups. Schizophr Bull 2000; 26: 179–92.
3. Fowler I, Carr V, Carter N, et al. Patterns of current and lifetime substance use in schizophrenia. Schizophr Bull 1998; 24: 443–5.
4. Cantor-Graae E, Nordstrom LG, McNeil TF. Substance abuse in schizophrenia: A review of the literature and a study of correlates in Sweden. Schizophr Res 2001; 48: 69–82.
5. Buckley PF. Prevalence and consequences of the dual diagnosis of substance abuse and severe mental illness. J Clin Psychiatry 2006; 67(Suppl 7)): 5–9.
6. Spencer C, Castle D, Michie P. An examination of the validity of a motivational model for understanding substance use among individuals with psychotic disorders. Schizophr Bull 2002; 28: 233–47.
7. Regier D, Farmer N, Rae D, et al. Comorbidity of mental disorders with alcohol and other drug abuse. J Am Med Assoc 1990; 264: 2511–18.

8. Mueser KT, Bennet M, Kushner MG. Epidemiology of substance use disorders among people with chronic mental illness. In: Lehman AF, Dixon LB. eds. Double Jeopardy: Chronic Mental Illness and Substance Use Disorders. Switzerland: Harwood Academic Publishers, 1995.

9. Morgan VA, Waterus A, Jablenski A, et al. People Living with Psychosis 2010. Report on the Second Australian National Survey. Canberra: Commonwealth of Australia, 2011.

10. Jablensky A, McGrath JJ, Herrman H, et al. Psychotic disorders in urban areas: an overview of the study on low prevalence disorders. Aust NZ J Psychiatry 2000; 34: 221–36.

11. Linszen DH, Dingemans PM, Lenior ME. Cannabis abuse and the course of recent-onset schizophrenic disorders. Arch Gen Psychiatry 1994; 51: 273–9.

12. Caspari D. Cannabis and schizophrenia: results of a follow-up study. Eur Arch Psychiatry Clin Neurosci 1999; 249: 45–9.

13. Arsenault L, Cannon M, Witton J, Murray R. Cannabis as a potential causal factor in schizophrenia. In: Castle D, Murray R. eds. Marijuana and Madness. Cambridge: Cambridge University Press, 2004: 186–97.

14. Castle DJ, Ames FR. Cannabis and the brain. Aust NZ J Psychiatry 1996; 30: 179–83.

15. Cantor-Graae E, Nordstrom LG, McNeil TF. Substance abuse in schizophrenia: A review of the literature and a study of correlates in Sweden. Schizophr Res 2001; 48: 69–82.

16. Dixon L. Dual diagnosis of substance abuse in schizophrenia: prevalence and impact on outcomes. Schizophr Res 1999; 35: 93–100.

17. Krystal JH, D'Souza CD, Madonick S, Petrakis IL. Toward a rational pharmacotherapy of comorbid substance abuse in schizophrenic patients. Schizophr Res 1999; 35: S35–49.

18. Owen R, Fischer E, Booth B, et al. Medication noncompliance and substance abuse among patients with schizophrenia. Psychiatr Serv 1996; 47: 853–58.

19. RachBeisel J, Scott J, Dixon L. Co-occurring severe mental illness and substance use disorders: a review of recent research. Psychiatr Serv 1999; 50: 1427–33.

20. Cuffel BJ, Shunway M, Chouljian TL, MacDonald T. A longitudinal study of substance use and community violence in schizophrenia. J Nerv Ment Dis 1994; 182: 704–8.

21. Carey M, Weinhardt L, Carey K. Prevalence of infection with HIV among the seriously mentally ill: review of research and implications for practice. Prof Psychol 1995; 26: 262–8.

22. Rosenberg SD, Drake RE, Brunette MF, Wolford GL, Marsh BJ. Hepatitis C virus and HIV co-infection in people with severe mental illness and substance use disorders. AIDS 2005;19(Suppl 3): S26–33.

23. Drake R, Antosca L, Noordsy D, et al. New Hampshire's specialised services for the dually diagnosed. New Dir Youth Dev 1991; 50L: 57–67.

24. Bartels S, Teague G, Drake R, et al. Substance abuse in schizophrenia: Service utilisation and costs. J Nerv Ment Dis 1993; 181: 227–32.

25. Siegfried N. A review of comorbidity: major mental illness and problematic substance use. Aust NZ J Psychiatry 1998; 32: 707–17.

26. Horsfall J, Cleary M, Hunt GE, Walter G. Psychosocial treatments for people with co-occurring severe mental illness and substance use disorders (dual diagnosis): a review of empirical evidence. Harv Rev Psychiatry 2009; 17: 24–34.

27. Schaub M, Franghaenal K, Stohler R. Reasons for cannabis use: patients with schizophrenia verses matched healthy controls. Aust NZ J Psychiatry 2008; 42: 1060–65.

28. Schofield D, Tennant C, Nash L, et al. Reasons for cannabis use in psychosis. Aust NZ J Psychiatry 2006; 40: 570–4.

29. Spencer C, Castle D, Michie P. An examination of the validity of a motivational model for understanding substance use among individuals with psychotic disorders. Schizophr Bull 2002; 28: 233–47.

30. Dixon L. Dual diagnosis of substance abuse in schizophrenia: prevalence and impact on outcomes. Schizophr Res 1999; 35: 93–100.
31. Drake RE, Mercer-McFadden C, Muesser KT, et al. Review of integrated mental health and substance use treatment for patients with dual disorders. Schizophr Bull 1998; 24: 589–608.
32. Essock SM, Mueser KT, Drake RE, et al. Comparison of ACT and standard case management for delivering integrated treatment for co-occurring disorders. Psychiatr Serv 2006; 57: 185–96.
33. Green AL, Drake RE, Brunette MF, Noordsy DL. Schizophrenia and cooccurring substance use disorder. Am J Psychiatry 2007; 164; 402–8.
34. Cleary M, Hunt GE, Matheson SL, et al. Psychosocial interventions for people with both severe mental illness and substance misuse (Cochrane Review). Cochrane Database Syst Rev 2009.
35. DrakeRE O'Neal EL, Wallach MA. A systematic review of psychosocial interventions for people with co-occuring severe mental and substance use disorders. J Subst Abuse Treat 2008; 34: 123–38.
36. Drake R, Mueser K. Psychosocial approaches to dual diagnosis. Schizophr Bull 2000; 26: 105–18.
37. James W, Castle DJ. Addressing cannabis abuse in peoples with psychosis. In: Castle D, Murray R. eds. Marijuana and Madness. Cambridge: Cambridge University Press, 2004: 186–97.
38. James W, Preston NJ, Koh G, et al. A group intervention which assists patients with dual diagnosis reduce their drug use: a randomized controlled trial. Psychol Med 2004; 34: 983–90.
39. Marlatt G, Gordon J. Relapse Prevention: Maintenance Strategies in the Treatment of Addictive Behaviours. New York: Guildford Press, 1985.
40. Miller W, Rollnick S. Motivational Interviewing: Preparing People to Change Addictive Behaviour. New York: Guildford Press, 1991.
41. Ziedonis D, Fisher W. Assessment and treatment of comorbid substance abuse in individuals with schizophrenia. Psychiatr Ann 1994; 24: 477–83.
42. Kavanagh D. An intervention for substance abuse in schizophrenia. Behav Change 1995; 12: 20–30.
43. Graham HL. The role of dysfunctional beliefs in individuals who experience psychosis and use substances: implications for cognitive therapy and medication adherence. Behav Cogn Psychother 1998; 26: 193–208.
44. Spencer C, Castle D, Michie P. An examination of the validity of a motivational model for understanding substance use among individuals with psychotic disorders. Schizophr Bull 2002; 28: 233–47.
45. James W, Preston NJ, Koh G, et al. A group intervention which assists patients with dual diagnosis reduce their drug use: a randomized controlled trial. Psychol Med 2004; 34: 983–90.
46. Barrowclough C, Haddock G, Tarrier N. Randomised controlled trial of motivational interviewing, cognitive behavior therapy, and family intervention for patients with comorbid schizophrenia and substance use disorders. Am J Psychiatry 2001; 158: 1706–13.
47. Haddock G, Barrowclough C, Tarrier N, et al. Randomized controlled trial of cognitive behavior therapy and motivational interviewing for schizophrenia and substance use: 18-month, carer and economic outcomes. Br J Psychiatry 2003; 183: 418–24.
48. Krystal JH, D'Souza CD, Madonick S, et al. Towards a rational pharmacotherapy of comorbid substance use in schizophrenic patients. Schizophr Res 1999; 35: S35–49.

49. Wobrock T, Soyka M. Pharmacotherapy of schizophrenia with comorbid substance use disorder: reviewing the evidence and clinical recommendations. Prog Neuropsychopharmacol Biol Psychiatry 2008; 32: 1375–85.
50. Green AI, Salomon MS, Brenner MJ, Rawlins K. Treatment of schizophrenia and cororbid substance use disorder. Curr Drug Targets CNS Neurol Disord 2002; 1: 129–39.
51. Kalyoncu A, Misral H, Pektas O, et al. Use of lamotrigine to augment clozapine in patients with resistant schizophrenia and comorbid alcohol dependence: a potent anti-craving effect? J Psychopharmacol 2005; 19: 301–5.

chapter 8

Management of acute behavioral disturbance in psychosis

David J. Castle, Nga Tran, Peter Bosanac, and Deirdre Alderton

This chapter outlines an approach to the management of acute behavioral disturbance in psychosis. It should be recognized at the outset that there are different reasons for people with psychotic illnesses to become acutely behaviorally disturbed, and potentially violent to themselves or others. The management of such scenarios requires an evaluation of the factors that might be contributing, and, where possible, an early intervention aimed at diffusing the situation prior to dangerous escalation.

"Organic" causes of acute behavioral disturbance

One often-missed cause of acute behavioral disturbance in psychosis is the intercession of "organic" factors, including head injury, metabolic and endocrine disturbances, and epileptic seizures. The patient might be experiencing an organic delirium, resulting in confusion, fear, and subsequent aggression. Intoxication with alcohol and illicit substances should be considered; withdrawal states (e.g., delirium tremens) might also be operating. Prescribed medications can also play a part here, for example, anticholinergic delirium associated with agents such as chlorpromazine or benztropine, and withdrawal states associated with benzodiazepines. Recognition and treatment of the delirium is crucial in such cases, and merely administering further medications can compound rather than resolve the problem.

Delirium usually has an acute or subacute onset and a fluctuating course. The clinical features include the following (1):

- Impaired attention
- Disorientation in time, place, and person
- Fluctuating concentration/attention span
- Rambling speech

- Emotional lability
- Worsening toward evening
- Visual hallucinations

The management of delirium has been reviewed by Meagher (2), and includes identification and treatment of the underlying cause, ensuring the safety of the individuals and their environment, and optimizing environmental stimulation. Medications used in delirium should not be ones that might worsen the patient's mental state. In particular, antipsychotics with potent central anticholinergic properties (e.g., chlorpromazine) should probably be avoided. Haloperidol is widely used in clinical practice, in doses of 1–2 mg orally, intramuscularly, or intravenously depending on the clinical state; it is repeatable after 30 minutes if not initially effective (2).

Although haloperidol continues to be the "gold standard" medication for the treatment of delirium, studies of risperidone, olanzapine, and quetiapine have attested to their successful use, given their relatively benign side-effect profile, and lack of negative impact on cognition. A review of 13 studies of atypical antipsychotics in the treatment of delirium (3) strongly supported the use of risperidone, olanzapine, and quetiapine in this setting. A review by Ozbolt et al. (4) also showed that risperidone, the most thoroughly studied atypical antipsychotic, was more effective than olanzapine; and quetiapine appeared to be a safe and effective alternative to high-potency antipsychotics in the treatment of delirium in elderly patients, with a lower extrapyramidal side-effect (EPSE) burden. Olanzapine has intrinsic anticholinergic activity (chap. 1) and this may theoretically exacerbate delirium in some particularly susceptible patients, so should be closely monitored in such settings (5). Quetiapine, with its very low incidence of EPSEs, showed a similar improvement and better tolerance for the treatment of delirium at doses of 50–200 mg daily (6–10). Aripiprazole (5–30 mg per day), likewise, has evidence to support its utility in the treatment of delirium (11–13). Data on amisulpride (14) and ziprasidone (15) are sparse; ziprasidone has potential arrhythmia-inducing properties that might mitigate its use in medically compromised patients. Further studies are required to elucidate the precise place of these particular atypical antipsychotics in managing delirium.

Benzodiazepines, such as lorazepam (2–4 mg orally, or parenterally, every 4 hours), are particularly useful in delirium related to alcohol and other substances (2), but can aggravate other deliria and should be used with caution. Respiratory function should be monitored, particularly with parenteral use.

Acute behavioral disturbance in psychosis

In the absence of delirium, patients with psychotic disorders do have a propensity to acute behavioral disturbance under certain circumstances. In schizophrenia, the behavioral disturbance is often mediated by fear, as the patient may feel persecuted, or believe he/she is being followed and spied

Box 8.1   Predictors of aggression in psychosis.

Young men
History of sociopathy/forensic history
Delirium, head injury
Alcohol intoxication
Illicit substance use
Psychosis, expressly if persecutory beliefs command hallucinations
Past aggression/violence

upon; thus, the intervention of police or mental health services can compound matters, and result in desperate acts of self-protection. In mania, the picture is different, with irritability and explosiveness often in response to apparently trivial events, or grandiose dismissiveness.

It serves well to recognize such factors, so that initial management does not inadvertently escalate matters. One should also be aware of those parameters associated with aggression in people with psychosis, as outlined in Box 8.1. Past aggression is probably the most powerful of all these predictors.

Signs of behavioral disturbance

Clinicians will come to recognize certain factors that are markers or predictors of imminent aggression in people with psychosis. These include pacing, agitation, angry gestures, closing of personal space, raised angry voice, and shouting. Verbal threats should always be taken seriously; one should be particularly wary if the patient is making specific threats toward a particular person, and consider withdrawing that person from the situation.

There is a gradation of acute behavioral disturbance from mild through moderate to severe. A useful approach is to grade the level of arousal using a standardized scale, such as that shown in Box 8.2. The virtue of this is that all staff can be using the same benchmarks, making assessment and communication easier, as well as guiding interventions and monitoring efficacy of each particular intervention. This brief scale has been validated against the "gold standard" but longer PANSS Excited Scale, with excellent correlation (kappa 0.83) (16).

Managing acute behavioral disturbance: nonpharmacological strategies

It is important to ensure that the staff members are well informed and feel safe—a fearful patient will be reassured by the sense that the staff are calm and know what they are doing. It is crucial that consistent messages are given to

Box 8.2 Acute arousal[a] scale (based on "patient arousal rating scale," fremantle hospital & health service).

5. Highly aroused, violent towards self, others, or property

4. Highly aroused and possibly distressed or fearful

3. Moderately aroused, agitated, becoming more vocal and unreasonable or hostile

2. Mildly aroused, pacing, still willing to talk reasonably

1. Settled, minimal agitation

0. Asleep or unconscious

[a]Symptoms of "arousal" include noisy, distressed, agitated, behavioral disturbance (increased motor activity, intrusive, and disinhibited), verbally abusive, physically abusive (to self, others, or property), and fearful.

the patient, so it is best to have a single nominated staff member who does the talking, and other attendant staff should be briefed as to what signal or words might indicate that physical restraint should be implemented, if required.

If possible the patient should be taken into an unstimulating environment, away from other patients, but the staff should ensure that an exit can be accessed easily. Support staff should be close by, but unobtrusive. Anything that might be used as a weapon (e.g., pens, pagers, mobile phones and so on) should be removed. The nominated staff member should talk in an even voice and not raise it. Speech should be slow and clear, other people present should be introduced, and everything that is going on should be explained. Sudden movements should be avoided. The patient should be reassured that the staff members want to help him/her, and will try to work with them toward a mutually acceptable outcome (17).

If *physical restraint* is required, then sufficient support staff should be close by and be aware of what their role will be. Security personnel or the police should be called in where indicated, and also need to be fully briefed about the clinical situation and what is expected of them. If possible, tasks for the restraint should be allocated ahead of time (e.g., arms, leg, and head) and a key word signaling the restraint to designated staff. Medications intended for administration should be drawn up in advance and the person to administer them selected. The patient should be talked to throughout, offering reassurance and explanation, and trying to obtain cooperation. Staff and the patient should be offered debriefing afterward (18).

The use of *seclusion* is somewhat controversial. It has been defined as "placement of a patient, alone, in a specially designated lockable room from which he or she can be observed through a window" (19). Potential benefits of seclusion include control and safety for the individual, other patients, and staff;

Box 8.3   The Pennsylvania program.

Six Core Strategies (National Executive Training Institute 2005)
- Leadership toward organizational change
- Using data to inform practice
- Workforce development
- Use of specific seclusion/restraint reduction tools
- Involvement of consumers
- Debriefing techniques

"time out" in a low-stimulus environment; and as a way of avoiding excessive use of medication. There are downsides, including the potential for perception of seclusion as punitive, or a violation of patient's rights (20). It can also reignite in the patient traumatic memories from their past, and arguably constitutes a traumatic event in itself.

Some centers have aimed for a "zero seclusion" policy and claim that this can be achieved without any increased risk to staff. The Pennsylvania State Hospital System's Seclusion and Restraint Reduction Program resulted in a substantial decrease in the rates (from 4.2 to 0.3 episodes per 1000 patient-days) and duration (from 10.8 to 1.3 hours) of seclusion with no significant changes in rates of staff injuries (21). The elements of this program are shown in Box 8.3.

On balance, the judicious use of seclusion can, in our view, be a safe and effective adjunct to the management of the acutely behaviorally disturbed patient, but its use should be kept to a minimum and closely monitored. Also, a standardized debriefing process should be in place; this affords the opportunity for both staff and the patient to ventilate feelings about the event, to work through some of the associated negative emotions, and plan for how better to deal with such situations in the future, should they arise. An example of a debriefing form for use in this context is shown in Figure 8.1.

Managing acute behavioral disturbance: pharmacological strategies

Rapid, effective, and safe psychopharmacological intervention is often required in the management of acute agitation. Box 8.4 highlights the desired targets of medication for the treatment of such acute scenarios.

Typical antipsychotics have a long history of use in the management of acute behavioral disturbance in people with psychotic disorders. However, *cardiac conduction problems*, including the risk of sudden cardiac death (notably

1 About a day ago we needed to take some actions to make things safe for you and other people here.

   Do you remember that?   Yes ❑   No ❑

2 Do you remember what happened?   Yes ❑   No ❑

   Details: _ .

   _

3 Do you know reasons why?   Yes ❑   No ❑

   Why?:_ _

   _

4 Do you believe it was necessary?   Yes ❑   No ❑

   Why?:_ _

   _

5 Do you know what medication was used?   Yes ❑   No ❑

   Please specify: _

Figure 8.1   *The 24–48 hour post-intervention patient debriefing form.*

Box 8.4   Desirable properties of medication in acute agitation.

Immediate effect
Available of different formulations: IM, rapid dissolving tablets, liquids
Calming effect without sedation
Limited side effects
Safety in overdose
Patient preference or history of response to a particular medication
Ease of switching to a continuation antipsychotic post acute phase

with droperidol), has led many clinicians to move away from their use, expressly at high doses. A more prevalent set of problems associated with typical antipsychotics are EPSEs (chap. 1). These are of particular concern in the acute setting, with high doses and rapid uptitration often being used. *Acute dystonias* are very frightening for the patient and laryngeal dystonia can prove fatal; immediate treatment with anticholinergic agents, either intramuscularly or intravenously, is required. *Akathisia* is extremely uncomfortable for the patient, and can feed the sense of agitation. *Neuroleptic malignant syndrome* is a rare but potentially fatal side effect, and is again more common in the context of high doses of typical antipsychotics (chap. 1). Awareness of these potential outcomes should lead to the monitoring of the patient in terms of mental state, EPSEs, pulse and blood pressure. Serial electrocardiograms and blood tests, including creatine phosphokinase levels should be performed where clinically indicated, and whenever high cumulative doses of antipsychotic agents have been administered.

Oral agents

The role of the atypical antipsychotics in the management of acute behavioral disturbance in psychosis has now been supported by the 2005 U.S. "Expert Consensus" Survey (22). In clinical trials, oral risperidone has been found to be as effective as, but better tolerated than, IM haloperidol when used alone or in combination with lorazepam in the rapid control of acute psychotic agitation (23). Baker et al. (24) reported a rapid decrease of agitation in patients with acute psychosis who were treated with rapid initial dose escalation of oral olanzapine (up to 40 mg/day). The availability of liquid or rapidly dispersible forms of these agents has been seen as a bonus in the acute setting. A recent systemic review (25) identified seven trials of oral antipsychotic therapy alone (two trials) or in combination with IM lorazepam (five trials), showing that haloperidol (5–15 mg), olanzapine (10–20 mg), risperidone (2–6 mg), and quetiapine (300–800 mg) are effective in the treatment of acute agitation. Aripiprazole, used in monotherapy or in combination with benzodiazepine displayed similar efficacy to olanzapine in agitated schizophrenia patients during a 5-day, randomized, double-blinded trial (26); there is also a parenteral form of aripiprazole available in some countries (see below) (27). To our knowledge, amisulpride has not been formally evaluated in terms of the immediate acute context, though it does have the potential benefit of tranquilization without marked sedation. The role of asenapine in this clinical scenario requires further study but potential advantages include sublingual administration and sedation with initial doses.

A novel, *breath-actuated delivery device* using the Staccato system containing loxapine has been put to test by Lesem and colleagues (28). Findings from this study showed promising results in reducing acute agitation within 10 minutes after inhalation in individuals with schizophrenia. Further investigation of this new loxapine formulation is warranted. A randomized, placebo-controlled study of *nicotine replacement therapy* (21 mg nicotine transdermal patch vs. placebo patch) for the reduction of agitation and aggression in smokers with schizophrenia (29) also suggests that smoking status should be included in the assessment of agitation and nicotine replacement included in the treatment of those (many) schizophrenia patients who are smokers.

Parenteral agents

If parenteral agents are required (Fig. 8.1) atypicals are again preferable to typical agents given tolerability characterized by fewer EPSEs and induction of dysphoria (30), and possibly less distress and trauma associated with the acute episode (31). For example, Wright et al. (32) compared IM olanzapine and IM haloperidol in the treatment of acute agitation, and demonstrated a faster onset of action with olanzapine, and a lower risk of EPSEs (33). IM ziprasidone also compares favorably with haloperidol in acute behavioral disturbance, and appears to be well tolerated and safe (34). Furthermore, IM ziprasidone may be more cost effective than typical antipsychotics in the acute setting in light of a reduced incidence of acute adverse events that often require extended periods of observation (35). Aripiprazole IM may also have a specific antiagitation effect rather than nonspecific sedation (27).

In terms of *efficacy*, head-to-head comparisons with IM haloperidol have shown that IM olanzapine reduced agitation more rapidly in one study (32), was more efficacious in the initial 90 minutes in another (36), but required additional medication in others (37,38); IM ziprasidone had a quicker response time in one study (39) and had a greater response rate in other studies (31,39,40). In a review of nine RCTs, none of which were head-to-head comparisons (41), the number needed to treat acute agitation at 2 hours for IM ziprasidone and IM olanzapine was significantly less than for IM aripiprazole.

In terms of *safety*, IM olanzapine was associated with fewer EPSEs (42) than IM haloperidol, including concurrent comparison with zuclopenthixol acetate in a large naturalistic study (43) and similar cardiac tolerability (44,45). IM ziprasidone required less anticholinergic medication for EPSEs in one study (46), had fewer EPSEs in two other studies (34,47) and showed a clinically insignificant increase in the QTc interval in another (48). IM aripiprazole had fewer EPSEs in one study (49). In a large database for IM olanzapine (50), most of the serious adverse events and mortality occurred with co-prescribed benzodiazepines and (in three quarters) other antipsychotics. As a precaution, benzodiazepines and olanzapine should not be administered parenterally within 2 hours of each other.

Indicative dosing guidelines for antipsychotic medication use in the acute setting are shown in Table 8.1.

An algorithmic approach to pharmacological management of acute behavioral disturbance in psychosis

As outlined above, the 1995 U.S. "Expert Consensus" Survey (22) regarding the most appropriate goals of emergency interventions and best choice of specific antipsychotic agents, concluded that the atypical antipsychotics are now preferred for the management of agitation in the setting of primary psychotic illnesses. Most clinicians agree that calming the patient without sedation as the most appropriate goal of emergency intervention since it will allow them to participate in further assessment and treatment. This is also consistent with the most recent Clinical Guidelines on Schizophrenia from the National Institute for Clinical Excellence (51) in the United Kingdom.

Table 8.1 Dosing guidelines for treatment of clinically significant acute agitation

Medication	Minimum–maximum single dose (mg)	Maximum total daily dose in the first 24 hr (mg)	Minimum dose interval (min)
Aripiprazole	5–10	30	120
Aripiprazole IM	5.25–15 Initial dose: 9.75 mg; subsequent dose after 2 hr, with no more than 3 doses in any 24 hr Maximum combined oral and IM doses per 24 hr: 30 mg	30	
Diazepam	5–15	60	75
Haloperidol	2.5–10	50	60
Haloperidol IM	2.5–10	35–40	60
Lorazepam	1–3	10–12	60
Lorazepam IM	0.5–3	10–12	60
Olanzapine	5–20	40	90
Olanzapine IM	5–10: Maximum 3 doses per any 24 hr and a minimum of 2 hr should elapse between each injection Lower dose 2.5–7.5 mg may be considered for geriatric, debilitated patients, or patients predisposed to hypotensive reactions, or when clinical factors warrant IM benzodiazepines should not be given concomitantly (or within two hours) of olanzapine IM	30	120
Quetiapine	50–200	600–800	75
Risperidone	1–3	7	75
Ziprasidone IM	10–20 10–20 mg increments 10 mg dose every 2 hr Or 20 mg dose every 4 hr	40	90

The aim is for rapid tranquilization rather than rapid neuroleptization (52). Although antipsychotic activity probably begins to accrue within 24 hours of treatment with antipsychotic agents (53), full antipsychotic efficacy may take some days to weeks to be established. High doses or cumulative doses of anti-psychotics should be avoided where possible, not least because of the risk of EPSEs or cardiac dysrhythmias.

Benzodiazepines may be used alone or as adjunctive medications in certain settings, for example where sedation is required and a relatively nonsedating antipsychotic is being used. There is some evidence that a benzodiazepine used in conjunction with an antipsychotic might have a greater benefit than either agent used alone (54). Several clinical studies showed a trend toward enhanced symptom reduction, such as agitation/aggression, with lorazepam combined with risperidone (55) or oral zuclopenthixol (56). Lorazepam, which is not cumulative with repeated doses or in hepatic impairment, is the preferred benzodiazepine, but the IM form is not available in all countries.

Any pharmacological intervention for acute behavioral disturbance should be tailored to the particular clinical situation and the efficacy monitored closely. Thus, the use of a scale such as that shown in Box 8.2 can guide the intervention and ensure consistency of approach. Figure 8.2 shows an algo-rithmic approach to the management of acute behavioral disturbance in psy-chosis, with interventions graded according to the degree of arousal. It should be noted that this algorithm reflects our own particular clinical experience in an Australian context. Other centers have preferences for other medications, and evidence is available to support the use of aripiprazole (26,27) in these settings; and parenteral lorazepam is not available in all jurisdictions.

These guidelines have been modified and refined with serial clinical audits, although effective in the vast majority of cases, are only guidelines and can be modified in particular clinical situations. For example, good response to a par-ticular agent in the past would support its use again, while benzodiazepines which cause respiratory depression should probably be avoided in patients with severe respiratory problems. Care should be taken with patients who have had an adverse reaction to an agent in the past; a history of neuroleptic malignant syndrome is of particular concern.

Finally, it will be noted that intravenous (IV) administration is not advocated, largely because of the potential for respiratory depression and arrest or cardiac conduction problems with this route. However, the IV route might be justified in certain clinical scenarios such as emergency departments, where strict moni-toring is mandated and resuscitation equipment is immediately available (57). Midazolam, droperidol, olanzapine, and combinations thereof have been effec-tively used intravenously in the emergency department setting (58).

Ideally the patient should be offered oral medication in the first instance (59) and consent should be attempted for any intervention. If a restraint and a forced injection are required, certain criteria need to be met, including that the patient is detained under the local Mental Health Act (a single restraint

GUIDELINES FOR PHARMACOLOGICAL MANAGEMENT
OF ACUTE AROUSAL & AGITATION IN PSYCHOSIS

STEP 1 - (Arousal level 2-3)
Mildly aroused, pacing, still willing to talk reasonably.
Moderately aroused, agitated, becoming more vocal, unreasonable or hostile.

ORAL

(Benzodiazepines) **Lorazepam 1-2.5mg** or **Diazepam 5-10 mg**
OR
(Atypical Options) **Olanzapine 5-10mg** or **Risperidone 1-2mg** (if less sedation required)
Review after 30-60 minutes, repeat if necessary.
If still ineffective, consider Step 2

PRECAUTIONS:
Lower doses should be considered in the elderly patients with low body weight, dehydration or no previous exposure to antipsychotic medication.
Monitor respiratory function when benzodiazepines are administered parenterally
Monitor postural blood pressure 30 min post-dose.
Monitor ECG, K & Mg if using high doses of antipsychotics, notably Ziprasidone.

STEP 2 - (Arousal level 3-4)
Moderately aroused, agitated, becoming more vocal, unreasonable and hostile.
Highly aroused, possibly distressed and fearful.

ORAL

(Atypical options) **Olanzapine 10-20mg** or **Risperidone 2-4mg** (if less sedation required)
PLUS
(Benzodiazepines) **Lorazepam 1-2.5 mg** or **Diazepam 5-10 mg**
Review after 30-60 minutes, repeat if necessary.
If still ineffective, consider Step 3

N1 Create opportunity and environment for patient to express fears, frustration, anger, etc. **(Ventilation)**
N2 Explore with patient what interventions/solutions would assist them to gain control **(Redirection)**
N3 Assess "time out" opportunity for patient to regain control (5-15min duration) **(Time Out)**
N4 If clinical situation warrants, patient may require restraint **(Restraint)**
N5 If required to place client in a safe environment seclusion might be considered. Explanation to be given to patient and staff **(Seclusion)**
The patient should be afforded the opportunity to debrief about the episode, at a reasonable interval.

STEP 3 - (Arousal level 4-5)
Refusing oral medication, moderately aroused, agitated, becoming more vocal, unreasonable and hostile. Highly aroused, distressed and fearful; violent toward self, others or property.

INTRAMUSCULAR

(Atypical options) **Olanzapine 10mg** repeated if necessary every 2 hours to a maximum of 40mg daily
or
Ziprasidone Mesilate: 10 mg every 2 hours or 20 mg every 4 hours, up to a maximum dose of 40 mg per day
(Benzodiazepines) **Clonazepam 1-2 mg** or if more rapid but shorter effect is required, consider **Midazolam 0.1mg/kg**
NOTE SPECIAL PRECAUTIONS: requires respiratory monitoring and availability of resuscitation equipment
Note: Clopixol acuphase might be used as per separate protocol, as a treatment regime (NOT prn*)

ALERTS:
EPSEs must be monitored and treated.
Anticholinergic agents NOT to be used routinely but 'as required' (PRN): Benztropine 2mg IM may be used for acute dystonias (Max 6 mg/24 hrs).
Combined use of Olanzapine IMI plus a benzodiazepine is potentially dangerous: *a gap of 2 HOURS IS REQUIRED BETWEEN THEIR IM USES.*
Ziprasidone: contraindicated if QTc 500ms Special precaution if QTc ≥450ms (male) & ≥470ms (female), recent myocardial ischaemia, heart failure & caution with concomitant benzodiazepines.
IM Midazolam should only ever be prescribed by a consultant and special precautions MUST be followed.
Clopixol acuphase should be prescribed as a course, *NOT just a PRN.*

NOTE: these guidelines are reflective of the local Australian context: other jurisdictions might have other preferred medications (eg. Lorazepam is the preferred IM benzodiazepine but is not universally available)

Figure 8.2 Guidelines for the treatment of acute arousal and agitation in psychosis. These guidelines reflect the author's clinical experience in an Australian context. Options are not detailed here, but those which have clinical and research support include aripiprazole (see text).

WARD	WEIGHT (kg)	AGE

Total number of medication charts ....
Chart numbers ....

Patient's name ....Unit no ....
Christian name ....
Address ....
....
Sex ....Birth date ....Age ....

Step 1	MEDICATION	Dose	Route	Additional information Check for effect after	
Date	Dr print name	Dr sign		Pharm	Imprest DD

Step 2	MEDICATION	Dose	Route	Additional information Check for effect after	
Date	Dr. print name	Dr. sign		Pharm	Imprest DD

Step 3	MEDICATION		Dose	Route	Additional information Check for effect after		
Date	Dr print name		Dr sign		Pharm		Imprest DD

Step	Date	Time	1st rating	Dose given	Route	Nurse	Check	2nd rating	Time	Nurse's signature

Note: based on charts used at Fremantle Hospital, Western Australia

Figure 8.3 *The cumulative medication chart.*

and forced medication may be permissible under duty of care, but this should be done only under exceptional circumstances). It should be noted that in patients experiencing their first episode of psychosis (i.e., neuroleptic naïve), and in the elderly, those with medical conditions, or those with a history of adverse reactions to antipsychotics, doses should be lowered. Ethnic variation in drug response and propensity to side effects should also be borne in mind when administering these agents, as there is racial variation in metabolism of antipsychotic medications via cytochrome P 450 (CYP 450) enzymes, especially CYP2D6, CYP2C9, and CYP2C19. Patients from certain ethnic groups

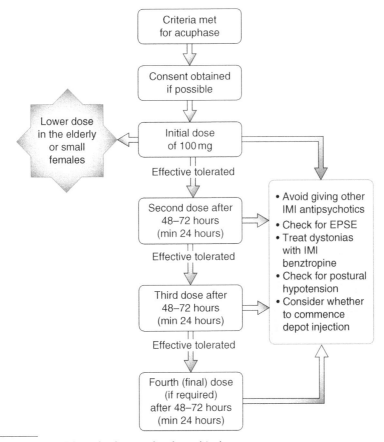

Figure 8.4 *Guidelines for the use of zuclopenthixol acetate.*

thus often require and respond to lower doses of psychotropic medications (60,61). The administration of medication should be closely monitored, and the efficacy or otherwise of particular interventions assessed at set time periods, which should be stipulated by the prescribing doctor (usually 30 minutes for IM medications and 60 minutes for oral medication). A pro forma for the documentation of such information is shown in Figure 8.3. This also allows a rapid appraisal of total medication use over a period of time.

The role of zuclopenthixol (clopixol) acuphase

One particular agent which has a special place in the management of acute behavioral disturbance in psychosis is zuclopenthixol (Clopixol Acuphase Lundbeck) (62,63). This agent (not available in some countries) is essentially a short-acting depot, with an effect lasting some 24–48 hours. It is very sedating, and the fact that it is relatively long lasting means that the requirement for numerous repeated injections in reduced, relative to shorter-acting agents. Ideally, acuphase should be used as a course of three to four injections, at least 24 hours apart, as detailed in Figure 8.4 and Box 8.5. The patient needs to be monitored, particularly with respect to blood pressure (it can cause profound

---

Box 8.5   Guidelines for the use of clopixol acuphase (zuclopenthixol acetate).

Initial treatment of acute arousal and agitation in psychosis is described in Figure 8.2

Acuphase should be considered as a treatment course rather than simply a PRN for acute arousal. An effort should be made, where feasible, to obtain verbal informed consent from the patient. It should not usually be used for first-episode patients

Suitable patients for the prescription of acuphase

- Have required Step-3 injections as per guidelines in Figure 8.2 more than once and have had sufficient time for assessment of response and/or side effects to previously injected drugs (minimum of 30–60 minutes)
- Have previously received acuphase and have shown a good tolerability and response to it

Prescribing information for acuphase

- Usual dose is 100 mg every 48–72 hours
- Females, neuroleptic naïve patients and the elderly may require lower doses (25 or 50 mg)
- Large young men may require higher doses (up to 150 mg)
- A course of injections would usually be prescribed (e.g., 100 mg every 48–72 hours.) Maximum dose is 400 mg over 2 weeks or 4 injections (whichever comes first)
- At least 24 hours must elapse between acuphase injections
- Review carefully for EPSEs and treat rigorously if they occur
- Monitor blood pressure carefully (hypotension may occur)

Sedative effects of acuphase

- Sedation may initially be seen between 15 and 90 minutes after injection and peaks after 8 hours
- Effects last up to 72 hours
- The first injection is usually the most sedating

Patients in whom caution is advised

- Are concurrently receiving other antipsychotics
- Are sensitive to EPSE's
- Have pre-existing cardiac disease
- TAKE CARE IF THE PATIENT IS STRUGGLING (dangerous if given accidentally into a vein)

postural hypotension) and EPSEs. Acuphase should be considered a treatment rather than an emergency intervention *per se*, and an attempt should be made to gain consent from the patient (64).

Conclusions

Acute behavioral disturbance is not uncommon in psychiatric settings, potentially endangering both patients and staff. It is important to try to understand what drives the arousal, and to intervene before matters escalate. The 2005 Expert Consensus Survey strongly endorsed the goal of emergency treatment as being to calm the patient without oversedation.

Pharmacotherapy with atypical antipsychotics alone or in combination with a benzodiazepine has proven to be as least efficacious as typical agents in the amelioration of agitation and psychosis in the emergency setting, and is mostly well tolerated in terms of their EPSE profile. Pharmacological interventions need to be administered in a structured and safe manner, and the effects and side effects carefully monitored.

Acknowledgements

We wish to acknowledge the role played by the staff of the Psychiatric Intensive Care Unit and Fremantle Hospital, Western Australia, and staff at the Royal Melbourne, Austin, and St Vincent's Hospitals in Melbourne in developing and piloting many of the strategies suggested here.

References

1. Meagher D. Delirium: the role of psychiatry. Adv Psychiatr Treat 2001; 7: 433–42.
2. Meagher DJ. Delirium: optimising management. BMJ 2001; 322: 144–9.
3. Boettger S, Breitbart W. Atypical antipsychotics in the management of delirium: a review of the empirical literature. Palliat Support Care 2005; 3: 227–37.
4. Ozbolt LB, Paniagua MA, Kaiser RM. Atypical antipsychotics for the treatment of delirious elders. J Am Med Dir Assoc 2008; 9: 18–28.
5. Lim CJ, Trevino C, Tampi RR. Can Olanzapine cause delirium in the elderly? Ann Pharmacother 2006; 40: 135–38.
6. Schwartz TL, Masand PS. Treatment of delirium with quetiapine. Primary care companion. J Clin Psychiatry 2000; 2: 10–12.
7. Kim KY, Bader GM, Kotlyar V, Gropper D. Treatment of delirium in older adults with quetiapine. J Geriatr Psychiatry Neurol 2003; 16: 29–31.
8. Sasaki Y, Matsuyama T, Inoue S, et al. A prospective, open-label, flexible-dose study of quetiapine in the treatment of delirium. J Clin Psychiatry 2003; 64: 1316–21.
9. Pae CU, Lee SJ, Lee CU, Lee C, Paik IH. A pilot trial of quetiapine for the treatment of patients with delirium. Hum Psychopharmacol 2004; 19: 125–7.

10. Devlin JW, Roberts RJ, Fong JJ, et al. Efficacy and safety of quetiapine in critically ill patients with delirium: a prospective, multicenter, randomized, double-blind, placebo-controlled pilot study. Crit Care Med 2010; 38: 419–27.

11. Boettger S, Friedlander M, Breitbart W, Passik S. Aripiprazole and haloperidol in the treatment of delirium. Aust NZ J Psychiatry 2011; 45: 477–82.

12. Alao AO, Moskowitz L. Aripiprazole and delirium. Ann Clin Psychiatry 2006; 18: 267–9.

13. Straker DA, Shapiro PA, Muskin PR. Aripiprazole in the treatment of delirium. Psychosomatics 2006; 47: 385–91.

14. Lee KU, Won WY, Lee HK, et al. Amisulpride versus quetiapine for the treatment of delirium: a randomized, open prospective study. Int Clin Psychopharmacol 2005; 20: 311–14.

15. Leso L, Schwartz TL. Ziprasidone treatment of delirium. Psychosomatics 2002; 43: 61–2.

16. Castle D, Daniel J, Knott J, et al. Development of clinical guidelines for the pharmacological management of behavoural disturbance and aggression in people with psychosis. Australas Psychiatry 2005; 13: 247–52.

17. Stevenson S. Heading off violence with verbal de-escalation. J Psychosoc Nurs Ment Health Serv 1991; 29: 6–10.

18. Brown T. Psychiatric emergencies. Adv Psychiatr Treat 1998; 4: 270–6.

19. Kikpatrick H. A descriptive study of seclusion: the unit environment, patient behaviour, and nursing interventions. Arch Psychiatr Nurs 1989; 3: 3–9.

20. Wynaden D, Orb A, McGowan S, et al. The use of seclusion in the year 2000: what has changed? Collegian 2001; 8: 19–25.

21. Smith G, Davis R, et al. Pennsylvania state hospital system's seclusion and restraint reduction program. Psychiatr Serv 2005; 56: 1115–22.

22. Allen MH, Currier GW, Carpenter D, Ross RW, Docherty JP. Expert consensus panel for behavioral E. The expert consensus guideline series. Treatment of behavioral emergencies 2005. J Psychiatr Pract 2005; 11(Suppl 1): 5–108.

23. Allen MH, Currier GW. Use of restraints and pharmacotherapy in academic psychiatric emergency services. Gen Hosp Psychiatry 2004; 26: 42–9.

24. Baker RW, Kinon BJ, Maguire GA, Liu H, Hill AL. Effectiveness of rapid initial dose escalation of up to forty milligrams per day of oral olanzapine in acute agitation. J Clin Psychopharmacol 2003; 23: 342–8.

25. Zeller SL, Rhoades RW. Systematic reviews of assessment measures and pharmacologic treatments for agitation. Clin Ther 2010; 32: 403–25.

26. Kinon BJ, Stauffer VL, Kollack-Walker S, et al. Olanzapine versus aripiprazole for the treatment of agitation in acutely ill patients with schizophrenia. J Clin Psychopharmacol 2008; 28: 601–7.

27. Currier GW, Citrome LL, Zimbroff DL, et al. Intramuscular aripiprazole in the control of agitation. J Psychiatr Pract 2007; 13: 159–69.

28. Lesem MD, Tran-Johnson TK, Riesenberg RA, et al. Rapid acute treatment of agitation in individuals with schizophrenia: multicentre, randomised, placebo-controlled study of inhaled loxapine. Br J Psychiatry 2011; 198: 51–8.

29. Allen MH, Debanne M, Lazignac C, et al. Effect of nicotine replacement therapy on agitation in smokers with schizophrenia: a double-blind, randomized, placebo-controlled study. Am J Psychiatry 2011; 168: 395–9.

30. Battaglia J. Pharmacological management of acute agitation. Drugs 2005; 65: 1207–22.

31. Cañas F. Management of agitation in the acute psychotic patient — Efficacy without excessive sedation. Eur Neuropsychopharmacol 2007; 17: S108–S14.

32. Wright P, Birkett M, David SR, et al. Double-blind, placebo-controlled comparison of intramuscular olanzapine and intramuscular haloperidol in the treatment of acute agitation in schizophrenia. Am J Psychiatry 2001; 158: 1149–51.
33. Wright P, Lindborg SR, Birkett M, et al. Intramuscular olanzapine and intramuscular haloperidol in acute schizophrenia: antipsychotic efficacy and extrapyramidal safety during the first 24 hours of treatment. Can J Psychiatry 2003; 48: 716–21.
34. Brook S, Walden J, Beneltia I. Ziprasidone and haloperidol in the treatment of acute exacerbation of schizophrenia and schizoaffective: comparison of intramuscular and oral formulation in a 6-week, randomized, blinded assessment study. Psychopharmacology (Berl) 2005; 178: 514–23.
35. Zimbroff DL, Allen MH, Battaglia J, et al. Best clinical practice with ziprasidone intramuscular: update after 2 years of experience. CNS Spectr 2005; 10(Suppl 11): 1–15.
36. Hsu WY, Huang S-S, Lee B-S, Chiu N-Y, Chiu NY. Comparison of intramuscular olanzapine, orally disintegrating olanzapine tablets, oral risperidone solution, and intramuscular haloperidol in the management of acute agitation in an acute care psychiatric ward in Taiwan. J Clin Psychopharmacol 2010; 30: 230–4.
37. Raveendran NS, Tharyan P, Alexander J, Adams CE. Rapid tranquillisation in psychiatric emergency settings in India: pragmatic randomised controlled trial of intramuscular olanzapine versus intramuscular haloperidol plus promethazine. BMJ 2007; 335: 865–73.
38. Freeman Dj, DiPaula BA, Love RC. Intramuscular haloperidol versus intramuscular olanzapine for treatment of acute agitation: a cost-minimization study. Pharmacotherapy 2009; 29: 930–6.
39. Preval H, Klotz SG, Southard R, Francis A. Rapid-acting IM ziprasidone in a psychiatric emergency service: a naturalistic study. Gen Hosp Psychiatry 2005; 27: 140–4.
40. Citrome L, Brook S, Warrington L, et al. Ziprasidone versus haloperidol for the treatment of agitation. Ann Emerg Med 2004; 44: S22.
41. Citrome L. Comparison of intramuscular ziprasidone, olanzapine, or aripirazole for agitation: a quantitative review of efficacy and safety. J Clin Psychiatry 2007; 68: 1875–85.
42. Chandrasena R, Dvorakova D, Lee SI, et al. Intramuscular olanzapine vs. intramuscular short-acting antipsychotics: safety, tolerability and the switch to oral antipsychotic medication in patients with schizophrenia or acute mania. Int J Clin Pract 2009; 63: 1249–58.
43. Downey LV, Zun LS, Gonzales SJ. Frequency of alternative to restraints and seclusion and uses of agitation reduction techniques in the emergency department. Gen Hosp Psychiatry 2007; 29: 470–4.
44. Lindborg SR, Beasley CM, Alaka K, Taylor CC. Effects of intramuscular olanzapine vs. haloperidol and placebo on QTc intervals in acutely agitated patients. Psychiatry Res 2003; 119: 113–23.
45. Houston JP, Centorrino F, Cincotta S, et al. An observational study of intramuscular olanzapine treatment in acutely agitated patients with bipolar I disorder or schizophrenia. Ann Emerg Med 2006; 48(Suppl)): 126.
46. Fernando C, Perez-Sola V, Gutierrez-Fraile M, et al. Sequential IM/oral ziprasidone and haloperidol in agitated patients with schizophrenia: a naturalistic comparison. Eur Neuropsychopharmacol 2009; 19(Suppl 3): S480–1.
47. Brook S, Lucey JV, Gunn KP, et al. Intramuscular ziprasidone reduced symptoms and was well tolerated in acute psychosis. Evid Based Ment Health 2001; 4: 3.
48. Miceli JJ, Tensfeldt TG, Shiovitz T, et al. Effects of high-dose ziprasidone and haloperidol on the QTc interval after intramuscular administration: a randomized,

single-blind, parallel-group study in patients with schizophrenia or schizoaffective disorder. Clin Ther 2010; 232: 472–91.

49. Tran-Johnson TK, Sack DA, Marcus RN, et al. Efficacy and safety of intramuscular aripiprazole in patients with acute agitation: a randomized, double-blind, placebo-controlled trial. J Clin Psychiatry 2007; 68: 111–19.

50. Marder SR, Sorsaburu S, Dunayevich E, et al. Case reports of postmarketing adverse event experiences with olanzapine intramuscular treatment in patients with agitation. J Clin Psychiatry 2010; 71: 433–41.

51. National Institute of Clinical Excellence. Violence – the short term management of disturbed/violent behaviour in in-patients psychiatric settings and emergency departments. NICE 2005; Guideline No 25.

52. Macpherson R, Anstee B, Dix R. Guidelines for the management of acutely disturbed patients. Adv Psychiatr Treat 1996; 2: 194–201.

53. Kapur S, Arenovich T, Agid O, et al. Evidence for onset of antipsychotic effects within the first 24 hours of treatment. Am J Psychiatry 2005; 162: 939–46.

54. Veser FH, Veser BD, McuMullan JT, Zealberg J, Currier GW. Risperidone versus haloperidol, in combination with lorazepam, in the treatment of acute agitation and psychosis: a pilot, randomized, double-blind, placebo-controlled trial. J Psychiatr Pract 2006; 12: 103–8.

55. Lejeune J, Larmo I, Chrzanowski W, et al. Oral risperidone plus oral lorazepam versus standard care with intramuscular conventional neuroleptics in the initial phase of treating individuals with acute psychosis. Int J Clin Psychopharmacol 2004; 19: 259–69.

56. Hovens JE, Dries PJ, Melman CT, Wapenaar RJ, Loonen AJ. Oral risperidone with lorazepam versus oral zuclopenthixol with lorazepam in the treatment of acute psychosis in emergency psychiatry: a prospective, comparative, open-label study. J Psychopharmacol 2005; 19: 51–7.

57. Knott JC, Taylor DM, Castle DJ. Randomized clinical trial comparing intravenous midazolam and droperidol for sedation of the acutely agitated patient in the emergency department. Ann Emerg Med 2006; 47: 61–7.

58. Chan E, Taylor D, Phillips G, et al. May I have your consent? Informed consent clinical trials – feasability in emergency situation. J Psychiatr Intensive Care 2011; 7: 109–13.

59. Currier GW, Medori R. Orally versus intramuscularly administered antipsychotic drugs in psychiatric emergencies. J Psychiatr Pract 2006; 12: 30–40.

60. Zhou SF. Polymorphism of human cytochrome P450 2D6 and its clinical significance: part II. Clin Pharmacokinet 2009; 48: 761–804.

61. Rosemary J, Adithan C. The pharmacogenetics of CYP2C9 and CYP2C19: ethnic variation and clinical significance. Curr Clin Pharmacol 2007; 2: 93–109.

62. Barnes CW, Alderton D, Castle D. The development of Clinical Guidelines for the use of Zuclopenthixol Acetate. Australas Psychiatry 2002; 10: 54–8.

63. Gibson Roger C, Fenton M, da Silva Freire Coutinho E, Campbell C. Zuclopenthixol acetate for acute schizophrenia and similar serious mental illnesses. Cochrane Database Syst Rev 2004: [Available from: http://www.mrw.interscience.wiley.com/cochrane/clsysrev/articles/CD000525/frame.html].

64. Fitzgerald P. Long acting antipsychotic medication, restraint and treatment in the management of acute psychosis. Aust NZ J Psychiatry 1999; 33: 660–6.

chapter 9

Managing the violent behaviors associated with the schizophrenic syndrome

Paul E. Mullen and Danny H. Sullivan

There is a statistically and clinically significant correlation between having a schizophrenic syndrome, and increased rates of antisocial behavior in general and violence in particular (1–6). Studies of homicide offenders consistently indicate that between 5 and 10% will have a schizophrenic disorder (Table 9.1). True rates of schizophrenia among homicide offenders are likely to be at the higher end of these estimates, as nearly all the studies have systematic biases which underestimate the level of the association.

Follow-up studies of large numbers of those with schizophrenia confirm the high levels of violent offending, including killing (7–10). Up to 10% of homicide offenders may have schizophrenia but the annual risk of a patient with schizophrenia committing a homicide is only in the region of 1 in 10,000, and for acquiring a conviction for violence, 1 in 150 (7). Minor forms of assault are more common (5–10% per year) but they are often conceptualized by clinicians not as illness-related but as contextual, 'personality based', or intoxication driven; these attributions may be bolstered by rigid categorical diagnostic systems or forensic formulations required for the legal system. The problems created by the antisocial behavior are further obscured from clinicians because so many who offend are subsequently invisible behind prison walls, where schizophrenia is 10 times more common than would be expected by chance (11).

There are three ways in which violence can be reduced among those with schizophrenia. The *population level* involves using knowledge of what mediates violence in those with schizophrenia to direct therapy and management of all those with the condition. At the *individual level*, risk assessments are needed to identify those at sufficiently high probability of acting violently to

Table 9.1 Studies from a range of countries using a range of methodologies all suggesting that homicide offenders are about 10 times more likely to have schizophrenia than would be expected by chance

Authors	Country	Number of Homicides	Homicides with Schizophrenia	Odds ratio (95% CI)
Hafner & Boker (1982) (17)	Western Germany	3367	8.0%	12.7 (11.2–14.3)
Eronen et al. (1996)	Finland	1037	6.1%	9.7 (7.4–12.6)
Wallace et al. (1998) (3)	Victoria, Australia	168	7.2%	10.1 (5.5–18.6)
Erb et al. (2001)	Germany	290 (incl. attempted)	10.0%	16.1 (11.2–12.5)
Schanda et al. (2004)	Austria	1087	5.4%	8.8 (6.7–11.5)

require specific intervention; to target such treatment to the dynamic and alterable risk factors (e.g., current living conditions) as opposed to static risk factors (e.g., gender and prior offending); finally, to managing risk *at the point where violence is imminent* (usually in the inpatient situation).

What mediates between the schizophrenic syndrome and violent behavior?

Box 9.1 provides a summary and model of factors that mediate violence in schizophrenia. Each of these factors is addressed in detail and their interactions are modeled in Figure 9.1.

Substance abuse

Epidemiological evidence supports a strong association between substance abuse and criminal behavior in those with schizophrenia (7,12–15). Correlations and associations do not necessarily reflect causal relationships. A study of 2861 patients first admitted to hospital over a 25-year period with schizophrenia and matched to community controls demonstrated that although over these years the rate of known substance abuse in patients rose from 8% to 27%, the rate of convictions for violence increased only modestly (from 6% to 10%) in line with the increase among controls (1–3%) (7). This study suggested that over the last 30 years, those with schizophrenia and a propensity to violence have increasingly turned to substance abuse, rather than violence having

Box 9.1   Mediators of violence in schizophrenia.

Substance abuse
Psychotic symptoms
Vulnerabilities associated with the illness
    Predating onset
    A result of active illness
    Related to treatment
Developmental factors
Social factors
Personality factors

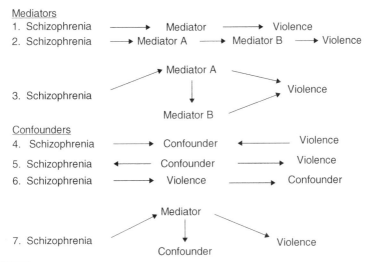

Figure 9.1   *Mediators have a causal relationship with schizophrenia and in turn increase the probability of violence and/or are causally related to a third factor which increases the risk of violence (1–3). Confounders either have a causal but unrelated relationship with both schizophrenia and violence or are the product of both schizophrenia and violence without mediating any connection between the two (4–6). Cofounders can also be related to mediators without relating directly to either schizophrenia or violence (7). In practice many factors operate partly as mediators and partly as confounders of the relationship.*

increased proportionately with community levels of substance abuse. This interpretation is supported by the work of both the groups of Tengström (16) and Vevera (9).

Although reducing rates of substance abuse in those with schizophrenia is an important therapeutic goal central to improving symptom control and quality of life, and will almost certainly decrease antisocial behavior, it is unlikely to be a panacea for propensities to violence. This is particularly so given the fact that the best effective management for substance use among those with schizophrenia remains problematic, as outlined in chapter 7.

Active symptoms

There is a substantial body of clinical experience and literature which supports a connection between active symptoms and antisocial behavior, though not all studies support the role of specific phenomena such as delusions and hallucinations (5,17–19). Although the role of active symptoms in the violence of schizophrenia has, in our opinion, been overestimated, that they have a role is undoubted. The evidence, for example, of an association between delusional jealousy and attacks on the partner is overwhelming, and persecutory delusions, hallucinations, and nonspecific psychotic agitation may all on occasion precipitate violence (20,21).

There is a growing support for a two-type model of violence in schizophrenia. (22,23). These are shown in Box 9.2. The majority of violence in the schizophrenic population is attributable to Type 2, though it is possible that among homicide offenders Type 1 are overrepresented. Interestingly, this typology may overlap with the associations which differentiate between antisocial behaviors limited to adolescence and those which persist through the life course (24).

Consequences of the psychopathology of schizophrenia

Schizophrenia psychopathology can impact on the risk of violent behavior through the following:

• Vulnerabilities *pre-dating* the onset of active symptoms, including developmental difficulties, dissocial traits, educational failure, increasing rates of conduct disorder, and early-onset substance abuse. The latter is of note as a common error is to diagnose a drug-induced psychosis in those with schizophrenia whose abuse has preceded their obvious psychotic symptoms.

Box 9.2   The two-type model of violence in schizophrenia.

Type 1 typically have organized delusional systems which are related to the violence, do not have prominent histories of conduct disorder or adult delinquency, usually commit their first violent offence after entering treatment, almost always attack a carer or acquaintance, and perhaps most importantly are in other senses similar to related patient cohorts

Type 2 tend to have disorganized clinical syndromes, have histories of conduct disorder and early-onset substance abuse, usually a history of multiple violent and nonviolent offences prior to diagnosis, commit domestic and nondomestic violence, and are on many measures more similar to offenders than to patients

- Vulnerabilities acquired as a result of *active illness*, including positive symptoms, personality deterioration, executive dysfunction, social dislocation, substance abuse, incarceration, and unemployment.
- Vulnerabilities related to *treatment*, such as for akathisia and neuroleptic-induced deficit syndrome, and erosion of social skills due to isolation from mainstream community life.

Developmental factors

Those with a schizophrenic syndrome at increased risk of violence frequently have a history of developmental problems, poor parenting, and disadvantage during childhood and early adolescence (25,26). A history of conduct disorder in childhood is far commoner in this group. So strong is the relationship that it works both ways, with those with a history of conduct disorder having an increased risk of developing schizophrenia later in life (27).

Current social context

Those with schizophrenia often fail to establish work and adult social roles even prior to the recognition of their disorder. Once established, schizophrenia is profoundly associated with unemployment (28), which usually brings in its wake financial insecurity and social decline. This tends to encourage a drift into a marginal existence characterized by poor housing, if not homelessness, in socially disorganized neighborhoods where substance abuse, interpersonal conflict, and crime are commonplace. Location of accommodation is associated with violence: the risk of violence in those with major mental disorders is demonstrably and dramatically increased in those discharged from hospital into a high-crime neighborhood (29,30).

Personality factors

There is now good evidence for personality factors mediating criminality in schizophrenia (31–35). Those with the schizophrenic syndrome may become irritable, dissocial, entitled, grandiose, suspicious, and negative; they may be unconcerned (or blind) to the feelings and interests of others, and fail to learn from experience. Psychopathic traits have been found more often in those with schizophrenia who are violent, with particular correlations between violence and those measures connected to social deviance and antisocial attitudes (35,36). Central to the emergence of violence are both the nature of the person in whom psychosis manifests, and the deleterious effects of the schizophrenic process on their personality.

What is to be done?

The links which mediate between schizophrenia and violence at a population level are represented schematically in Figure 9.2. But how can we break these links?

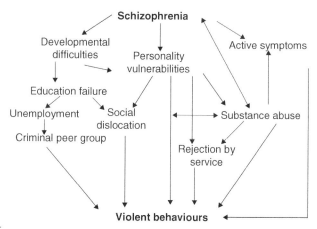

Figure 9.2 *The major mediators between having schizophrenia and behaving violently are illustrated. The very complexity of the nexus between illness and violence offers multiple opportunities for intervening to break the links.*

Box 9.3   Risk assessment.

(a) *Simple.* The high-risk group will include a large number of young men with a childhood history of conduct disorder, antisocial and violent behavior in adolescents, substance abuse, unemployment, and a disorganized lifestyle

(b) *Clinical.* Risk is dramatically increased in those who are angry and suspicious, lacking insight and rejecting therapy, threatening and feckless. Specific delusional syndromes, in particular delusional jealousy, dramatically increase risks, as do personality traits such as callousness and entitlement

(c) *Multidisciplinary.* No professional group has a monopoly on the knowledge required to evaluate risk and each should have appropriate input. Current ward behavior, social context, mental state, personality and intellectual evaluations, and above all a thorough history are central

(d) *Systematic.* There are many risk assessment instruments of widely varying probity. The best define high-risk groups using dynamic as well as static variables, thus allowing recognition of factors to be targeted for intervention. Their prime function for the clinician is to direct attention to known correlates of violent behavior. Instruments can define high-risk groups. What they cannot do is tell you with acceptable error rates the chances of any particular individual in that high-risk group being violent. This makes them good as tools for needs assessment, and poor as justifications for punitive controls. Instruments like the HCR 20 have a place in structuring the professional's approach to risk assessment, while at the same time leaving a place for common sense and clinical knowledge (38)

Culture change in generic services

The mental health community has to start by accepting the fact that violent and antisocial behaviors are among the potential complications of having a schizophrenic syndrome. Many services take violent behavior as grounds for exclusion from services. We would argue instead that the research evidence reflects that violent behavior should define increased need for service provision (37) rather than abandonment. With recognition that risk of violence is core business, comes the possibility of remediation. As long as the problem of violence is minimized, diverted onto other services, or dismissed as "not illness related," there can be no progress in reducing its occurrence. Those at high risk of behaving violently, though they constitute less than 10% of those with schizophrenia, need to be prioritized for management. But how can the high-risk population be recognized?

The assessment of risk

Many psychiatric services exclude angry young men with substance use problems and forensic issues. Opportunities for early intervention are lost, negative attitudes toward services are engendered in patients, and those of this group at risk of violence either avoid services or are denied such services. Risk assessment should commence at the point of triage, when high-risk patients may be excluded for spurious reasons or before adequate information exists to determine how best to intervene. Risk assessment is not an arcane art, and a practical guide is provided in Box 9.3.

General principles of management

Many high-risk patients will be young, substance abusing, rejecting of treatment, and disorganized. Extended admissions of more than a month are required to enforce a sufficient period of abstinence from cannabis and other drugs of abuse to even begin effective treatment of schizophrenic symptoms. Few such patients will be adherent to medications once discharged, nor likely to remain in supervised accommodation of their own accord, but community treatment orders can facilitate compliance, along with other interventions to enhance and monitor compliance with treatment. The responsivity principle (37) requires that high-risk patients receive more intensive intervention, such as assertive case management. However, coercion is unlikely to succeed in the long term, and indeed it is at times of confrontation or disagreement that violence is most likely to occur.

Social interventions

High-risk patients on leaving hospital need to be placed in stable accommodation in low-crime neighborhoods. This simple and obvious recommendation is rendered hopelessly idealistic by local resistance to locating any accommodation for the mentally ill, let alone mentally abnormal offenders, in more stable neighborhoods. The evidence that marginalization is associated with increased offending has not altered parochial thinking despite strong overall community interests in reducing offending.

In the short term, patients also need regular support from consistent clinicians with whom they have positive relationships, and activities and structure in their lives. In the medium term, programs to enhance social interaction and integration with family when possible, to develop work-related skills and provide recreational and sporting activities become the focus. If this population does not acquire a structured and satisfying lifestyle in the long term, be that around vocational activities, recreation or social groups, then they will remain at risk of relapse into substance abuse, downward social drift, and crime. Discharge planning should explicitly factor in goals to ameliorate those social disadvantages which serve as perpetuating factors in violence risk.

Psychological management

Developmental disruptions, genetic predispositions, and the illness process may, singly or in combination, leave some people with schizophrenia with personality traits and attitudes which might be termed criminogenic. Reducing the possibility of future violence depends to a significant degree on modifying these factors and the behaviors they generate.

Skepticism persists about managing severe personality disorders especially when associated with a schizophrenic syndrome. Partly this reflects the failure of such approaches as dynamic psychotherapies, therapeutic communities, casework, and simplistic behavioral therapies. Personality disorders *per se* may indeed be untreatable but many of their elements, as found in schizophrenic syndromes, are open to modification and improvement. It is possible to improve interpersonal skills, anger control, assertiveness, victim empathy, and to reduce the cognitive distortions which support violent behaviors (39,40). The goal is not the idealistic creation of a benign and prosocial personality, but rather to develop sufficient skills to minimize the deleterious effects of disordered personality on everyday interactions (41,42).

Pharmacological management

The primary psychotic illness requires adequate pharmacological treatment (chap. 1). Adherence is a key issue in this group (also chap. 10) and *depot antipsychotic medication* is often preferable and may facilitate the maintenance of clinical input which otherwise may diminish over time. The available depot antipsychotics are reviewed in chapter 1. The evidence for antipsychotic medication as having a specific antiaggressive effect favors clozapine (43) and in settings where adherence can be monitored or assured, this is the preferable alternative.

Other adjunctive medications may also be used to reduce potential for violence. *Benzodiazepines* may be useful in the short term, but in the longer term may create potential for conflict in dependent patients seeking escalation of dosage; alprazolam, flunitrazepam, and clonazepam should be used with caution due to the occasional emergence of aggression and behavioral disinhibition. *Antiepileptic drugs* may be of benefit, possibly through added sedation, although their toxicity and tolerability limit use, and there are few methodologically rigorous or sustained trials to support their use: carbamazepine, valproate, topiramate, and phenytoin have been used. *Lithium* has demonstrated efficacy in reducing in aggression in personality disorder and organic conditions, but may not be tolerated. *Serotonergic antidepressants* have also been put to test, but with little evidence of violence reduction except when this is a manifestation of depression.

Substance abuse

The assessment and management of drug and alcohol abuse among those with schizophrenia has perforce become a major priority. In those at high risk of violence, substance abuse is most often present and its effective control is a prerequisite for any other management. This issue is covered in more detail by Lubman et al. (44) and in chapter 7.

Restructuring therapeutic goals and service systems

Mental health services, particularly when under pressure, tend to focus on symptom control, which involves a primarily biomedical approach focused on medication. Whether this is ever sufficient is doubtful but in those at high risk of violence it is totally inadequate as all but a holding measure. Substance abuse, personality vulnerabilities, and social context need—if not equal priority with symptom control—at least to be a major part of the management process. If managing the criminogenic and substance abuse issues is to have a chance of success in this group, it has to involve not just adding a few special programs but creating a total immersion for the patient in the drive for change (16).

On how not to confront violence in inpatient settings

Violence most often occurs in the context of either fear or anger. Instrumental violence where a conscious choice is made to employ intimidation or assault to gain a particular end is unusual although not uncommon in those with psychotic disorders.

  In our experience fear mostly spurs violence among those with a schizophrenic disorder. Anxiety and fear are linked but phenomenologically separable. *Anxiety* is about the bringing forward into the present of threats from the future. Anxiety is about what may happen. *Fear* is the response to a danger in the present. It is about what is happening now. Anxiety directs behavior to avoid a future possibility. Fear directs behavior to responding to a present danger. Anxiety is less likely to precipitate a confrontation with those believed to be a threat though it can occasionally motivate a pre-emptive strike. Fear encourages either flight or fight. Situations which reduce the ability to flee will increase the probability of fight. Situations which make attack difficult can encourage withdrawal. Once anxiety reaches a certain level it readily transmutes into fear. High levels of anxiety are usually present in those with acute psychotic symptoms. This is particularly marked following admission when patients have to cope with a sudden change in their situation and a set of unfamiliar expectations and potential threats. When admission has been coerced, the level of anxiety often compounded by anger will be increased.

The psychotic state will color the patient's experiences but it is important not to forget the feeling of powerlessness and confusion when thrust into a new environment among strangers will be stressful for anyone. Explaining, orienting, and introducing, not once and quickly, but with care and repeatedly, can address some of the reality-based anxieties and fears. If patients are able to verbalize their fears this provides the opportunity for discussing them (not simply dismissing or reassuring). Attempts need to be made to deal first with their roots in the real situation and then, and only then, with the misperceptions and false beliefs. The patient may be so highly aroused that effective communication becomes impossible. At this point psychopharmacological assistance may become useful (chap. 8). The problems with benzodiazepines are well known. The advantages of their use in the highly aroused patient should not be forgotten. They are acceptable in most patients, and more than acceptable, which is part of the problem. Orally they act reasonably rapidly. Withdrawal states are not infrequently part of the problem with recently admitted patients and benzodiazepines can assist with this aspect of management. They are, however, only a short-term solution to an immediate crisis. Only when the patient feels less threatened will the risks of a violent response be reduced.

Anger is usually produced by the judgment that the individual has suffered an injustice, humiliation, or undeserved injury. It is a response to perceived harm. Anger escalates when the individuals feel their grievances being ignored, trivialized, or compounded. Humiliation is particularly problematic for patients for whom well-intentioned acts and comments aimed at giving help can be experienced as demeaning because they emphasize their own dependent and powerless position. Anger is most likely to explode into violence when it is confronted by a response involving an actual or implied threat. Anger demands acknowledgment, apology, and restitution. Restitution, particularly in response to grievances based in false beliefs, is rarely practical, but what can often be provided are acknowledgment and a response which is accommodating rather than confrontational. De-escalation does not always work. The penultimate response is to confront the patient with sufficient staff to make clear to them, if that is possible, that they would be wiser to withdrawal. Restraint is the ultimate response and though sometimes necessary is always a failure of management. These issues are addressed in more detail in chapter 8.

Anger often merges gradually. Anger will generate threats before attack in many cases. This is why threats must always be taken seriously. If someone takes the trouble to threaten you, then you should, even as a matter of good manners, acknowledge the threat and that it frightened you (even if it didn't). Not to offer a response or to make a threat in return (e.g., "you will end up in seclusion") is to challenge the patient to make good on their threat. Acknowledging the threat, and that it had the desired effect of frightening is the first stage in exploring the reasons for the anger which produced the threat. Not all threats reflect anger but it is usually clear which is anger based.

Managing violence in the inpatient context is similar in principle to managing violence in patients with schizophrenia in the community. First try and minimize as many of the risk factors facilitate violence. Second, continue to assess the current probability of violence to allow intervention aimed at the risk factors thought to be currently driving an increase in the violent potential. Finally respond to the immediate threat of violence. In the inpatient setting the emphasis is on detecting the signs of escalating fear and anger and managing them before they explode into violence.

It is not possible to prevent all violence in those with schizophrenia. The objective is to reduce its occurrence and mitigate its impact on the patient and others.

Conclusions

The violent behavior associated with the schizophrenic syndrome makes a socially significant contribution to violence in our communities but also lays waste to the lives of those individuals. A 10% or so of those with a schizophrenic

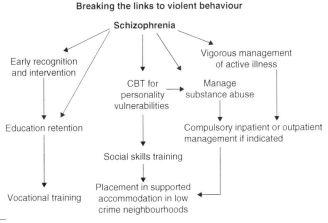

Figure 9.3   *Illustrates some of the interventions which could reduce the strength of the association between having schizophrenia and behaving violently. All interventions depend on accepting that it is the services duty to manage the violence which can emerge from schizophrenia as well as those with schizophrenia who are also substance abusing, delinquent, and objecting.*

syndrome from which the perpetrators of most of the serious violence will emerge are essentially identifiable in advance. A structured program to manage the criminogenic personality and behavioral factors, substance abuse, social dislocation, together with active symptoms could prevent the progress to violence (Fig. 9.3). Such systems of care have the potential to significantly reduce serious criminal violence, including homicide, reduce the number of prisoners with schizophrenia, stop the ever-escalating demand for forensic psychiatric beds, and, most important of all, improve the lives of many of the most disturbed and disadvantaged of those with schizophrenia.

References

1. Hodgins S. Mental disorder, intellectual deficiency, and crime – evidence from a birth cohort. Arch Gen Psychiatry 1992; 49: 476–83.
2. Hodgins S, Mednick S, Brennan PA, et al. Mental disorder and crime: evidence from a Danish birth cohort. Arch Gen Psychiatry 1996; 53: 489–96.
3. Wallace C, Mullen PE, Burgess P, et al. Serious criminal offending and mental disorder. Br J Psychiatry 1998; 172: 477–84.
4. Angermeyer MC. Schizophrenia and violence. Acta Psychiatr Scand Suppl 2000; 102: 63–7.
5. Arseneault L, Moffitt T, Caspi A, Taylor P, Silva P. Mental disorders and violence in a total birth cohort: results from the Dunedin Study. Arch Gen Psychiatry 2000; 57: 979–86.
6. Walsh E, Buchanan A, Fahy T. Violence and schizophrenia: examining the evidence. Br J Psychiatry 2001; 180: 490–5.
7. Wallace C, Mullen PE, Burgess P. Criminal offending in schizophrenia over a 25 year period marked by deinstitutionalization and increasing prevalence of comorbid substance use disorders. Am J Psychiatry 2004; 161: 716–27.
8. Soyka M, Morhart-Klute V, Schoech H. Delinquency and criminal offences in former schizophrenic inpatients 7–12 years following discharge. Eur Arch Psychiatry Clin Neurosci 2004; 254: 289–94.
9. Vevera J, Hubbard A, Vesely A, Papezova H. Violent behaviour in schizophrenia – Retrospective study of four independent samples from Prague, 1949 to 2000. Br J Psychiatry 2005; 187: 426–30.
10. Fazel S, Buxrud P, Ruchkin V, Grann M. Homicide in discharged patients with schizophrenia and other psychoses. Schizophr Res 2010; 123: 263–9.
11. Fazel S, Danesh J. Serious mental disorder in 23,000 prisoners: a systematic review of 62 surveys. Lancet 2002; 359: 545–50.
12. Swanson JW, Swartz MS, Elbogen EB. Effectiveness of atypical antipsychotic medications in reducing violent behaviour among persons with schizophrenia in community based treatment. Schizophr Bull 2004; 30: 3–20.
13. Steadman HJ, Mulvey EP, Monahan J, et al. Violence by people discharged from acute psychiatric inpatient facilities and by others in the same neighbourhoods. Arch Gen Psychiatry 1998; 55: 393–401.
14. Soyka M. Substance misuse, psychiatric disorder and violent and disturbed behaviour. Br J Psychiatry 2000; 176: 345–50.
15. Steele J, Darjee R, Thomson LDG. Substance dependence and schizophrenia in patients with violent and criminal propensities. J Forensic Psychiatry Psychol 2003; 14: 569–84.

16. Mullen PE. Schizophrenia and violence: from correlations to preventative strategies. Adv Psychiatr Treat 2006; 12: 239–48.
17. Hafner H, Boker W. Crimes of Violence by Mentally Abnormal Offenders. (trans. H. Marshall) Cambridge: Cambridge University Press, 1982.
18. Taylor PJ. Motives for offending among violent and psychotic men. Br J Psychiatry 1985; 147: 491–8.
19. Appelbaum PS, Robbins PC, Monahan J. Violence and delusions: data from the MacArthur Violence Risk Assessment Study. Am J Psychiatry 2000; 157: 566–72.
20. Mullen PE. Jealousy and the emergence of violent and intimidating behaviours. Crim Behav Ment Health 1996; 6: 199–205.
21. Foley SR, Kelly BD, Clarke M, et al. Incidence and clinical correlates of aggression and violence at presentation in patients with first episode psychosis. Schizophr Res 2005; 72: 161–8.
22. Steinert T, Voellner A, Faust V. Violence and schizophrenia: two types of criminal offenders. Eur J Psychiatry 1998; 12: 153–65.
23. Ge X, Donnellan MB, Wenk E. Differences in personality and patterns of recidivism between early starters and other serious male offenders. J Am Acad Psychiatry Law 2003; 31: 68–77.
24. Moffitt TE, Caspi A. Childhood predictors differentiate life-course persistent and adolescence-limited antisocial pathways among males and females. Dev Psychopathol 2001; 13: 355–75.
25. Schanda H, Foldes P, Topitz A, et al. Premorbid adjustment of schizophrenic criminal offenders. Acta Psychiatr Scand 1992; 86: 121–6.
26. Fresan A, Apiquian R, De la Fuente-Sandoval C, et al. Premorbid adjustment and violent behaviour in schizophrenic patients. Schizophr Res 2004; 69: 143–8.
27. Gosden NP, Kramp P, Gabrielsen G, et al. Violence in young criminals predicts schizophrenia: a 9 year register based follow-up of 15 to 19 year old criminals. Schizophr Bull 2005; 31: 759–68.
28. Perkins R, Rinaldi M. Unemployment rates among patients with long-term mental health problems: a decade of rising unemployment. Psychiatr Bull 2002; 26: 295–8.
29. Logdberg B, Nilsson L-L, Levander MT, Levander S. Schizophrenia, neighbourhood, and crime. Acta Psychiatr Scand 2004; 110: 92–7.
30. Silver E. Extending social disorganisation theory: a multilevel approach to the study of violence among persons with mental illness. Criminology 2000; 38: 1043–74.
31. Tengström A, Hodgins S, Kullgren G. Men with schizophrenia who behave violently: the usefulness of an early- versus late-start offender typology. Schizophr Bull 2001; 27: 205–18.
32. Nolan KA, Volavka J, Mohr P, Czobor P. Psychopathy and violent behaviour among patients with schizophrenia or schizoaffective disorder. Psychiatr Serv 1999; 50: 787–92.
33. Moran P, Walsh E, Tyrer P, et al. Impact of comorbid personality disorder on violence in psychosis. Br J Psychiatry 2003; 183: 182–34.
34. Moran P, Hodgins S. The correlates of comorbid antisocial personality disorder in schizophrenia. Schizophr Bull 2004; 30: 791–802.
35. McGregor K, Castle D, Dolan M. Schizophrenia spectrum disorders, substance misuse, and the four-facet model of psychopathy: the relationship to violence. Schizophr Res 10.1016/j.schres.2011.09.010.
36. Fullam RS, Dolan M. The criminal and personality profiles of patients with schizophrenia and psychopathic traits. Pers Individ Dif 2006; 40: 1591–602.
37. Andrews DA, Bonta J. The Psychology of Criminal Conduct. Cincinnati: Anderson, 1998.
38. Webster CD, Douglas KS, Eaves D, Hart SD. HCR -20 Assessing Risk for Violence [Version 2]. British Columbia: Simon Fraser University, 1997.

39. Novaco RW. Remediating anger and aggression with violent offenders. Leg Criminol Psychol 1997; 2: 77–88.
40. Renwick SJ, Black L, Ramm M. Anger treatment with forensic hospital patients. Leg Criminol Psychol 1997; 2: 103–16.
41. McGuire J. Offender Rehabilitation and Treatment: Effective Programs and Policies to Reduce Re-offending. Chichester: John Wiley, 2003.
42. Hollin CR. Handbook of Offender Assessment and Treatment. Chichester: John Wiley, 2003.
43. Citrome L, Volavka J, Czobor P, et al. Effects of clozapine, olanzapine, risperidone, and haloperidol on hostility among patients with schizophrenia. Psychiatr Serv 2001; 52: 1510–14.
44. Lubman DI, King JA, Castle DJ. Treating comorbid substance abuse in schizophrenia. Int Rev Psychiatry 2010; 22: 191–201.
45. Eronen M, Tiihonen J, Hakola P. Schizophrenia and homicidal bevavior. Schizophr Bull 1996; 22: 83–9.
46. Erb M, Hodgins S, Freese R, et al. Homicide and schizophrenia: maybe treatment does have a preventive effect. Crim Behav Ment Health 2001; 11: 6–26.
47. Schanda H, Knecht G, Schreinzer D, et al. Homicide and major mental disorders: a 25 year study. Acta Psych Scand 2004; 110: 98–107.

chapter 10

Understanding and enhancing adherence to treatment in people with schizophrenia

Peter Hayward, Diane Agoro, Sarah Swan, and Til Wykes

Medication is clearly a critical part of the treatment of people with schizophrenia. Regrettably, as in many other conditions, patients do not always take their medication in the doses and regimens prescribed, and this can have adverse consequences, including psychotic relapse. This chapter outlines the extent of this problem and suggests ways to understand and manage it. We do not here specifically address the role of long-acting injectable antipsychotics in ensuring people receive their medication: this is addressed in chapter 1. Suffice to say here that even such strategies should be used in as collaborative and noncoercive manner as possible.

Definitions

Traditionally, the term "compliance" has been used to refer to the degree to which a patient follows medical advice and complies with treatment recommendations. A patient who takes his medication is said to be "compliant," while one who refuses or forgets is called "noncompliant," or described as showing "poor compliance." It has been suggested that these labels promote a one-sided view of the consultation process: the doctor offers wise and correct advice and the sensible patient obeys without question. The term "adherence" has been advocated recently as suggesting a more active role for the patient, while the Royal Pharmaceutical Society of Great Britain (1) advocates the term "concordance" as promoting the idea of collaboration between the patient and the prescriber. Ideally, the consultation process and the devising of treatment recommendations, whether they involve pharmacological, psychosocial, or other types of treatment, should be a process of collaborative empiricism where the patient is treated as an equal partner. There is some empirical evidence that this approach leads to superior treatment outcome and a greater patient satisfaction; more importantly, this approach respects the autonomy of the patient. How to ensure adherence in practice is what we will expand on throughout this chapter.

Factors affecting adherence

A variety of factors can either promote or undermine treatment adherence (Box 10.1). As a rule, adherence to treatment regimens is far lower for most medical conditions, than professionals might wish. It has been suggested that only around half of patients adhere to a variety of long-term treatment regimens, for illnesses including heart disease, asthma, and AIDS. Consider for a moment the well-established rules of a healthy lifestyle: avoidance of alcohol, tobacco, and fattening foods; regular exercise; low levels of stress; daily flossing of the teeth; etc.: do you always adhere to all these practices?

People in general tend to take treatment when they are in distress, while preventive interventions are often forgotten. This is, of course, especially true of patients who do not believe that they are ill, but have other explanations for their problems, such as paranoid or grandiose delusional beliefs. Low IQ and disorganized thinking may interfere with adherence, especially if medication regimens are complicated. Side effects may also be a problem, although a patient may find one particular side effect intolerable and another much less problematic. One patient might find a certain symptom intolerable and another one mildly annoying, while a second patient reacts in exactly the opposite way. Patients with psychiatric conditions are more likely to adhere to long-term treatments if they see benefit in them, if the treatments are easily available and uncomplicated, and if they are offered in a pleasant and convenient setting by professionals who they like and who show them respect and offer them other kinds of practical help. Most importantly, the treatments should be effective and provide benefits that outweigh their side effects.

Besides the factors that are outlined in Box 10.1, there are others that affect adherence. These include insight, reactance, and stigma, which are described in detail.

Insight

Traditionally, the term "insight" is used to mean the correct understanding, by the patient, of his illness. This terminology has been criticized as meaning, in practice, that insight consists of agreeing with the doctor. For many of those with long-term mental illness, their beliefs and experiences seem

Box 10.1   Factors affecting adherence.

The Person
Cultural and family values
Experiences of illness and treatment
Support network and milieu
Personality
Psychological reactance
Intelligence
Views of illness

The Treatment
Therapeutic alliance
Treatment setting
Effectiveness
Complexity
Side effects
Stigma

The Illness
Delusional beliefs
Positive aspects of illness experience
Depression/anxiety
Cognitive impairment
Lack of motivation

obviously true, significant, and even in some cases life-enhancing. To perceive oneself as extraordinarily important or in intimate contact with a famous or attractive person might be seen as very desirable and even to be persecuted by enemies with strange powers might be seen as better than being completely ignored by everyone. While some sufferers may well find the belief that their experiences are "just an illness" as comforting, others may see it as demeaning, or may well prefer other types of explanations. Some measures of insight actually use treatment adherence as one part of the construct (2), but it is important to note that having "good insight" does not necessarily mean that one will adhere to treatment. The opposite can also be true—patients may adhere to a treatment regimen while denying the illness for which it was prescribed (3).

Reactance

The concept of reactance, which has strong theoretical links with that of nonadherence, has been used to describe the tendency for people to react negatively to pressure and coercion. Some people, when told forcibly that they must do something, go along, while others will react in exactly the opposite way; the latter are said to be high in reactance (4). Moore et al. (5) found that a scale measuring psychological reactance was a good predictor of treatment adherence. This would suggest that, for those high in reactance, adherence to treatment could best be achieved by a nonconfrontational approach, by convincing the patient to choose freely to receive treatment. Unfortunately, many patients undergo their first experience of psychiatric treatment involuntarily, by being detained in hospital. This will often be a highly distressing experience that, whether or not such hospitalization was objectively necessary, will create a legacy of antagonism and resentment in the person detained.

Stigma

There is strong research evidence that lay people hold stigmatizing, prejudiced views about the mentally ill, and that these views discourage sufferers from seeking treatment (6). The lay public seems to know relatively little about those with serious mental illness, but to see such people as bizarre, difficult, unhygienic, and dangerous. Further, lay people often define mental illness in terms of treatment received rather than symptoms exhibited. Thus, most people will be slow to accept that they have a stigmatized condition. Labeling in this context becomes very important; we do not have to insist that a person accepts our diagnostic label, or even our label of "illness," in order for them to benefit from treatment. To say that a treatment "relieves stress" or "might help you to cope better" might well be more acceptable to many people, and these statements are also true. If a patient and a professional agree on a treatment approach, does it really matter if they disagree on a diagnostic label?

Promoting adherence

Failure to adhere to prescribed medication is often said to be one of the major causes of relapse among sufferers from severe mental illness. At the same time, a growing body of research is demonstrating that the principles of cognitive–behavioral therapy (CBT) can be used successfully to promote adaptive functioning in a variety of psychiatric conditions including schizophrenia, paranoid psychosis, and other forms of serious mental illness (chap. 2). In spite of this, relatively little effort has been made to use CBT techniques to enhance adherence to treatment regimens. Some of the pioneers in the field of CBT for psychosis have suggested the application of such techniques in this area (7–9), and a few empirical trials suggest that such approaches can improve adherence and decrease relapse rates (10–14). However, negative results have also been reported (15). In spite of this, we believe that the CBT approach points the best way to better understanding and concordance between patient and health professional. This is because CBT is, by its very nature, a collaborative enterprise, seeking an agreed model of the difficulties to be addressed and the ways of alleviating those difficulties. In applying such an approach to patients with major mental illness, or, for that matter, any condition requiring medical treatment, the goal should not be to "get them to take their tablets" but first to create a good treatment alliance, and then to persuade patients to consider various treatment options (16). Based on these ideas, our own trials of the so-called "Compliance Therapy" (10,11) produced some promising results, but further research has not borne out its effectiveness, at least as a short-term "stand alone" therapy (17). In spite of this, we believe that the guiding principles of such a therapy can produce beneficial results if incorporated in standard forms of pharmacotherapy.

As explained in Kemp et al. (10), we conceptualized the process of building adherence in three stages. The first is to elicit the patient's concerns and problems, and to try to understand his or her model of the root of these difficulties. Initially a review of illness history may be useful; although, it goes without saying that it is not helpful to insist that the patient has an illness. Many patients see their problems as external or due to "stress" or "pressures of circumstance" rather than as mental illness. Kingdon and Turkington (7) with their idea of the "normalizing rationale" are very helpful in this situation: they tell patients that their symptoms are very common, and can be seen in many people under conditions of excessive stress, thus avoiding the stigma that a label of major mental illness carries. The first goal is thus to find a rationale that is acceptable to the patient, so that the idea of medication can be introduced as a possible coping strategy to deal with ongoing problems (18).

The second key step with any patient is to ask him/her to consider the advantages and disadvantages of taking medication. Most psychotropic medications have a wide variety of disagreeable side effects, and other issues, such as diagnosis and stigma, may be very important for particular individuals. However, most patients will also be able to pick out advantages in particular medications, ranging from improved sleep to better relationships with loved ones. To avoid reactance, as noted above, the patients must always feel that the final choice is theirs. If a patient chooses not to take medication, it is important to maintain a good therapeutic relationship, so that if he/she encounters future difficulties, he/she may be open to reconsidering this decision. The advantage of this approach is that it enhances the therapeutic alliance, which has been shown to be an important predictor of adherence (19).

A useful tool at this point can be some form of self-monitoring (20). A simple form can be developed between the patient and professional, allowing the patient to monitor the patient's mental state and side effects. A trial period can be suggested, and when it is over, both the patient and the clinician will have clear evidence as to the effectiveness or otherwise of the particular medication. Formally devised instruments may be less helpful than a simple form that focuses on the patient's own self-chosen problems (Fig. 10.1).

If medication proves effective, and the patient is well, a new problem arises: as noted above, many people find it hard to adhere to regimens of preventative medication, because people are not motivated to take medication when they feel well. This is the third stage of building adherence. The professional should offer advice on this point and encourage the use of long-term prophylactic treatment, pointing out both the arguments in favor and the problems many people encounter. Some evidence suggests that longer-term interventions focused on

Feeling anxious and threatened

| Much better | A bit better | Same | A bit worse | Much worse |

Poor Sleep

| Much better | A bit better | Same | A bit worse | Much worse |

Restlessness

| Much better | A bit better | Same | A bit worse | Much worse |

Ability to Concentrate

| Much better | A bit better | Same | A bit worse | Much worse |

Feeling that the 'world depends on me'

| Much better | A bit better | Same | A bit worse | Much worse |

Dry mouth

| Much better | A bit better | Same | A bit worse | Much worse |

Feeling that 'The television is talking to me'

| Much better | A bit better | Same | A bit worse | Much worse |

Tired/no energy

| Much better | A bit better | Same | A bit worse | Much worse |

Figure 10.1   *Bill's personal checklist.*

Box 10.2   Enhancing adherence.

Key principles
Emphasize personal choice and responsibility
Focus on patient's key concerns, personal goals, fears, and worries
Express empathy for patient's problems and dilemmas
Support self-efficacy
Key techniques
Regular summarizing
Inductive questioning to elicit patient's own concerns
Explore pros and cons of treatment options
Use normalizing rationale to combat stigma
Focus on patient's own long-term goals
Approaches to avoid
Lecturing/preaching
Insisting on particular diagnostic labels
Debating with the patient
Laying down the law

the barriers to long-term adherence can be of benefit in many cases (17). However, many patients will probably stop their medication at some point and fall ill again. Such an outcome does not mean that we have failed. The establishment of a good, collaborative relationship should improve long-term engagement with services for most patients. Some patients may not be able to take prophylactic medication at all; for them, short-term medication during acute episodes may be the best option.

We offer a brief summary of some of the key elements in a collaborative approach outlined in Box 10.2. We hope that evidence as to the benefits of this approach will continue to accumulate. In any case, many sufferers, and many professionals, find it to be both helpful and congenial. More research in this neglected field could help to find new ways to foster collaboration between patient and prescriber.

References

1. Royal Pharmaceutical Society of Great Britain. From Compliance to Concordance: Achieving Shared Goals in Medicine Taking. London: RPSGB, 1997.
2. David AS. Insight and psychosis. Br J Psychiatry 1990; 156: 798–808.
3. Staring AB, Van der Gaag M, Duivenvoorden HJ, et al. Why do patients with schizophrenia who have poor insight still take antipsychotics? Memory deficits as moderators between adherence belief and behaviour. J Psychiatr Pract 2011; 17: 320–9.
4. Fogarty JS. Reactance theory and patient noncompliance. Soc Sci Med 1997; 45: 1277–88.
5. Moore A, Sellwood W, Stirling J. Compliance and psychological reactance in schizophrenia. Br J Clin Psychol 2000; 39: 287–95.
6. Hayward P, Bright JA. Stigma and mental illness: a review and critique. J Ment Health 1997; 6: 345–54.
7. Kingdon DG, Turkington D. Cognitive Behavioural Therapy of Schizophrenia. New York: Guilford, 1994.
8. Nelson H. Cognitive Behavioural Therapy with Schizophrenia. Cheltenham: Stanley Thornes, 1997.
9. Beck JS. A cognitive therapy approach to medication compliance. In: Kay J. ed Integrated Treatment of Psychiatric Disorders. Review of Psychiatry. Vol. 20 Washington, D.C: American Psychiatric Association, 2001: 113–41.
10. Kemp R, David A, Hayward P. Compliance therapy: an intervention targeting insight and treatment adherence in psychotic patients. Behav Cogn Psychother 1996; 24: 331–50.
11. Kemp R, Kirov G, Everitt B, et al. Randomised controlled trial of compliance therapy: 18-month follow-up. Br J Psychiatry 1998; 172: 413–19.
12. Swanson A, Pantalon MV, Cohen KR. Motivational interviewing and treatment adherence among psychiatric and dually diagnosed patients. J Nerv Ment Dis 1999; 187: 630–5.
13. Hayashi N, Yamashina M, Igarashi Y, et al. Improvement of patient attitude toward treatment among inpatients with schizophrenia and its related factors: Controlled study of a psychological approach. Compr Psychiatry 2001; 42: 240–6.
14. Dolder CR, Lacro JP, Leckband S, Jeste DP. Interventions to improve antipsychotic medication adherence: review of recent literature. J Clin Pharmacol 2003; 23: 389–99.

15. O'Donnell C, Donohoe G, Sharkey L, et al. Compliance therapy: a randomised controlled trial in schizophrenia. BMJ 2003; 327: 1–4.
16. Perkins RE, Repper JM. Compliance or informed choice. J Ment Health 1999; 8: 117–29.
17. Barkhof E, Meijer CJ, de Sonneville LMJ, et al. Interventions to improve adherence to antipsychotic medication in patients with schizophrenia- A review of the past decade. Eur Psychiatry 2011; 27: 9–18.
18. Beck EM, Cavelti M, Wirtz M, et al. How do socio-demographic and clinical factors interact with adherence attitude profiles in schizophrenia? A cluster-analytical approach. Psychiatry Res 2011; 187: 55–61.
19. Day JC, Bentall RP, Roberts C, et al. Attitudes towards antipsychotic medication: the impact of clinical variables and relationship with health professionals. Arch Gen Psychiatry 1990; 62: 717–24.
20. Randall F, Wood P, Day J, et al. Enhancing appropriate adherence with neuroleptic medication: two contrasting approaches. In: Morrison AP. ed. A Casebook of Cognitive Therapy for Psychosis. Hove, UK: Brunner-Routledge, 2002.

chapter 11

Psychological interventions to help people with psychiatric disabilities succeed at work

Morris D. Bell and Jimmy Choi

Inactivity and loss of productive function generally accompany severe psychiatric disorders (e.g., schizophrenia, other psychotic disorders, mood disorders, and post-traumatic stress disorder). Yet, surveys (1) indicate that more than 75% of people with these disorders wish to return to productive activity of some kind. Vocational services such as supported employment (SE) have helped people with severe and persistent mental illness to obtain community-based competitive jobs by finding appropriate opportunities, often with accommodation and supportive services. SE is now regarded as an evidence-based practice (2). A manualized version of SE for severe mental illness (SMI) populations called Individual Placement and Support (IPS) has advanced the implementation of SE. A toolkit is available to assist in implementation (1).

While SE appears superior to other types of vocational services for SMI, employment outcomes remain modest (3). Moreover, rates of employment are significantly worse for those with schizophrenia diagnosis (4) which suggests that this large subsample of people with SMI may need interventions that target illness-specific features related to their work impairments.

Therefore, SE only partially addresses the problem. It may provide appropriate supports and work opportunity, but patients' work disability remains apparent. People with SMI in SE continue to have difficulty performing their job tasks and often their interpersonal problems disrupt their work. In this chapter, we review psychological interventions to enhance work services, each of which addresses illness-related deficits that may not be sufficiently overcome through on-the-job supports.

Work behavior feedback groups with goal setting

Participants receiving work services meet in a weekly group (usually 4–8 workers with a facilitator) for approximately 1 hour to review on-site evaluations of members' work performance and to problem solve and set performance goals for the following week. We (M. Bell, G. Bryson, P. Lysaker, W. Zito, T. Greig, J. Fiszdon, and J. Choi) have developed these groups in a number of different settings that include transitional and SE programs.

To provide systematic feedback, we created the Work Behavior Inventory (WBI) as a standardized work performance assessment instrument (5). The WBI is rated by a trained vocational counselor who observes workers on the job and interviews their supervisors. The WBI scales include Work Habits, Work Quality, Social Skills, Cooperativeness, and Personal Presentation. Research findings indicate that work performance measured by the WBI has a significant relationship to subsequent work outcomes.

In the workers' meetings, half the members receive feedback each week, but all participate in problem solving and goal setting. The facilitator encourages a process of accurate empathy in which true achievement is acknowledged and praised and problems are realistically confronted. A good deal of social learning occurs as members help each other and learn from each other's experiences. Each week, members report on their progress toward their individual goals and set new goals, often based on the WBI feedback they have received. Goals might include on-the-job behaviors such as increasing hours of work, being more punctual, being tidier in appearance, taking fewer breaks, or approaching a co-worker about having lunch together. In programs that begin with transitional employment with an expectation of moving on to competitive employment, goals might also include preparing a resume, networking for another job, or going to a job interview.

There are several important reasons for believing that regular work performance feedback and goal setting are especially important for psychiatrically impaired veterans. First, severe psychiatric disorders often impair people's ability to perceive themselves and others accurately. Feedback provides information to workers about their work habits and work quality; and importantly, it evaluates their social skills, personal presentation, and cooperativeness on the job. These interpersonal behaviors are crucial for vocational success, yet they are not usually addressed directly by supervisors or co-workers in helpful ways. Left alone, these problems can build up until there is a critical incident leading to job loss. Regular and systematic feedback can provide many people with psychiatric disorders a social prosthesis for their impairments in reading cues from their social environment about their interpersonal behaviors, while goal setting and problem solving can often successfully address these issues.

Second, motivation, sense of purpose, and self-confidence can be profoundly affected by psychiatric disorders. Regular feedback provides workers with a psychiatric disorder continual reassurance about what they are doing, whether it is right, as well as what they need to improve on. Since feelings of worthlessness often lead these workers to believe that others are seeing them as inadequate, getting accurate feedback about how they are viewed by their supervisors can reduce mistrust and provide greater confidence in dealing with people at work. As goals are set and attained, workers develop greater feelings of self-efficacy and become more willing to attempt new challenges.

Finally, research literature from industrial and organizational psychology strongly supports the effectiveness of work feedback and goal setting for improving individual and organizational productivity. A review of the literature (6) on motivation and experiments in work feedback and goal setting concluded that "goal-setting theory is among the most valid and practical theories of employee motivation in organizational psychology."

We studied this intervention with 74 patients with schizophrenia in a transitional work program, who were randomized to receive work performance feedback and goal-setting or usual services. Those receiving feedback showed greater overall improvement in work performance, and particularly on WBI Social Skills, Cooperativeness, and Personal Presentation. They also worked significantly more hours and weeks during the 6-month transitional work period. Additionally, they showed greater improvements on the intrapsychic dimension of the Quality of Life scale (QLS) (7) that reflects increased motivation, a sense of purpose, and enjoyment of life. In subsequent studies that employ cognitive–behavioral therapy or cognitive remediation (to be described later), we have included the work feedback and goal-setting groups as part of the rehabilitation services. We did so because we feel that other psychological interventions combine easily with these groups and that these feedback and goal-setting groups may be necessary to generalize the effects of these other interventions.

The indianapolis vocational intervention program: A cognitive–behavioral approach

The Indianapolis Vocational Intervention Program (IVIP) offers participants engaged in work activity a weekly group and individual intervention that target beliefs and behaviors which might interfere with their abilities to sustain work. In the IVIP model, groups are generally used to teach participants didactic material. Individual sessions are used to apply what they learned to weekly work experience.

Overall, both group and individual sessions of the IVIP are based on the principles of cognitive–behavioral therapy. The group lasts generally 30–40 minutes and involves three activities: (*i*) teaching the week's didactic material; (*ii*) assisting participants to put the didactic material into practice with some type of application exercise; and (*iii*) giving work feedback to participants. The IVIP didactic curriculum is organized into four 2-week modules (total of eight sessions). These are presented in order and repeated at least three times during participants' 6-month program. The content of each of these modules is summarized in Table 11.1. During the didactic presentation, the scheduled material is presented both abstractly and applied to participant's actual work experiences using a wide variety of exercises. These include scripted, videotaped, and spontaneous role-play, practicing progressive muscle relaxation, and generating in-session thought records.

Work feedback, the last aspect of the intervention section, is derived from the WBI. WBI feedback is given to participants every other week for the first 8 weeks and then monthly. The final section of the group session is the 10 to 15-minute wrap-up during which the group leader asks participants to summarize what they have learned and/or to identify what made the most impact on them.

The individual counseling component of the IVIP is an opportunity for participants to review and apply didactic materials from groups and to learn to identify and conceptualize concerns using the cognitive behavioral model. Before the therapy session begins, participants rate the strength of their conviction and extent of impact for up to four beliefs that participants and therapists have collaboratively identified. Next, participants report the extent to which they worked on and accomplished a mutually agreed upon between-session assignment and give a brief update of the previous work week including any mental health concerns. The therapist also reviews the written practice assignment from the preceding group session.

The IVIP was created to help persons with schizophrenia spectrum disorders learn to identify and monitor their own thoughts and behaviors regarding work and to give them an optimal chance for success. It was developed in response to the observation that due to several factors associated with mental illness, including stigma, many people with schizophrenia view themselves as having limited competence, relatively low value in the eyes of others in their community and little chance of success at work, even with assistance. They may believe they have little ability to influence their lives and a personal narrative in which failure in social and vocational contexts is expected (8).

To date one randomized controlled study has examined the impact of the IVIP on work outcomes (9,10). In this study, 100 participants with schizophrenia or schizoaffective disorder were offered a 6-month job placement and were randomized to receive IVIP (n = 50) or support services matched for treatment intensity (n = 50). Participants in the IVIP group worked significantly more hours and weeks than those in the support group and had better average work performance on the WBI. Baseline and follow-up scores indicated the IVIP group sustained initial levels of hope and self-esteem through follow-up while the support group experienced declines. This study thus provides initial evidence that the IVIP can assist persons to persist at work and to sustain their hope and enthusiasm over time. This has also been illustrated by one case report to date (11).

Table 11.1   Description of indianapolis vocational intervention program group didactic modules

Module title	Session number and title	Session objectives (Examples of concepts and skills to be addressed)
Thinking and Work	1. Thinking Errors and Work	Recognize impact of negative thinking
		Identify automatic thoughts that impact work
	2. Modifying Self-Defeating Thinking	Modify dysfunctional cognitions using 4-A model[a]
		Apply 4-A model to participants' work experiences
Barriers to Work	3. Problem Solving Barriers to Work	Identify existing or potential barriers to work
		Employ steps of problem solving to work barriers
	4. Coping with Emotions	Define emotional states that threaten work
		Learn cognitive–behavioral therapy skills to manage difficult emotions
Workplace Relationships	5. Accepting and Learning from Feedback	Differentiate between constructive and destructive criticism
		Apply steps for responding to feedback at work
	6. Effective Self-Expression	Learn assertive communication principles
		Practice giving feedback in work settings effectively
Realistic Self-Appraisal	7. Thinking about Capabilities and Limitations	Identify thinking errors compromising self-appraisal
		Identify strengths, limitations, and necessary accommodations
	8. Managing Success	Define failure and success via the cognitive model
		Modify dysfunctional cognitions regarding work failures

[a]The 4-A model emphasizes the connections between being "aware," "answering," "acting," and "accepting."

Workplace fundamentals: A social skills approach

The UCLA Social and Independent Living Skills Program is a manualized social skills training intervention for persons with SMI. Similar to other modules in the package, Wallace and Tauber (12) developed the Workplace Fundamental Skills Module, which focuses on social skills in the workplace that may supplement SE. Instruction is provided utilizing the behavioral teaching techniques outlined in Table 11.2. Skills are generally taught in weekly group sessions lasting about 90 minutes with participants finishing the module in 12–24 sessions.

The overall goal of the module is to teach nine specific skills grouped into three skill sets on how to sustain employment. Skill Set One identifies key procedures in the workplace (e.g., break times and paydays). This skill set teaches how to identify and obtain information about investments made by the participant at work, called "Gives" (time, tools, relationships, etc.), and rewards they receive when they work, called "Gets" (pay, satisfaction, etc.). In Skill Set Two the participants are taught to "be on the alert for problems" so they can examine their work environment and develop a profile of potential problem areas, called "Sweats" (getting along with co-workers, difficult job task, etc.). Skill Set Three is about preventing and solving problems identified in the previous set. Participants are taught how to use a general problem-solving method to prevent and solve work-related problems in areas of mental and physical health, substance abuse, interactions with supervisors and co-workers, work performance, and motivation.

The empirical literature behind the UCLA Social and Independent Living Skills Program is substantial, with the programs translated into over 15 languages by independent investigators, adapted to numerous ethnic cultures on every continent, and disseminated all over the world to hospitals, in- and outpatient programs, community centers, and day treatment programs. The Workplace

Table 11.2 Behavioral teaching techniques in the UCLA social and independent living skills program

- Introduction to skill sets
- Videotape demonstration
- Role-playing with clinician and peers
- Step-by-step problem solving to resolve lack of resources to implement skills (e.g., money, time etc.)
- Problem solving to resolve disparity between learned skills and unexpected outcomes
- In-vivo assignments to practice skills outside the group under the trainer's supervision
- Homework assignments designed to generalize skills to the workplace

Fundamentals Module (WFM) is, however, relatively new and investigations are only currently emerging regarding its validation and efficacy. Only two published empirical studies (12,13) have reported findings on the module in relation to SE and provide tentative support of its efficacy. In a yet to be published study by Tauber and Wallace (in preparation), 42 employed participants were randomly assigned to WFM + IPS or IPS only. Over the course of 18 months, participants who received WFM along with IPS had fewer job turnovers (p < 0.013) and were significantly more satisfied with their jobs (p < 0.009). The initial literature on the WFM and the soundness of its basic principles suggest that targeting social skill problems while on the job may have a place in augmenting SE.

Neurocognitive enhancement therapy: A cognitive remediation approach

Neurocognitive Enhancement Therapy (NET) was developed by our group (Bell and Wexler) to address directly impairments in elemental cognitive processes that may interfere with new learning, such as that occurs in vocational rehabilitation. NET is primarily comprised of computer-based training tasks with graduated levels of difficulty that challenge cognitive abilities often compromised in mental illness (e.g., attention, memory, and executive function). We have used several sources for the cognitive training exercises, and several other software packages are either available or in development. Our first studies primarily used the Psychological Software Services CogReHab software that was originally developed for people with compromised brain function and modified by us for use in people with schizophrenia. In more recent studies we have also used auditory and visual training software developed by Posit Science (www.positscience.com). Cognitive training tasks include those targeting simple attention, complex attention and response inhibition, verbal and visual memory, language-mediated cognition, category formation, planning, and strategy.

The approach is to have some exercises that narrowly target specific cognitive processes (e.g., visual reaction time), which may have associations to specific brain areas, and to have other types of exercises that use many integrated brain processes. The curriculum of exercises begins with primary sensory processing and discrimination and builds to more complex tasks. Subjects graduate to a more difficult level when they achieve and sustain a prescribed level. Cognitive training occurs in the "Cog Lab," an attractive learning center with multiple computer work stations. Efforts are made to create an upbeat, reinforcing environment with postings of individual accomplishments and sometimes small prizes for achieving various levels of success. While little is known about how much training is needed, we encourage participants to practice these exercises every day for an hour and believe that at least 40 sessions is probably the minimum necessary to achieve clinical benefit, although it takes more than 100 hours to complete the entire curriculum of exercises.

We have incorporated these cognitive training sessions into a comprehensive rehabilitation program that includes the work performance feedback and goal setting group described earlier, with the addition of specific feedback about their cognitive functioning on the job. This feedback is based upon the Vocational Cognitive Rating Scale that is rated along with the WBI. Fuller descriptions of these interventions are available elsewhere (14,15).

This intervention was developed to address the common cognitive impairments in schizophrenia and other psychotic disorders, which have been identified as rate-limiting factors in social and occupational domains. Over the past few years, a number of studies have found that specific cognitive deficits predicted work performance and outcomes (16). Evidence of brain plasticity offers a scientific foundation for cognitive remediation. There are several examples of clinical applications of neuroplasticity outside of psychiatry. These include Constraint-Induced Movement Therapy (CIMT) (17) in post-stroke hemiparesis rehabilitation and auditory discrimination training for people receiving hearing aids (18) or who have central auditory processing disorder or dyslexia (19,20). In schizophrenia and other mental illnesses, the basic mechanisms of overcoming learned nonuse and facilitating use-dependent cortical reorganization may have application.

Several literature reviews of cognitive remediation have been published most recently (21), and most conclude that the literature favors clinical benefit of one type or another. We have conducted two randomized clinical trials that combine our NET training with work services. The first was performed at the VA Connecticut Healthcare System and involved 6 months of NET plus work therapy (WT) compared with WT alone (N = 145). The second was at the Connecticut Mental Health Center and involved a year of active intervention that included NET plus a hybrid vocational program of transitional and SE (NET + SE) compared with SE alone (N = 76). Participants in both studies were diagnosed with schizophrenia or schizoaffective disorder and were in outpatient treatment. Details of method are available elsewhere (15,22).

We found that participants receiving NET improved on training tasks and that almost half of those with significant clinical deficits on working memory tasks reached normal levels of performance by the conclusion of the training (23). We tested the generalization of the training to similar but untrained tasks on neuropsychological testing and found significantly greater improvement for those receiving NET at the conclusion of the training (22). These improvements endured for 6 months after the end of the active training (24). We also have unpublished evidence that those receiving NET showed greater improvement in work performance (WBI scores) and cognitive performance on the job (VCRS scores) during the active interventions. Most importantly, work outcomes were better for those receiving NET with their work services. In the VA study, those in NET + WT worked significantly more hours (p < 0.05) and earned more money during the 6 months following the intervention.

In the Connecticut Mental Health Center study, we found that NET + SE led to significantly more hours worked (p < 0.05) during the 12 months after the intervention (transitional and competitive employment combined hours) and significantly higher rates (p < 0.05) of competitive employment (15). In an extension of that study (N = 174), we found that cognitive training differentially benefited those with poor community function at baseline: they were more than twice as likely to obtain competitive employment over 2 years if they had NET + SE (50%) compared with those who only received SE (22.7%). For those with better community functioning at baseline, both groups had competitive employment rates of 55% (25).

Taken together, these findings suggest that cognitive training can have significant functional benefits when included in a comprehensive rehabilitation program that affords opportunity to acquire practical new learning. We believe that cognitive training improves cognitive processing and thereby makes it possible for participants to gain more from other forms of rehabilitation.

McGurk and colleagues (26) published the first small (N = 44) effectiveness study combining SE with cognitive training. They call their program "Thinking Skills for Work." Clients with SMI who had had a previous job failure were randomized to receive SE or SE augmented with their program. Results were remarkable. Those receiving the cognitive augmentation showed a significantly greater improvement on cognitive functioning and on depression and autistic preoccupation scores on the PANSS. They also worked more hours and earned higher wages. Most importantly, 69.6% achieved competitive employment as compared with only 4.8% of those receiving SE alone (p = 0.000).

Conclusions

Those looking for ways to improve the lives of people recovering from persistent and SMI may find excitement and hope in the programs that have been presented in this report. SE and other work services offer opportunities for community reintegration through the constructive social roles that working provides. For some, working may lead to reduced symptoms, greater self-esteem, and a higher quality of life.

The four interventions that we have described address overlapping but distinct areas of impairment that accompany mental illness and that may be barriers to achieving work success. Each of these approaches has a sound rationale and at least some evidence of efficacy. Most have a manual or a systematic description that makes it possible to replicate the methods in other settings.

There is every reason to believe that a comprehensive approach to vocational rehabilitation could combine these interventions to the benefit of the patient. We are not yet at the point where we can be prescriptive about exactly what methods to apply to which patients, and some of these interventions may be better suited to some settings than to others. Yet, there is sufficient evidence to warrant clinicians and vocational specialists using their own judgment to enhance their existing work services with these approaches. It is hoped that these interventions will allow people with mental illness to more speedily and effectively reintegrate into their community so that they may lead more satisfying lives.

References

1. Becker D. Supported Employment Toolkit. Lebanon, NH: Psychiatric Research Center, 2002.
2. Bond GR, Becker DR, Drake RE, et al. Implementing supported employment as an evidence-based practice. Psychiatr Serv 2002; 52: 313–22.
3. Cook JA, Leff HS, Blyler CR, et al. Results of a multisite randomized trial of supported employment interventions for individuals with severe mental illness. Arch Gen Psychiatry 2005; 62: 505–12.
4. Razzano LA, Cook JA, Burke-Miller JK, et al. Clinical factors associated with employment among people with severe mental illness: findings from the employment intervention demonstration program. J Nerv Ment Dis 2005; 193: 705–13.
5. Bryson GJ, Bell MD, Lysaker PH, Zito W. The Work Behavior Inventory: a scale for the assessment of work behavior for people with severe mental illness. Psychiatr Rehabil J 1997; 20: 47–55.
6. Locke EA, Latham GP. Building a practically useful theory of goal setting and task motivation. A 35-year odyssey. Am Psychol 2002; 57: 705–17.
7. Heinrichs DW, Hanlon TE, Carpenter WT Jr. The Quality of Life Scale: an instrument for rating the schizophrenic deficit syndrome. Schizophr Bull 1984; 10: 388–98.
8. Lysaker PH, Bond G, Davis LW, Bryson GJ, Bell MD. Enhanced Cognitive Behavioral Therapy for vocational rehabilitation in schizophrenia: Effects on hope and work. J Rehabil Res Dev 2005; 42: 673–82.
9. Lysaker PH, Davis LW, Bryson GJ, Bell MD. Effects of cognitive behavioral therapy on work outcomes in vocational rehabilitation for participants with schizophrenia spectrum disorders. Schizophr Res 2009; 107: 186–91.
10. Lysaker PH, Buck KD. Narrative enrichment in the psychotherapy for persons with schizophrenia: a single case study. Issues Ment Health Nurs 2006; 27: 233–47.
11. Davis LW, Lysaker PH, Lancaster RS, Bryson GJ, Bell MD. The Indianapolis Vocational Intervention Program: a cognitive behavioral approach to addressing rehabilitation issues in schizophrenia. J Rehabil Res Dev 2005; 42: 35–45.
12. Wallace CJ, Tauber R. Supplementing supported employment with workplace skills training. Psychiatr Serv 2004; 55: 513–15.
13. Mueser KT, Aalto S, Becker DR, et al. The effectiveness of skills training for improving outcomes in supported employment. Psychiatr Serv 2005; 56: 1254–60.
14. Bell MD, Bryson GJ, Greig TC, Fiszdon JM, Wexler BE. Neurocognitive enhancement therapy with work therapy: productivity outcomes at 6- and 12-month follow-ups. J Rehabil Res Dev 2005; 42: 829–38.
15. Wexler BE, Bell MD. Cognitive remediation and vocational rehabilitation for schizophrenia. Schizophr Bull 2005; 31: 931–41.
16. McGurk SR, Meltzer HY. The role of cognition in vocational functioning in schizophrenia. Schizophr Res 2000; 45: 175–84.
17. Taub E, Morris DM. Constraint-induced movement therapy to enhance recovery after stroke. Curr Atheroscler Rep 2001; 3: 279–86.

18. Stecker GC, Bowman GA, Yund EW, et al. Perceptual training improves syllable identification in new and experienced hearing aid users. J Rehabil Res Dev 2006; 43: 537–52.
19. Cohen W, Hodson A, O'Hare A, et al. Effects of computer-based intervention through acoustically modified speech (Fast ForWord) in severe mixed receptive-expressive language impairment: outcomes from a randomized controlled trial. J Speech Lang Hear Res 2005; 48: 715–29.
20. Merzenich MM, Jenkins WM, Johnston P, et al. Temporal processing deficits of language-learning impaired children ameliorated by training. Science 1996; 271: 77–81.
21. Wykes T, Huddy V, Cellard C, McGurk SR, Czobor P. A meta-analysis of cognitive remediation for schizophrenia: methodology and effect sizes. Am J Psychiatry 2011; 168: 472–85.
22. Bell MD, Bryson GJ, Greig TC, Corcoran C, Wexler BE. Neurocognitive enhancement therapy with work therapy: effects on neuropsychological test performance. Arch Gen Psychiatry 2001; 58: 763–8.
23. Bell MD, Bryson GJ, Wexler BE. Cognitive remediation of working memory deficits: durability of training effects in severely impaired and less severely impaired schizophrenia. Acta Psychiatr Scand 2003; 108: 101–9.
24. Fiszdon JM, Bryson GJ, Wexler BE, Bell MD. Durability of cognitive remediation training in schizophrenia: performance on two memory tasks at 6-month and 12-month follow-up. Psychiatry Res 2004; 125: 1–7.
25. Bell MD, Corbera S, Wexler BE. Cognitive remediation and competitive employment: differential benetis for schizophrenia patients with poor community function. In: Paper presented at the Schizophrenia International Research Society Annual Meeting. Florence, Italy, 2012.
26. McGurk SR, Mueser KT, Pascaris A. Cognitive training and supported employment for persons with severe mental illness: one-year results from a randomized controlled trial. Schizophr Bull 2005; 31: 898–909.

chapter 12

Enhancing socialization in people with schizophrenia

Anna W. Lui and Shirley M. Glynn

A diagnosis of schizophrenia often entails difficulties in social and/or occupational functioning. While positive symptoms (i.e., hallucinations, delusions) and negative symptoms (i.e. amotivation, apathy, asociality, anhedonia) can certainly be distressing in and of themselves, the deleterious effect they have on both community adjustment and subjective quality of life cannot be overestimated (1–5). Cognitive impairments (problems in concentration, attention, and memory) in schizophrenia are also highly related to poorer functional outcomes (chap. 4) (6,7).

Individuals with schizophrenia are less likely to be employed (chap. 11) (8) and to marry (9). They often have difficulty parenting their children (10–13), may have constrained social networks (14), are more likely to be homeless than the general population (15), and are at heightened risk for the development of depression and anxiety (chap. 5) (16,17). While long-term studies of prognosis in schizophrenia are hopeful (18), the diagnosis can cause great dysfunction in diagnosed persons' lives, especially in their adolescence and young to middle adulthood.

Improving socialization requires adequate interpersonal skills *and* opportunities to utilize these skills. In this chapter, we first discuss the development of the social skills training movement for schizophrenia and other psychiatric disorders. We then present the efficacy data for these types of interventions. We next outline the practical difficulties in generalizing skill use to "the real world," highlighting the impact of limited opportunities for application. We also discuss the role of societal and self-stigma in influencing socialization opportunities and efforts for persons with schizophrenia. We posit that interventions targeted at combating internalized feelings of shame and defeat about mental illness may improve participation and benefits accruing from traditional social skills-building programs. We then briefly discuss the recovery movement and the role of peer support in addressing socialization issues. Finally, we represent some new methodologies to strengthen socialization skills and the potential impact of social network media on enhancing socialization and combating stigma.

The development of the social skills training movement in schizophrenia

As outlined in chapter 1, the advent of effective antipsychotic medications in the 1950s brought optimism to the field of schizophrenia treatment (19,20). However, it subsequently became clear that pharmacological treatment alone does not usually restore individuals with schizophrenia to the level of functioning typically found in their non-ill counterparts (21). There are likely many reasons for this disparity. Persisting negative symptoms, which are less amenable to the impact of antipsychotic agents (22,23) are often reflected in asociality and amotivation, and can impact on social and vocational functioning (chap. 3). Even if medications adequately control positive and negative symptoms, persons who have been ill during much of their adolescence and early adulthood often have missed critical opportunities to master developmental tasks such as moving from home, meeting a partner, and initiating a career. Decades later, with the lapse of time, the potential atrophy of any skills they did possess, and constrained social and vocational opportunities, it can be very difficult for many individuals to accomplish these goals even if their symptoms have lessened.

During the 1960s and 1970s, a variety of psychosocial interventions began to be developed to be implemented in concert with medications to minimize symptoms and/or improve community adjustment in schizophrenia. One of the best studied of these interventions is social skills training (24), which is grounded in behavioral principles originally established in animal laboratories and then extended to humans. Early studies demonstrated that, similar to persons without psychotic disorders, the behavior of persons with psychotic disorders could be shaped using behavioral principles such as extinction, rehearsal, reinforcement, prompting, and shaping (25). Mental health professionals began using this knowledge to develop treatment programs, which incorporated learning principles to reduce problematic behaviors and promote pro-social behaviors in persons with serious and persisting psychiatric illnesses, including schizophrenia.

Social skills have been classified as "receiving" (accurately perceiving the facial expression, body language, and speech of another), "processing" (using systematic logic to understand what is being conveyed while avoiding errors such as jumping to conclusions, or personalizing), and "sending" capacities (clearly reflecting in speech and behavior the response to the information processed) (26). Traditional social skills training focuses on improving the ability to deliver an intended communication ("sending skills"): most early programs placed relatively less emphasis on helping participants perceive and understand the nuances of others' speech or nonverbal behavior ("receiving" and "processing" skills); and, if they attempted to accomplish this at all, tended to do this in an unsystematic manner.

Social skills training programs are described in detail in a number of comprehensive texts, including those by Bellack and colleagues (27) and Liberman and colleagues (28). They typically target nonverbal (eye contact, proximity), paralinguistic (voice tone, speech latency), and linguistic behavior (clear, comprehensible speech), with a goal of helping individuals develop the communication skills necessary to meet instrumental and affiliative goals. These interventions are often offered in a group format in order to provide individuals with modeling opportunities and multiple sources of feedback and opportunities to generalize behaviors. In-session work is augmented with out-of-session assignments to strengthen generalization to non-clinic settings.

Social skills training strategy is now widely used in the treatment of schizophrenia. In addition to standing on its own, social skills training is often a key component of other interventions. For example, communication skills is an explicit component of family psychoeducational programs (e.g., behavioral family therapy: see chap. 15) (29,30) and it is often an implicit aspect of other recovery-oriented programs such as supported employment (chap. 11) (31) and illness management and recovery (the facilitator coaching the consumer how to interact effectively with the treatment team) (32). A comprehensive set of modules, incorporating social skills training to address diverse issues such as workplace behavior, medication-taking, and dating and intimacy, have been developed as part of the UCLA Social and Independent Living Skills program (chap. 11) (33). Controlled research has demonstrated that participants can learn the skills taught in the modules (34), irrespective of symptom level, and that participants make gains in social adjustment (35).

The efficacy of social skills training in schizophrenia

In considering the efficacy of social skills training in schizophrenia, one must make an informed decision—in what domains are the benefits of social skills training likely to be observed? This is a more complicated question than it might first appear. Early social skills trials in schizophrenia typically involved single case or small studies and investigated whether the skills could even be learned (36,37). Consistent with a behavioral approach, the emphasis was on assessing change in the behavioral domain targeted (that is, if you are teaching someone how to initiate a conversation, you will then measure their skill in beginning a conversation). However, with the heightened emphasis on relapse prevention as an important goal in an increasingly deinstitutionalized population, researchers also began to investigate whether participation in social skills training programs actually impacted on clinical outcomes (24). This study was typically grounded in an application of the stress–vulnerability model of schizophrenia (38,39), with the idea being that a competent use of social skills would reduce ambient stress, and hence relapse.

A series of meta-analyses on the impact of social skills training in schizophrenia has shown that skills can be learned and maintained in the laboratory, but that generalization to the community rarely occurs spontaneously; it typically must be programmed (40–44). Use of the skills in the community likely results in the improved social functioning which has been established in individuals provided with specific generalization training (45). However, the data on the impact of social skills training on relapse or clinical status are less conclusive (40,42,46). Given that these programs do not regularly target changes in symptoms, these limited results are perhaps not surprising and emphasize how critical it is to link interventions with likely domains of impact.

Improving social skills in the community

In considering how socialization in the community can be enhanced in persons with serious and persisting psychiatric illnesses, three issues become apparent: (*i*) the complexity of the task; (*ii*) the role of the recovery movement in our understanding of the issues; and (*iii*) the availability of new social cognition interventions which may improve outcomes. Each of these will be addressed in detail.

The complexity of enhancing socialization in schizophrenia
Environmental factors
One of the primary challenges in helping people with schizophrenia improve their socialization is limited opportunities to use skills. Even in the general population, social isolation is a common circumstance due to the decline in civic engagement (47). The erosion of social networks, according to Putnam, is most recognizable by the dwindling memberships in many civic engagements from PTA meetings to bowling leagues. Church attendance, one of the most common associational membership in the United States, has also been declining compared with the early 1990s (48). The proportion of persons living alone in the United States has increased from 17% in 1970 to 28% in 2011 (49). Americans are also working longer hours, compared to their counterparts in other countries (50). Self-reports of loneliness are common, particularly among the elderly and ethnic minorities (51,52), although the availability of the Internet may somewhat mitigate this problem (53).

In light of the difficulty in making social connection in the general population, it is not surprising that social dysfunction and isolation are also common in schizophrenia. Societal stigma against people with serious psychiatric illnesses is well-documented (54,55). Unfortunately, in addition to symptoms and stigma, persons with schizophrenia may confront many practical obstacles to increasing their socialization. Those receiving some kind of disability compensation are usually on very modest budgets, which often do not provide extra income to go to concerts, movies, ballgames, or other social events. Funds are often limited for hobbies which require any financial outlay. Transportation and/or lack of a car may be a limiting factor.

Persons living in supervised residential settings may have limited opportunities to interact with others who are not disabled. When there are chances to interact with the general public, people with schizophrenia often also confront challenges in participating effectively in the social schema (56) that dictate many interpersonal interactions. For example, in many initial social interactions, individuals typically inquire about each others' jobs and families. Disabled persons who are not in the workforce and/or may have limited contact with their kin can have difficulty fielding such questions. During times of symptom exacerbations, even the persons' hygiene and grooming may be compromised.

Unfortunately, the spontaneous and unstructured nature of many social interactions makes transfer of skills learned in clinic to the environment particularly challenging. Furthermore, the voluntary nature of these interactions typically means that the use of a "coach" or "support person" (akin to the types of interventions used in supported employment programs) to facilitate social engagement is very difficult. The onus is often on the person with schizophrenia to create the opportunities to interact with others and then to use their skills competently during these opportunities. This can be a formidable task, particularly for a person with a high level of negative symptoms.

One possibility to circumvent this gap is to assist the person with schizophrenia to develop *hobbies* or *leisure time activities*, rather than *specific interpersonal connections* through increasing environmental support. Here, a support person in the community can play a pivotal role in helping the individual acquire any supplies needed for the activity (e.g., inexpensive yarn for knitting and rentable kayaks), identify opportunities and/or locations to participate in the activity (e.g., a nearby knitting shop and a local pond), and facilitate connection with these venues. Of course, opportunities for social interaction present themselves during each of these activities, but they are part of the process, rather than the outcome. We have used a community-based support person, in conjunction with a formal independent living, social, and problem-solving skills training program from the UCLA modules, to improve overall community adjustment in our test of In-Vivo Amplified Skills Training (45) in persons with schizophrenia and schizoaffective disorder. Similarly, Tauber and colleagues (57) found that the addition of indigenous supporters (residential treatment staff, family friends, etc.) to problem solve generalization difficulties can increase the interpersonal problem-solving skills and community functioning benefits accruing from participation in a comprehensive social and independent living skills program.

Nevertheless, there is much work to be done in the area. One of the disturbing features of the community-based care movement in schizophrenia is that we now have a whole generation of persons with the illness who have had few or no hospitalizations and are acutely attuned to the activities and lives of their non-ill peers. As they progress in their recoveries, they often look with longing at the (apparent) ease with which their non-ill friends make friends, date, move from home, attend school, and pursue careers. The high levels of stigma surrounding the serious and persisting psychiatric illnesses (58), as well as distressing psychiatric symptoms, can render these tasks very formidable for person with schizophrenia.

Personal factors

From a humanistic perspective, the onset of schizophrenia often disrupts the self-actualizing process at a crucial time when the person is forming and striving toward a meaningful adult identity (chap. 17). Psychotic experiences and disruptions in cognition often interrupt this process, and thereby contribute negative internal experiences to this new identity. Among those who have to confront social stigma, negative interpersonal interactions, and lack of social support and resources, their sum experiences may further trigger a social downward drift, reinforcing this negative self-perception.

While mindful of recovery-oriented perspectives to empower patients, clinicians must acknowledge the struggles of individuals with schizophrenia to engage in social life. A growing body of recent research has been examining the impact of self-stigma (59) and defeatist beliefs (60) on real-world functioning. For example, though neurocognitive deficits contribute to skill-based functional impairment in schizophrenia, they only account for a moderate amount of variance in community functioning (61). Negative symptoms, such as anhedonia, avolition, and hopelessness, directly interfere with social functioning and have been moderately resistant to psychosocial interventions (62). Prompted by a lack of a clear relational construct between cognitive impairment, negative symptoms, and social functioning, Grant and Beck examined these connections in a sample of individuals with predominantly negative symptoms and found personal defeatist beliefs to be the mediating link (63).

Negative self-perception may limit the benefits of socialization interventions targeting behavioral skills alone. Interventions directly addressing self-attitudes and beliefs may be an important prerequisite to increasing the efficacy of these skills-based interventions. As recommended by the Schizophrenia Patient Outcomes Research Team (PORT) (64), interventions such as social skills training, supportive employment, and assertive community treatment have solid evidence in improving social functioning. However, there remain a subset of individuals who consistently avoid or lack the motivation to engage in social activities, and they continue to perform poorly in real-world functioning. Interventions that specifically target these negative beliefs may be required. Lysaker and colleagues (65) have written of the potential value of individual psychotherapy in helping persons with schizophrenia "make sense of" their lives and develop a more positive, consistent narrative of their personal stories. As discussed in chapter 2, a form of individual therapy which may promote this work is cognitive–behavioral therapy for psychosis, which has demonstrated a positive social functioning outcome in a number of studies (66–68), and often includes work on developing a conceptual formulation to understand the development of psychotic experiences within a life context and specific activities eliciting and changing defeatist beliefs (69).

Enhancing socialization in recovery-oriented care

Since the publication of the Surgeon General and President's *New Freedom Commission on Mental Health* report, the concept of recovery has assumed center stage in public policy and practice. Despite the lack of a uniform conceptualization, most in the field agree that recovery from a serious mental illness is a process which involves learning to accept the illness, acquiring a sense of hope about the future and discovering a renewed sense of self (70). Enhancing socialization and community functioning are obvious goals in recovery. To help one grow beyond the often catastrophic effects of schizophrenia, it is important to validate patients' struggles, to help them accept illness-related challenges, to reframe their personal narrative to move from a "victim" to a "survivor" stance, and to help them find the strength to re-engage in social life activities.

To normalize unusual experiences, peer group interventions such as the "Hearing Voices Network" (71) and programs like the Wellness Recovery Action Plan (WRAP) (72) may provide promise for recovery, because they build on peer experience in context with illness management skills, and de-emphasize biological etiological models of mental illness. However, evidence on the benefits of participation in peer group interventions has not (yet) been clearly established. Furthermore, unlike the well-established peer support model for alcohol or substance abuse, peer support group formats and conceptual foundation for serious mental illness vary widely, especially with regard to their adoption of an illness model of schizophrenia. Research on peer support is limited and inherently challenging to design and execute. Nonetheless, peer support has great potential in facilitating the development of personal, social, environmental, and spiritual connections that may help individuals with schizophrenia to confront the effects of discrimination and stigma. Peer-to-peer support programs may gain even more traction if they are centered on providing emotional, appraisal, and informational support as a precursor to participation in skills-based socialization programs. For example, Granholm et al. (68) suggest that enhanced therapist-guided peer support group interventions along with Cognitive–Behavioral Social Skills Training can have an impact on socially disinterested attitudes, and thus potentiate skills training to yield better community functioning.

Social cognition interventions

As discussed above, the emphasis in most social skills training programs in improving interpersonal "sending" skills, that is, helping individuals convey what they wish to convey with competent verbal, nonverbal, and paralinguistic behavior. However, to be a competent social being, one also has to perceive correctly the behavior of others ("receiving" skills) and then infer accurately their intent and disposition ("processing" skills). Persons with schizophrenia often have profound deficits in these areas. They may be unable to recognize facial expressions accurately (73) and/or they may commit logical errors in interpreting the behavior of others (74,75) and/or they may have limited perspective taking (76); these deficits all reduce their ability to interact effectively with others.

These perceiving and processing deficits are the realm of "social cognition," and there are now a number of studies documenting social cognition deficits in schizophrenia (77) as well as suggesting methods to remediate these difficulties (78–81). These interventions can be targeted at a component skill such as improving facial affect recognition (82) or they can be more comprehensive and address multiple deficits (79–81). These programs typically involve repeated practice, behavioral strategies, and presentation of ambiguous social stimuli to help individuals learn to identify and interpret accurately more subtle social cues. While research in this area is very preliminary, this specialized attention to the subtleties of interpersonal interactions will appear to be a critical component in enhancing socialization in schizophrenia.

Networking through social media

With the rapid growth of wireless technologies in computers and handheld devices, social networking sites (SNS) such as Facebook, LinkedIn, and Twitter have become popular venues for social connections. According to the Pew Research Center, 65% of online adults use SNS, and of those, 67% reported using SNS as a way to maintain contact with close ties and reconnect with old friends (83). Though SNS and other online communities (i.e., blogs and special interest sites) have varying monitoring mechanisms, usage of this medium is quite democratic. Other than a high percentage of young adult users between the ages of 18 and 29, the differences in usage by gender, ethnicity, and socioeconomic background are not significant (84). During the late 1990s, researchers and social critics were debating the effects of the Internet on social life. Kraut et al. (85) conducted a longitudinal survey of Internet users and found a disturbing trend that people were substituting their time using the Internet rather than engaging in social activities. However, in less than a decade, Kraut et al. (86) refuted their earlier hypothesis and found that Internet use actually has positive effects on psychological and physical well being, on social involvement, and on communication and knowledge.

Though promising, the use of this technology to enhance socialization for persons with serious mental illness is open to question. Reports of online cruelty and safety issues have generated some concerns about this medium (87). Exposure to on-line hostility could have a deleterious effect on self-esteem and self-image. While Kraut and colleagues found that Internet use predicted better psychosocial outcome, this effect was evident only for extroverts and those with existing social support, and not for introverts with less social support—the latter description might fit many persons with schizophrenia. A recent randomized controlled trial (88) evaluating the use of a professionally developed and monitored online illness education program (including discussion boards on which participants with schizophrenia and their families could post comments) found the Internet intervention led to a significant reduction of symptoms compared with a control group. However, another recent randomized controlled trial evaluating the Internet peer support for individuals with psychiatric disabilities (89) could not determine whether an *unmonitored* Internet support is helpful or harmful.

Overall, the democratizing nature of the Internet holds promise as an effective social networking medium, particularly as a way to combat the stigma of mental illness. For example, many mental health support sites, such as schizophrenia.com and National Alliance on Mental Illness (NAMI), already provide a forum for individuals to discuss their experience with psychosis and other issues related to their illness. Professional mental health organizations could adopt formal guidelines to promote the use of social media for support among their clients. Meanwhile, clinicians could familiarize themselves with various social media, and discuss strategies for navigating online resources and support with their clients.

Conclusions

Deficits in social skills and poor community adjustment are common in schizophrenia. Traditional social skills training programs have provided a platform to increase the interpersonal capacities of a person with schizophrenia. Nevertheless, the generalization of skills to the community has been problematic. New treatment innovations, focusing on using community supporters to provide opportunities to practice skills, addressing self-stigma, and targeting interventions to the breadth of deficits resulting from problems in social cognition, are very promising.

References

1. Norman RM, Malla AK, Cortese L, et al. Symptoms and cognition as predictors of community functioning: a prospective analysis. Am J Psychiatry 1999; 156: 400–5.
2. Norman RM, Malla AK, McLean T, et al. The relationship of symptoms and level of functioning in schizophrenia to general wellbeing and the quality of life scale. Acta Psychiatr Scand 2000; 102: 303–9.
3. Robinson DG, Woerner MG, McMeniman M, Mendelowitz A, Bilder RM. Symptomatic and functional recovery from a first episode of schizophrenia or schizoaffective disorder. Am J Psychiatry 2004; 161: 473–9.
4. Torgalsboen AK. Full recovery from schizophrenia: the prognostic role of premorbid adjustment, symptoms at first admission, precipitating events and gender. Psychiatry Res 1999; 88: 143–52.

5. Racenstein JM, Harrow M, Reed R, et al. The relationship between positive symptoms and instrumental work functioning in schizophrenia: a 10-year follow-up study. Schizophr Res 2002; 56: 95–103.
6. Green MF. What are the functional consequences of neurocognitive deficits in schizophrenia? Am J Psychiatry 1996; 153: 321–30.
7. Brekke JS, Raine A, Ansel M, Lencz T, Bird L. Neuropsychological and psychophysiological correlates of psychosocial functioning in schizophrenia. Schizophr Bull 1997; 23: 19–28.
8. Blyler CR. Understanding the employment rate of people with schizophrenia: different approaches lead to different implications for policy. In: Lezenweger MF, Hooley JM, eds. Principles of Experimental Psychopathology: Essays in Honor of Brendan A. Maher. Washington, DC: American Psychological Association, 2003: 107–15.
9. Hutchinson G, Bhugra D, Mallett R, et al. Fertility and marital rates in first-onset schizophrenia. Soc Psychiatry Psychiatr Epidemiol 1999; 34: 617–21.
10. Craig T, Bromet EJ. Parents with psychosis. Ann Clin Psychiatry 2004; 16: 35–9.
11. Miller LJ. Sexuality, reproduction, and family planning in women with schizophrenia. Schizophr Bull 1997; 23: 623–35.
12. Miller LJ, Finnerty M. Sexuality, pregnancy, and childrearing among women with schizophrenia-spectrum disorders. Psychiatr Serv 1996; 4: 502–6.
13. Mullick M, Miller LJ, Jacobsen T. Insight into mental illness and child maltreatment risk among mothers with major psychiatric disorders. Psychiatr Serv 2001; 52: 488–92.
14. Randolph ET. Social networks in schizophrenia. In: Mueser KT, Tarrier N, eds. Handbook in Social Functioning in Schizophrenia. Boston: Allyn and Bacon, 1998: 238–48.
15. Susser E, Struening EL, Conover S. Psychiatric problems in homeless men: lifetime psychosis, substance use, and current distress in new arrivals at New York City shelters. Arch Gen Psychiatry 1989; 46: 845–50.
16. Siris SG. Depression in schizophrenia: perspective in the era of "Atypical" antipsychotic agents. Am J Psychiatry 2000; 157: 1379–89.
17. Braga RJ, Mendlowicz MV, Marrocos RP, Figueira IL. Anxiety disorders in outpatients with schizophrenia: prevalence and impact on the subjective quality of life. J Psychiatr Res 2005; 39: 409–14.
18. Harding CM, Brooks GW, Ashikaga T, Strauss JS, Breier A. The Vermont longitudinal study of persons with severe mental illness: II. Long-term outcome of subjects who retrospectively met DSM-III criteria for schizophrenia. Am J Psychiatry 1987; 144: 727–35.
19. May P. Treatment of Schizophrenia: A Comparative Study of Five Treatment Methods: Science House. 1968.
20. May PR, Tuma AH, Dixon WJ, et al. Schizophrenia: A follow-up study of the results of five forms of treatment. Arch Gen Psychiatry 1991; 38: 776–84.
21. Wallace CJ. Community and interpersonal functioning in the course of schizophrenic disorders. Schizophr Bull 1984; 10: 233–57.
22. Alphs L. An industry perspective on the NIMH consensus statement on negative symptoms. Schizophr Bull 2006; 32: 225–30.
23. Kirkpatrick B, Fenton WS, Carpenter WT Jr, Marder SR. The NIMH-MATRICS consensus statement on negative symptoms. Schizophr Bull 2006; 32: 214–19.
24. Wallace CJ, Liberman RP. Social skills training for patients with schizophrenia: a controlled clinical trial. Psychiatry Res 1985; 15: 239–47.
25. Meichenbaum DH. The effects of instructions and reinforcement on thinking and language behavior of schizophrenics. Behav Res Ther 1969; 7: 101–14.
26. Donahoe CP, Carter MJ, Bloem WD, et al. Assessment of interpersonal problem-solving skills. Psychiatry 1990; 53: 329–39.
27. Bellack AS, Mueser KT, Gingerich S, Agresta J. Social Skills Training for Schizophrenia: A Step-by-Step Guide. New York: The Guilford Press, 2004.

28. Liberman RP, DeRisi WJ, Mueser KT. Social Skills Training for Psychiatric Patients. Needham Heights, MA: Allyn & Bacon, 1989.

29. Falloon IR, Boyd JL, McGill CW. Family Care of Schizophrenia: A Problem-solving Approach to the Treatment of Mental Illness. New York, NY: The Guilford Press, 1984.

30. Mueser KT, Glynn SM. Behavioral Family Therapy for Psychiatric Disorders. 2nd edn. Oakland, CA: New Harbinger Publications, Inc, 1999.

31. Becker DR, Drake RE. A Working Life for People with Severe Mental Illness. New York: Oxford University Press, 2003.

32. Mueser KT, Corrigan PW, Hilton D, et al. Illness management and recovery for severe mental illness: a review of the research. Psychiatr Serv 2002; 53: 1272–84.

33. Liberman RP, Wallace CJ, Blackwell G, et al. Innovations in skills training for the seriously mentally ill: the UCLA Social and Independent Living Skills modules. Innov Res 1993; 2: 43–59.

34. Eckman TA, Wirshing WC, Marder SR, et al. Technique for training schizophrenic patients in illness self-management: a controlled trial. Am J Psychiatry 1992; 149: 1549–55.

35. Marder SR, Wirshing WC, Mintz J, et al. Two-year outcome for social skills training and group psychotherapy for outpatients with schizophrenia. Am J Psychiatry 1996; 153: 1585–92.

36. Matson JL, Zeiss AM, Zeiss RA, Bowman W. A comparison of social skills training and contingent attention to improve behavioural deficits of chronic psychiatric patients. Br J Soc Clin Psychol 1980; 19: 57–64.

37. Hersen M, Bellack AS. A multiple-baseline analysis of social-skills training in chronic schizophrenics. J Appl Behav Anal 1976; 9: 239–45.

38. Zubin J, Spring B. Vulnerability: a new view of schizophrenia. J Abnorm Psychol 1977; 86: 103–26.

39. Nuechterlein KH, Dawson ME. A heuristic vulnerability/stress model of schizophrenic episodes. Schizophr Bull 1984; 10: 300–12.

40. Benton MK, Schroeder HE. Social skills training with schizophrenics: A meta-analytic evaluation. J Consult Clin Psychol 1990; 58: 741–7.

41. Corrigan PW. Social skills training in adult psychiatric populations: a meta-analysis. J Behav Ther Exp Psychiatry 1991; 22: 203–10.

42. Dilk MN, Bond GR. Meta-analytic evaluation of skills training research for individuals with severe mental illness. J Consult Clin Psychol 1996; 64: 1337–46.

43. Kopelowicz A, Liberman RP, Zarate R. Recent advances in social skills training for schizophrenia. Schizophr Bull 2006; 32: S12–23.

44. Kurtz MM, Mueser KT. A meta-analysis of controlled research on social skills training for schizophrenia. J Consult Clin Psychol 2008; 76: 491–504.

45. Glynn SM, Marder SR, Liberman RP, et al. Supplementing clinic-based skills training with manual-based community support sessions: effects on social adjustment of patients with schizophrenia. Am J Psychiatry 2002; 159: 829–37.

46. Pilling S, Bebbington P, Kuipers E, et al. Psychological treatments in schizophrenia: II. Meta-analyses of randomized controlled trials of social skills training and cognitive remediation. Psychol Med 2002; 32: 783–91.

47. Putnam R. Bowling Alone: The Collapse and Revival of American Community. New York, NY: Simon & Schuster, 2001.

48. Barna, Research, Group. The State of the ChurchVentura. CA: The Barna Group, 2000.

49. US Census Bureau. More Young Adults are living in Parent's Home. Census Bureau Report. Washington DC: US Department of Commerce, 2011.

50. The International Labor Organization. Key Indicators of the Labour Market. Geneva: The International Labor Organization, 2003: 857.

51. Heinrich LM, Gullone E. The clinical significance of loneliness: a literature review. Clin Psychol Rev 2006; 26: 695–718.
52. Locher JL, Ritchie CS, Roth DL, et al. Social isolation, support, and capital and nutritional risk in an older sample: ethnic and gender differences. Soc Sci Med 2005; 60: 747–61.
53. Morahan-Martin J, Schumacher P. Loneliness and social uses of the Internet. Comput Human Behav 2003; 19: 659–71.
54. Farina A, Felner RD. Employment interviewer reactions to former mental patients. J Abnorm Psychol 1973; 82: 268–72.
55. Stigma FA. Handbook of Social Functioning in Schizophrenia. In: Mueser KT, Tarrier N, eds. Boston: Allyn & Bacon, 1998: 247–79.
56. Corrigan PW, Wallace CJ, Green MF. Deficits in social schemata in schizophrenia. Schizophr Res 1992; 8: 129–35.
57. Tauber R, Wallace CJ, Lecomte T. Enlisting indigenous community supporters in skills training programs for persons with severe mental illness. Psychiatr Serv 2000; 51: 1428–32.
58. Crisp AH, Gelder MG, Rix S, Meltzer HI, Rowlands OJ. Stimatization of people with mental illnesses. Br J Psychiatry 2000; 177: 4–7.
59. Corrigan PW, Watson AC. Understanding the impact of stigma on people with mental illness. World Psychiatry 2002; 1: 16–20.
60. Horan WP, Rassovsky Y, Kern RS, et al. Further support for the role of dysfunctional attitudes in models of real-world functioning in schizophrenia. J Psychiatr Res 2010; 44: 499–505.
61. Green MF. What are the functional consequences of neurocognitive deficits in schizophrenia? Am J Psychiatry 1996; 153: 321–30.
62. Bustillo J, Lauriello J, Horan W, Keith S. The psychosocial treatment of schizophrenia: an update. Am J Psychiatry 2001; 158: 163–75.
63. Grant P, Beck A. Defeatist beliefs as a mediator of cognitive impairment, negative symptoms, and functioning in schizophrenia. Schizophr Bull 2009; 35: 798–806.
64. Dixon LB, Dickerson F, Bellack AS, et al. The 2009 schizophrenia PORT Psychosocial Treatment Recommendations and summary statements. Schizophr Bull 2010; 36: 48–70.
65. Lysaker P, Glynn S, Wilkniss S, Silverstein S. Psychotherapy and recovery from schizophrenia: a review of potential applications and need for future study. Psychol Serv 2010; 7: 75–91.
66. Dickerson F, Lehman A. Evidence-based psychotherapy for schizophrenia 2011 update. J Nerv Ment Dis 2011; 199: 520–6.
67. Tarrier N. Cognitive behaviour therapy for schizophrenia—a review of development, evidence and implementation. Psychother Psychosom 2005; 74: 136–44.
68. Wykes T, Steel C, Everitt B, Tarrier N. Cognitive behavior therapy for schizophrenia: effect sizes, clinical models, and methodological rigor. Schizophr Bull 2008; 34: 523–37.
69. Granholm E, Ben-Zeev D, Link PC. Social disinterest attitudes and group cognitive-behavioral social skills training for functional disability in schizophrenia. Schizophr Bull 2009; 35: 874–83.
70. Davidson L, O'Connell MJ, Tondora J, Lawless M, Evans A. Recovery in serious mental illness: a new wine or just a new bottle? Prof Psychol Res Pract 2005; 36: 480–7.
71. Welcome to the Hearing Voices Network USA (2011). [Retrieved: December 22, 2011]. [Available from: http://www.hearingvoicesusa.org/]
72. Cook JA, Copeland ME, Jonikas JA, et al. Results of a randomized controlled trial of mental illness self-management using wellness recovery action planning. Schizophr Bull 2011; doi: 10.1093/schbul/sbr012.

73. Mueser KT, Penn DL, Blanchard JJ, Bellack AS. Affect recognition in schizophrenia: A synthesis of findings across three studies. Psychiatry 1997; 60: 301–8.
74. Bentall RP, Corcoran R, Howard R, Blackwood N, Kinderman P. Persecutory delusions: a review and theoretical integration. Clin Psychol Rev 2001; 21: 1143–92.
75. Bentall RP, Swarbrick R. The best laid schemas of paranoid patients: autonomy, sociotropy and need for closure. Psychol Psychother 2003; 76: 163–71.
76. Langdon R, Coltheart M, Ward PB. Empathetic perspective-taking is impaired in schizophrenia: evidence from a study of emotion attribution and theory of mind. Cogn Neuropsychiatry 2006; 11: 133–55.
77. Couture SM, Penn DL, Roberts DL. The functional significance of social cognition in schizophrenia: a review. Schizophr Bull 2006; 32: S44–63.
78. Choi KH, Kwon JH. Social cognition enhancement training for schizophrenia: A preliminary randomized controlled trial. Community Ment Health J 2006; 42: 177–87.
79. Horan WP, Kern RS, Tripp C, et al. Effficacy and specificity of social cognitive skills training for outpatients with psychotic disorders. J Psychiatry Res 2011; 45: 1113–22.
80. Combs DR, Elerson K, Penn DL, et al. Stability and generalization of Social Cognition and Interaction Training (SCIT) for schizophrenia: six-month follow-up results. Schizophr Res 2009; 112: 196–7.
81. Roberts DL, Penn DL. Social cognition and interaction training (SCIT) for outpatients with schizophrenia: a preliminary study. Psychiatry Res 2009; 166: 141–7.
82. Wolwer W, Frommann N, Halfmann S, et al. Remediation of impairments in facial affect recognition in schizophrenia: efficacy and specificity of a new training program. Schizophr Res 2005; 80: 295–303.
83. Smith A. Why americans use social media. PEW Research Center. Published online 11-14-2011. [Available from: http://www.pewinternet.org/Reports/2011/why-Americans-Use-Social-Media.aspx].
84. Madden M, Zickuhr K. 65% of Online Adults Use Social Networking Sites. PEW Research Center. Published online 8–27-2011 [Available from: http://www.pewinternet.org/Reports/2011/Social-Networking-Sites.aspx].
85. Kraut R, Patterson M, Lundmark V, et al. Internet paradox. A social technology that reduces social involvement and psychological well-being. Am Psychol 1998; 53: 1017–31.
86. Kraut R, Kiesler S, Bonka B, et al. Internet paradox revisited. J Soc Issues 2002; 58: 49–74.
87. Lenhart A, Madden M, Smith A, et al. Teens' kindness and cruelty on social network sites. PEW Research Center. Published online 11–9-2011. [Available from: http://pewinternet.org/Reports/2011/Teens-and-social-media.aspx].
88. Rotondi AJ, Anderson CM, Haas GL, et al. Web-based psychoeducational intervention for persons with schizophrenia and their supporters: one-year outcomes. Psychiatr Serv 2010; 61: 1099–105.
89. Kaplan K, Salzer MS, Solomon P, Brusilovskiy E, Cousounis P. Internet peer support for individuals with psychiatric disabilities: a randomized controlled trial. Soc Sci Med 2011; 72: 54–62.

Chapter 13

The clinical needs of women with schizophrenia

Jayashri Kulkarni, Paul B. Fitzgerald, and Mary V. Seeman

Women with schizophrenia often have different clinical needs compared with men with the same diagnosis because of a number of important gender differences in the presentation, course, and outcome of schizophrenia. Women and men with schizophrenia can differ in premorbid functioning, psychotic triggers, and variation in the clinical manifestation of specific symptoms and in numerous dimensions of outcome. However, the treatment generally provided for people with schizophrenia is still largely gender-blind, thereby neglecting a number of needs specific to women. In order to optimize the outcomes for women with schizophrenia, treatments need to be tailored to meet their special needs.

Development of schizophrenia in women

Over the past decade, there has been considerable interest in the "prodrome" or pre-psychosis period (1). The onset of schizophrenia appears to result from a complex interaction between many factors, including genetic vulnerability, stressful or traumatic life events, vulnerable neural circuitry, brain structural changes such as hippocampal shrinkage (2), illicit substance use (amphetamines or cannabis), and the neurohormonal changes that come with puberty. Each of these factors is being actively studied, but we still have no clear understanding about the origins and development of schizophrenia.

While the etiology is uncertain, some gender differences appear to hold true across different countries and races. Earlier age at onset of schizophrenia is associated with poor premorbid functioning. Women tend to have a later age of first onset of schizophrenia with better premorbid functioning and better initial outcomes (3). Kraepelin initially described "dementia praecox" as a disorder of young men. Work done transnationally since then has continued to show that women present up to 5 years later than men with a first onset of psychosis (4). Debates still continue about the age of onset difference between the genders, and one of the confounding issues is the subtyping of schizophrenia. The most debilitating form of schizophrenia appears to be an early-onset type, which is accompanied by a relatively greater degree of neurodevelopmental deficit. Men appear to be overrepresented in this group (4). The still unanswered question then arises about whether the gender differences in age of onset are actually due to the sex of the person, or the subtype of schizophrenia.

Other gender differences in the development of schizophrenia have been described and key among these differences are symptoms. Women have been found to experience more paranoid symptoms (5) and are more likely to show depression than men. The presence of affective symptoms is linked to more favorable outcomes (6). Women with schizophrenia have been noted to be more likely to acknowledge illness and seek medical attention than men. This increased insight (7) may contribute to a better outcome for women.

Epidemiology of gender differences in schizophrenia

A very detailed research of sex differences in schizophrenia was done in the ABC Schizophrenia Study, conducted in Germany by Häfner and colleagues (8). A large population catchment area of 1.5 million people was surveyed and 232 people met the criteria for first symptom onset of schizophrenia spectrum disorders. Using rigorous methodology, which included obtaining data form informants and a range of supporting documents, Häfner (9) found a significant difference in the age of onset of schizophrenia, with men presenting on average 3–4 years earlier than women. This significant gender difference was found across many symptoms and extended to first admission to hospital. The ABC (age, beginning, course) Schizophrenia Study (10) also examined incidence rates and first admission rates over the life cycle. Female incidence rates increased more slowly than male rates and had one peak between 15 and 30 years and then a second smaller peak in the age group between 45 and 50 years. Other studies have also shown this gender difference in age of onset of schizophrenia, with a bimodal distribution of schizophrenia onset in women, and a unimodal one in men (11).

The estrogen protection hypothesis

The sex differences noted in the age of onset of schizophrenia, in particular the bimodal distribution of the incidence of new schizophrenia cases in women, led researchers to propose that estrogen may confer protection against the early onset of severe schizophrenia (12,13). Women were seen as vulnerable to relapses of schizophrenia or to suffer their first episode of illness during times when estrogen production diminishes:—during the monthly cycle, or postpartum, or at the perimenopause. Häfner (8) and Seeman (14) independently suggested the hypothesis that estrogen may have an effect in the developing brain, with estrogen actions delaying the onset of schizophrenia. Further rise in estradiol and other gonadal steroids during puberty is also hypothesized to reinforce the functional effect of estrogen.

The estrogen protection hypothesis rests on three main lines of work: epidemiological studies, basic science studies using animal models, and those using clinical studies. The hypothesis that estrogen has a protective effect in schizophrenia has a number of potential clinical treatment implications, which are explored in this chapter.

Basic science evidence for estrogen as a psychoprotectant

Estrogen's neuroprotective actions appear to be mediated by a wide range of actions, which include increased cerebral blood flow, antioxidant effects, and increased cerebral glucose utilization. There may also be slower, genomic effects, with subsequent permanent modification of neural circuits (15,16). There are at least two estrogen receptors (α and β), and imaging techniques have mapped their widespread distribution to brain areas including the hypothalamus, amygdala-hippocampal area, substantia nigra and subthalamic nucleus, cerebellum, and various areas of the cerebral cortex (17,18). Estrogen modulates multiple neurotransmitter systems, including the dopaminergic, serotonergic, cholinergic, and GABAergic pathways (19–21). Evidence from animal studies has shown that long-term estradiol treatment may preserve striatal dopamine concentrations by decreasing the affinity of the transporter for dopamine (22,23). Animal studies also have shown that long-term estradiol treatment can modulate brain serotonergic activity by increasing serotonin synthesis and its release in the dorsal raphe (24).

Clinical support for the estrogen protection hypothesis

Riecher-Rössler and colleagues (25) showed a correlation between symptoms of psychosis in women with schizophrenia and serum estrogen levels. They found, in a clinical population of 32 women with schizophrenia, that there was a significant inverse relationship between serum estrogen levels and psychopathology. Paranoid symptoms, ward behaviors, and psychosis symptoms in general were all worse when women were in their low serum estrogen menstrual phase. Riecher-Rossler's findings (26) have been confirmed in other studies that describe fluctuation in psychosis symptom severity across the menstrual cycle, with worsening of psychosis in low estrogen cycle phases (27–29).

Other evidence that psychotic symptoms worsen in low estrogen phases of the menstrual cycle includes a study conducted by Hallonquist et al. (27) and by Hoff et al. showing that specific cognitive performance is estrogen-level related (30).

Another important line of evidence for the role of estrogen as a neuroprotective agent comes from studies examining gender differences in response to antipsychotic medication treatment. Seeman's (31) careful review of the gender difference in response to antipsychotic treatment showed that women of childbearing age tend to have a more rapid and better response to medication than do men. Of note, Seeman (31) also reported that postmenopausal women tend to have poorer responses to medication than younger women, and are liable to illness exacerbation. These studies strongly suggest that estrogen provides an agonistic effect for antipsychotic medication (32).

Following these lines of evidence, clinical trials using estrogen as a treatment adjunct were started and have shown promising results. Kulkarni and colleagues (33) demonstrated that adding estradiol in oral form, or more efficaciously in transdermal form (34), can be associated with enhanced symptom response for women with schizophrenia. More recently, clinical trials conducted with a selective estrogen receptor modulator raloxifene have also shown promising results for women with schizophrenia (35), and add further evidence to the hypothesis that estrogen has a neuroprotective effect. Using estradiol treatment as an augmentation for women with persistent schizophrenia symptoms has clinical utility, provided caution is taken with breast and reproductive tissue monitoring (34). Clinically, estradiol augmentation can range from adjunctive use of the oral contraceptive pill to augmentation with transdermal estradiol in perimenopausal women. The potential uses of estrogen treatment in women with schizophrenia are listed in Box 13.1.

Management of schizophrenia in women

There are several important areas of clinical consideration in managing women with schizophrenia, which have been largely overlooked until the past decade. In this section we outline the management of sexual issues in women with schizophrenia, including pregnancy; menopause in women with schizophrenia; special medication management and long-term psychosocial recovery programs; and safety issues for women with schizophrenia.

Box 13.1 Potential clinical uses of estrogen augmentation in schizophrenia.

- Where the patient experiences an exacerbation of symptoms that clearly appears to relate to fluctuating hormonal levels through the menstrual cycle
- In women with resistant symptoms
- During life stages where estrogen levels are low (e.g., menopause)
- There may also be a role for estrogen in the treatment of tardive dyskinesia

Sexuality and women with schizophrenia

The preferred community-based treatment model for patients with schizo-phrenia provides socialization and sexual relationship opportunities. Studies conducted since the institution of policies favoring community treatment of patients with schizophrenia indicate that the illness does not directly limit the sexual interest or desire of patients, and most patients continue to be sexually active (36). However, side effects of antipsychotic medication, including seda-tion and gynecological effects of raised prolactin, may impact on sexual desire and behavior, as outlined in Box 13.2.

The quality of the sexual lives of women with schizophrenia is negatively impacted by many factors. Women with schizophrenia experience high rates of sexual abuse, often feel pressured to have sex, and all too often take part in sex-exchange behavior or other activities that place them at substantial risk for sexually transmitted diseases. These activities include engaging in sex with homosexual and bisexual partners and having more lifetime partners. In addi-tion, patients with schizophrenia report relatively poor levels of knowledge in regards to safe sex behavior and family planning issues (37).

Pregnancy and schizophrenia

The desire to reproduce is a basic human urge and women with schizophrenia are no different to other women in this regard. In the past, women with schizophrenia were either actively discouraged or, more likely their treating clinicians largely ignored the topic. Many women with schizophrenia had unplanned pregnancies (38).

Currently, discussions between women patients and their doctors rarely include planning pregnancies, since the control of psychosis symptoms tends to dominate the clinical interaction. While the clinician's concern is adequate parenting, the woman's concern is her wish to be a mother. The two views seem at odds with each other but they need not be if the pregnancy is planned. The current common use of atypical antipsychotic medications increases the risk of pregnancy, since the ovulation suppression that occurred with the

---

Box 13.2   Medication-related negative influences on sexual functioning in women with schizophrenia.

- Hyperprolactinemia leading to menstrual irregularities, diminished libido, and impaired sexual functioning
- Weight gain, resulting in a negative impact on body image
- Sedation
- Nocturnal urinary incontinence
- Concern regarding potential negative impact of medication on any offspring

"typical" or older antipsychotic medications is now less likely. Of the newer medications, risperidone is the one still associated with diminution of fertility through its elevation of prolactin release by the pituitary gland (chap. 1).

Clearly, there are many psychosocial issues that pregnant women with schizophrenia have to face, all of which clinicians need to address with their female patients. Overall, women with schizophrenia have poorer pregnancy-related outcomes (Box 13.3) (39). Some are related to exposure to antipsychotic medication during pregnancy, but multiple factors need to be considered, including poverty, inadequate housing, social isolation, poor nutrition, tobacco smoking, substance abuse, pregnancy stress, domestic abuse, exposure to infection, and poor antenatal health care.

A difficult problem is the lack of evidence-based information about safe antipsychotic medication use in pregnancy. There are two important goals. First is to ensure that the mother remains well during the pregnancy and the postnatal period. Second is to ensure that the developing baby does not suffer antipsychotic medication-induced malformations or developmental problems. Good antenatal care and the safe delivery of a healthy baby are important management goals to optimize outcomes for both the new mother and her baby. Enabling women with schizophrenia to mother their children well is a crucial role that clinicians need to work on, to optimize the mental health of the next generation. In Australia, we have established the National Register of Antipsychotic Medication in Pregnancy to collect data in this important area (40). We have been able to observe that stopping antipsychotics during pregnancy is not the answer—the outcomes are worse. In this situation, the pregnant women's mental health often deteriorates badly, which leads to hospitalization, multiple medications, and eventual separation of mother and baby due to the mother's continuing mental illness. The second-generation antipsychotic medications such as olanzapine, quetiapine, and risperidone

---

Box 13.3 Adverse side effects of antipsychotics, to which women are particularly prone.

- Parkinsonism
- Tardive dyskinesia
- Sexual dysfunction
- Gynecomastia and galactorrhea
- Menstrual irregularity
- Osteoporosis
- Cardiovascular effects
- QTc prolongation
- Weight gain
- Metabolic effects

seem relatively safe for use in pregnancy from our small database, so far. Much more data and longer-term follow-up of babies born to women who took antipsychotics during pregnancy is needed to understand which antipsychotics are safest in pregnancy. An evidence-based guideline showing which antipsychotic medication is safest in pregnancy is needed and the National Register of Antipsychotic Medication in Pregnancy data set is a start toward meeting this clinical need (41).

Pregnant women with schizophrenia need special antenatal care, particularly those with relapsing, severe illness. Education about nutrition, smoking cessation, ceasing illicit drug use, and minimizing alcohol intake during pregnancy are important issues for good antenatal care. Unfortunately, most health systems do not provide comprehensive, integrated care for women with schizophrenia. The communication between obstetric services and mental health systems can be inadequate, leading to difficult clinical situations and the possibility of postpartum psychosis relapse. The management of postpartum psychosis needs a holistic approach, with a special focus on keeping mother and baby together.

The safety of antipsychotics in breast-feeding is largely unknown. Most clinicians negotiate the issue of breast-feeding with the new mother. The desire of the new mother to breast feed her newborn to provide the best start in life for her baby is a strong motivator for breast-feeding. However, there are concerns about antipsychotic drug ingestion by the neonate and this clinical problem requires data to create evidence-based guidelines.

Looking after pregnant women with schizophrenia is, thus, complicated. There needs to be active support, parenting education, and family networking. Optimal physical health care is required. Children's services may need to be consulted because some women suffering from schizophrenia may either not be able to look after their babies or will need agency as well as family help.

Motherhood for women with schizophrenia is often complicated by single status, alienation from family of origin, poverty, and poor general health (42). These vulnerable mothers face the extra challenge of frequently enough mothering difficult-to-soothe, and possibly developmentally delayed children. Parenting help is a crucial aspect of schizophrenia treatment for women.

There are too few services that provide holistic care for the family unit when the mother has schizophrenia. Better management of women with schizophrenia who become mothers is a vital clinical issue that has impact on both the current population of ill women and future generations.

Menopause and women with schizophrenia

Menopause is associated with a number of new potential stressors including the death of previously supportive parents, aunts, and uncles; ill health of the patient or spouse; and the departure of children from the home (43). In addition, hormones may play an important role in mediating the course of schizophrenia at this age. The severity of schizophrenia levels off in men after their 40s. This may be related to the depletion of dopamine receptors with age, a decline that is more precipitous in men than in women. In women the pattern may differ (44), possibly related to the gradual diminution of the protective effect of estrogen.

Women with schizophrenia have been noted to deteriorate at this time with respect to worsening auditory hallucinations, delusions, and thought disorder (45). Perimenopausal women experience hot flushes, sleep disturbances, mood swings, and poor cognitive functioning, as well as worsening of psychotic symptoms (46). Deterioration in a middle-aged women's mental state may not be recognized as being largely due to menopause transition hormone shifts, and the treatment may mistakenly involve increased antipsychotic medications, hospitalizations, and added psychotropic medications (47).

Hormone replacement therapy (HRT) provides an alternative and perhaps a more effective approach to the treatment of menopause symptoms that may, in women with schizophrenia, include worsening psychosis. Of course, HRT carries its own risks (48,49) as the Women's Health Initiative study has indicated. Good medical care and ongoing monitoring will be needed if HRT is used as a treatment adjunct for menopausal women with schizophrenia. In the near future, there may be a role for augmentation of antipsychotics with selective estrogen receptor modulators (50), the so-called "brain estrogens" in peri- and postmenopausal women with schizophrenia (35).

Other physical health issues associated with the menopause such as weight gain, hypercholesterolemia, diabetes, osteoporosis and the possibility of an increased risk of breast cancer need ongoing medical monitoring. Many of these physical health issues can be exacerbated by antipsychotic medication; hence there is an even greater need for good physical health care and monitoring for women with schizophrenia as they enter the menopausal transition. Psychosocial issues related to being middle aged, such as fears of aging, loss of fertility, change in domestic situations, and other mid-life events also need assessment and appropriate action by treating clinicians.

Medication treatment for women with schizophrenia

Medications for schizophrenia have improved substantially over the past decade. However, there is still work to be done to tailor treatments specifically to women with schizophrenia. In general, women experience more adverse antipsychotic side effects than men (Box 13.3) (51). The vulnerability of women to adverse effects may be due to higher concentrations of free drug reaching target sites; an enhancement of dopamine blockade by estrogen; a longer duration of storage of neuroleptics in adipose tissue; a higher prevalence of immune reactions in women than in men; and a greater risk, in women, of drug–drug interactions because of women's greater likelihood of comorbid (and treated) illness (52,53).

Some side effects of antipsychotics may be of different significance to men and women. As a gross generalization, men are most disturbed by side effects that interfere with performance, especially sexual performance; women tend to be more disturbed by side effects which affect appearance, weight gain being an important one, especially to women (54).

Extrapyramidal side effects of antipsychotics in women
Extrapyramidal motor side effects are amongst the more common and disabling side effects of antipsychotics. Acute dystonia, long thought to be more prevalent among men, has been shown in a first-episode fixed dosed 10-week study, to occur more readily in women (55). As these authors point out, earlier clinical studies did not take into account the fact that young male patients were commonly prescribed higher doses than women, probably because they were *perceived* as more threatening and their behavior was seen as requiring higher, and more rapid dosing.

Historical studies have suggested that tardive dyskinesia is more common in female than male patients treated with antipsychotics (56). However, a more recent cohort study found tardive dyskinesia to be more common in elderly men, although its *severity* may be greater in women in their later years (57). There is also evidence that the severity and incidence of tardive dyskinesia peak in men at age 50–70 but continues to increase in women with age (56). The reasons for this are not fully understood.

Clinical trials
Attempts are being made worldwide to ensure that equal numbers of women and men enter randomized controlled trials of new medications to facilitate ensuing medication guidelines. In the past, this was a concern since many randomized controlled trials of antipsychotic medications were conducted in male-dominant populations. The 1988, the Food and Drug Administration recommendation about new drug trials needing to include equal gender numbers has had significant effect, but vigilance about this is still needed (58,59). Therapeutic guidelines still provide a range of dosing that commonly ignores the gender of the patient. In managing women with schizophrenia, clinicians need to factor in the gender, weight, and ethnicity of their patients in order to prescribe a correct, therapeutic dose of drug with minimal risk of the more important side effects.

Antipsychotic drug metabolism in women
Women have different drug metabolism and kinetics of antipsychotic medications than men (55), and if prescribed a dose based on male physiology,

unwanted side effects can occur. Antipsychotic medications are sequestered into adipose tissue differently in women, and different liver enzymatic actions can impact the availability of the drug to the central nervous system (CNS) (60). Gonadal steroids impact on the CNS and clearly affect the drug response different in men and women (61). As outlined earlier, tardive dyskinesia is seen more commonly in women than men (62). Weight gain is a troubling side effect of many antipsychotic drugs for men and women, but it appears to be worse for women with schizophrenia (63). Weight gain can predispose women to diabetes, which is an increasing health risk globally (64).

Hyperprolactinemia

Antipsychotic drugs that cause hyperprolactinemia pose special problems for women. Prolactin is a pituitary hormone that is normally elevated in breast-feeding women in order to facilitate lactation. It has potent antagonist impact on estrogen, progesterone, and testosterone production. Dopamine inhibition by antidopaminergic (antipsychotic) drugs increases prolactin (65). Hyperprolactinemia over a long period can increase the risk for osteoporosis in both women and men (65). Importantly in women, prolactin is secreted by breast tissue and is implicated in cell migration, especially to the lymphatic system. In a large cohort of nurses, it has been shown that women who had naturally higher prolactin levels are at a much greater risk of developing breast cancer than other women, with rapid progression of the disease (66). With artificial prolactin elevation, through the use of antipsychotic drugs, it is possible that increased lactotroph cell formation may increase the risk of breast cancer (67). Animal studies have reported a greater migration and axillary node spread of cancerous cells with long-standing hyperprolactinemia (68). Therefore, women taking antipsychotic drugs that cause hyperprolactinemia need ongoing breast monitoring and bone density scanning (69).

Hyperprolactinemia is also associated with sexual dysfunction, lowered libido, poor vaginal lubrication, and anorgasmia. Adding estrogen treatment or testosterone treatment to the antipsychotic medication may assist these sexual dysfunction problems in post- and premenopausal women (70,71). High prolactin levels can also cause anovulatory menstrual cycles and hence infertility, which may require changing medication if the woman wishes to become pregnant (72).

Weight gain and diabetes

As detailed in chapter 6, many antipsychotics are associated with weight gain and, as a frequent result, the development of diabetes mellitus. Atypical antipsychotics are associated with weight gain, hyperlipidemia and glucose intolerance (73). The impact of the peptide hormones leptin, ghrelin, and adinopectin are important in the regulation of weight and other metabolic factors. Leptin is produced by adipose cells and plays a key role in CNS feedback mechanisms to control appetite and metabolism (74). Antipsychotics such as clozapine and olanzapine have been shown to increase serum leptin, which in turn, creates an increase in adipose cells with a further rise in leptin (75). This effect is amplified in women, who on an average have more adipose tissue than men and a relatively elevated serum leptin (76). Although many interventions have been proposed and are under investigation to treat weight gain in this population, there is no clear solution to the problem of medication-related weight gain (chap. 6). Patients need to be carefully monitored and advised in advance as to the benefits of increased physical activity and appropriate dietary alterations. The capacity of patients, especially those with negative symptoms, to make lifestyle changes, however, may be relatively limited. Fortunately, it appears that some of the newer antipsychotic medications may not have weight gain side effects, but further clinical experience with such drugs is required before being able confidently to change antipsychotic regimens in order to prevent or reverse weight gain.

Specific antipsychotic medications, their known side effects and management recommendations in women are detailed in Table 13.1.

Treatment of affective symptoms

Women patients have briefer and fewer hospitalizations than men during their reproductive years and may have, during this period, a less severe course of illness (78,79). They also have more mood features, fewer negative symptoms, and better preserved social skills. Women initially presenting with what appears to be a nonaffective psychosis are more likely than men to be subsequently diagnosed with a mood disorder (80). Because of the frequent affective component to their illness, women with schizophrenia may respond to mood stabilizers, and, as a result, antipsychotic doses may be able to be kept relatively low. Many mood stabilizers have important pregnancy contraindications that are important to remember. Similarly, the use of antidepressant medication in addition to antipsychotic medication may be a common occurrence in the clinical management of women with schizophrenia. In this situation, drug interactions and the side-effect profiles of both classes of drugs need to be considered.

Psychological treatments for women with schizophrenia

Traditionally, psychological treatments have not been specially tailored for a particular gender. In view of the large number of women who have traumatic childhoods or have experienced sexual abuse prior to developing schizophrenia, it is important to appropriately use specialized techniques such as dialectical behavioral therapy (81). As outlined in chapter 2, the treatment of persistent symptoms with cognitive–behavioral therapy is a useful adjunctive

Table 13.1   Issues of side effects of some antipsychotics, education, and women with schizophrenia[a]

Antipsychotic medication	Major side effects for women	Recommendations
Haloperidol	Extrapyramidal side effects (EPSEs)	Concomitant use of benztropine
	Tardive dyskinesia with long-term use	Use lowest possible does of haloperidol to minimize movement disorder
Chlorpromazine	Excess sedation, weight gain, sun sensitivity, some EPSEs	Use intermittently for sedation at the lowest dose possible
Olanzapine	Weight gain	If weight gain is more than 10 kg and continues after 3 months, change the antipsychotic medication
	Increased rise of diabetes	Advise about diet and exercise; monitor serum glucose
Risperidone	Hyperprolactinemia leading to potential osteoporosis	Monitor prolactin levels, bone density; regular breast screening; consider adding estrogen or changing drug if level very high
	Theoretical increase in risk of breast cancer	Regular breast screening; genetic test for breast cancer risk; change antipsychotic if breast screening is abnormal, or if a high genetic risk of breast cancer
	Possible infertility	Change medication if conception is difficult
	Sexual dysfunction (decreased libido, poor lubrication, and anorgasmia)	Use of lubricants; consider adding testosterone/ estrogen/progesterone
Quetiapine	Weight gain	Advise about healthy diet and exercise. Change medication if weight gain continues
	Hyperlipidemia	Treat with anticholesterol medication, if dietary changes insufficient

(*Continued*)

Table 13.1   Issues of side effects of some antipsychotics, education, and women with schizophrenia[a] *(Continued)*

Aripiprazole	Agitation, insomnia	Administer drug in morning; lower the dose if needed
	Unexpected new behaviors e.g., addictions such as gambling	Consider change in medication
Ziprasidone	Sedation	Administer medication at night; lower the dose if possible
	Cardiac adverse effects/QT interval prolongation	Regular cardiac monitoring with EKG and echocardiogram
Asenapine	Insufficient clinical experience	
Clozapine	Weight gain	Dietary/exercise advice. If no other option, consider using metformin treatment
	Blood dyscrasias (agranulocytosis)	Regular blood monitoring (chap. 1)
	Cardiomyopathy, myocarditis	Regular EKGs and echocardiograms (chap. 1)
	Sialorrhea	Anticholinergic drugs

[a]The list is not an exhaustive one but provides examples of special medication issues faced by women with schizophrenia (77).

therapy (82). In working with women, specific empowerment issues may need to be addressed (83). Techniques aimed at coming to terms with illness, loss and understanding the social context of femininity are some of the newer approaches that address gender-specific issues.

The response to inpatient family intervention, in a well-designed randomized trial, has been shown to be superior in women relative to men (84), but illness duration may be an important confounder (85). Cognitive remediation techniques (chap. 11) are useful for work skilling programs for women. Women with longer-term schizophrenia may have specific difficulties about entering/re-entering the workforce and specific attention needs to be paid to upskilling women in areas such as computer technology, among other work domains.

It is rare for schizophrenia recovery programs to focus on parenting skills, but for women with schizophrenia who may have lost custody of their children due to their illness this is a key skill which may be needed to be taught in order to regain access to their children. While developing new recovery programs, the inclusion of mothering skills training should have a high priority (86).

Service provision for women with schizophrenia

Women with schizophrenia are being managed more and more out of the hospital setting, as community psychiatry has become the standard mode of service provision. However, people with schizophrenia do need hospitalization from time to time to treat acute psychosis relapses. Over time, the public sector psychiatry wards in many jurisdictions have come to house more acutely and severely ill patients. This raises many issues for women with schizophrenia. Women report more fear of being attacked and hurt so that safety issues on wards and in outpatient programs become important concerns for them (87).

In Western countries, most psychiatry wards contain men and women patients in the same ward setting. Women with schizophrenia sometimes have a history of domestic abuse and living in mixed gender wards with disinhibited male patients can create situations that may retraumatize them. Sexual and other assaults have occurred on inpatient units. Women inpatients experience the majority of such assaults (88). In 2006, the National Patient Safety Agency in the United Kingdom published a detailed analysis of mental health patient safety incidents between November 2003 and September 2005. There were 122 sexual assault incidents reported and key recommendations from this report resulted in the United Kingdom adopting a policy of gender segregation on psychiatric wards (88). This is a new trend in psychiatry ward design and will, it is hoped, improve the inpatient treatment experience for women with mental illness. Clinicians have a duty of care to manage their female patients safely and in an environment that promotes recovery.

It is increasingly recognized that the therapeutic relationships formed by patients with schizophrenia play an important role in the recovery process. Schizophrenia, and in particular negative symptoms, affects the capacity of patients to form and maintain interpersonal relationships that may buffer stressful life experiences. Female patients are often better able to form therapeutic relationships but may be more sensitive to frequent alterations in healthcare providers, a situation that often occurs in public mental health services.

Treating women with schizophrenia may require more personal involvement on the part of the clinician and more attention paid to the continuity of therapeutic relationships.

Longer–term outcomes

Overall, the severity of illness expression is less debilitating in women than men during the first decade following onset, but it worsens in subsequent years and eventually approximates to that of men (89). The marital rates of men, presumably reflecting the age of onset but also the contrasting roles that men and women assume during courtship, almost always have been shown to be lower than those of women (90). Homelessness, suicide, and being the victim of homicide are further outcome variables that are reported to favor women over men, but this may be culture specific (91).

Conclusions

There are many gender differences in the presentation of schizophrenia. Compared with men, women with schizophrenia tend to experience a later age of illness onset, differences in symptom presentation and differences in disease incidence and prevalence. Based on these epidemiological findings, several important biological hypotheses have been put forward to explain the differences. The "estrogen protection" hypothesis is a key one. Other hypothesis about the genetic transmission of schizophrenia stems from observing gender differences (92). Cognitive differences between the sexes are important bases for both the treatment and understanding of the etiology of schizophrenia (93).

There is now ample evidence to show that schizophrenia in women has a different course and outcome compared with men with this illness. There may also be gonadal hormone "triggers" for relapse in women (94).

Managing women with schizophrenia requires new approaches that have a clear gender focus. In this way, more specific, better tailored treatments for women with schizophrenia can be developed and implemented to provide better outcomes for women.

References

1. Yung AR, Nelson B, Thompson A, Wood SJ. The psychosis threshold in Ultra High Risk (prodromal) research: is it valid? Schizophr Res 2010; 120: 1–6.
2. Wood SJ, Berger GE, Lambert M, et al. Prediction of functional outcome 18 months after a first psychotic episode: a proton magnetic resonance spectroscopy study. Arch Gen Psychiatry 2006; 63: 969–76.
3. Walker E, Bollini A. Pubertal neurodevelopment and the emergence of psychotic symptoms. Schizophr Res 2002; 1: 17–23.
4. Angermeyer MC, Kuhn L. Gender differences in age at onset of schizophrenia. An overview. Eur Arch Psychiatry Neurol Sci 1988; 237: 351–64.
5. Beratis S, Gabriel J, Hoidas S. Age at onset in subtypes of schizophrenic disorders. Schizophr Bull 1994; 20: 287–96.
6. Lewine R. At issue: sex and gender in schizophrenia. Schizophr Bull 2004; 30: 755–62.
7. Gómez-de-Regil L, Kwapil TR, Blanqué JM, et al. Predictors of outcome in the early course of first-episode psychosis. Eur J Psychiatry 2010; 24: 87–97.
8. Hafner H, Hambrecht M, Loffler W, Munk-Jorgensen P, Riecher-Rossler A. Is schizophrenia a disorder of all ages? A comparison of first episodes and early course across the life-cycle. Psychol Med 1998; 28: 351–65.
9. Hafner H, an der Heiden W, Behrens S, et al. Causes and consequences of the gender difference in age at onset of schizophrenia. Schizophr Bull 1998; 24: 99–113.

10. Hafner H, Maurer K, Loffler W, et al. The epidemiology of early schizophrenia. Influence of age and gender on onset and early course. Br J Psychiatry 1994; 23(Suppl): 29–38.
11. Castle DJ, Wessely S, Murray RM. Sex and schizophrenia: effects of diagnostic stringency, and associations with and premorbid variables. Br J Psychiatry 1993; 162: 658–64.
12. Seeman MV, Lang M. The role of estrogens in schizophrenia gender differences. Schizophr Bull 1990; 16: 185–94.
13. Hafner H, Behrens S, De Vry J, Gattaz WF. An animal model for the effects of estradiol on dopamine-mediated behavior: implications for sex differences in schizophrenia. Psychiatry Res 1991; 38: 125–34.
14. Seeman MV. Gender differences in schizophrenia. Can J Psychiatry 1982; 27: 107–12.
15. Behl C. Oestrogen as a neuroprotective hormone. Nat Rev Neurosci 2002; 3: 433–42.
16. McEwen BS. Invited review: estrogens effects on the brain: multiple sites and molecular mechanisms. J Appl Physiol 2001; 91: 2785–801.
17. Taber KH, Murphy DD, Blurton-Jones MM, Hurley RA. An update on estrogen: higher cognitive function, receptor mapping, neurotrophic effects. J Neuropsychiatry Clin Neurosci 2001; 13: 313–17.
18. Ostlund H, Keller E, Hurd YL. Estrogen receptor gene expression in relation to neuropsychiatric disorders. Ann NY Acad Sci 2003; 1007: 54–63.
19. Kritzer MF, Kohama SG. Ovarian hormones differentially influence immunoreactivity for dopamine beta- hydroxylase, choline acetyltransferase, and serotonin in the dorsolateral prefrontal cortex of adult rhesus monkeys. J Comp Neurol 1999; 409: 438–51.
20. Bethea CL, Lu NZ, Gundlah C, Streicher JM. Diverse actions of ovarian steroids in the serotonin neural system. Front Neuroendocrinol 2002; 23: 41–100.
21. Dluzen D, Horstink M. Estrogen as neuroprotectant of nigrostriatal dopaminergic system: laboratory and clinical studies. Endocrine 2003; 21: 67–75.
22. Ohtani H, Nomoto M, Douchi T. Chronic estrogen treatment replaces striatal dopaminergic function in ovariectomized rats. Brain Res 2001; 900: 163–8.
23. Disshon KA, Boja JW, Dluzen DE. Inhibition of striatal dopamine transporter activity by 17beta-estradiol. Eur J Pharmacol 1998; 345: 207–11.
24. Amin Z, Canli T, Epperson CN. Effect of estrogen-serotonin interactions on mood and cognition. Behav Cogn Neurosci Rev 2005; 4: 43–58.
25. Riecher-Rossler A, Hafner H, Stumbaum M, Maurer K, Schmidt R. Can estradiol modulate schizophrenic symptomatology? Schizophr Bull 1994; 20: 203–14.
26. Riecher-Rossler A, Hafner H, Dutsch-Strobel A, et al. Further evidence for a specific role of estradiol in schizophrenia? Biol Psychiatry 1994; 36: 492–4.
27. Hallonquist J, Seeman M, Lang M, Rector N. Variation in symptom severity over the menstrual cycle of schizophrenics. Biol Psychiatry 1993; 33: 207–9.
28. Endo M, Daiguji M, Asano Y, Yaniashita I, Lakahaashi S. Periodic psychosis occurring in association with her menstrual cycle. J Clin Psychiatry 1978; 39: 456–61.
29. Bergemann N, Mundt C, Parzer P, et al. Estrogen as an adjuvant therapy to antipsychotics does not prevent relapse in women suffering from schizophrenia: results of a placebo-controlled double-blind study. Schizophr Res 2005; 74: 125–34.
30. Hoff AL, Kremen WS, Wieneke MH, et al. Association of estrogen levels with neuropsychological performance in women with schizophrenia. Am J Psychiatry 2001; 158: 1134–9.
31. Seeman MV. Current outcome in schizophrenia: women vs men. Acta Psychiatr Scand 1986; 73: 609–17.
32. Gattaz WF Vogel P, Riecher-Rossler A, Soddu G. Influence of the menstrual cycle phase on the therapeutic response in schizophrenia. Biol Psychiatry 1994; 36: 137–9.

33. Kulkarni J, de Castella A, Smith D, et al. A clinical trial of the effects of estrogen in acutely psychotic women. Schizophr Res 1996; 20: 247–52.
34. Kulkarni J, de Castella A, Fitzgerald PB, et al. Estrogen in severe mental illness: a potential new treatment approach. Arch Gen Psychiatry 2008; 65: 955–60.
35. Kulkarni J, Gurvich C, Lee SJ, et al. Piloting the effective therapeutic dose of adjunctive selective estrogen receptor modulator treatment in postmenopausal women with schizophrenia. Psychoneuroendocrinology 2010; 35: 1142–7.
36. Miller L. Sexuality, reproduction, and family planning in women with schizophrenia. Schizophr Bull 1997; 23: 623–35.
37. Miller LJ, Finnerty M. Family planning knowledge, attitudes and practices in women with schizophrenic spectrum disorders. J Psychosom Obstet Gynaecol 1998; 19: 210–17.
38. Dunsis A Smith GC. Consultation – liaison psychiatry in an obstetric service. Aust NZ J Psychiatry 1996; 30: 63–73.
39. Bennedsen BE, Mortensen PB, Olesen AV, Henriksen TB, Frydenberg M. Obstetric complications in women with schizophrenia. Schizophr Res 2001; 47:167–75.
40. Kulkarni J McCauley-Elsom K, Marston N, Gilbert H, et al. Preliminary findings from the National Register of Antipsychotic Medications in Pregnancy. Aust NZ J Psychiatry 2008; 42: 38–44.
41. Monash Alfred Psychiatry Research Centre M. NRAMP. 2010 [cited 2011]. [Available from: http://www.maprc.org.au/nramp]].
42. Seeman MV. Schizophrenia and motherhood. In: Göpfert M, Webster J, Seeman MV, eds. Parental Psychiatric Disorder: Distressed Parents and their Families. 2nd edn. Cambridge, U.K: Cambridge University Press, 2004: 161–71.
43. Seeman MV. Does menopause intensify symptoms in schizophrenia? In: Lewis-Hall F, Williams TS, Panetta JA, Herrera JM, eds. Psychiatric Illness in Women: Emerging Treatments and Research. Washington, DC: American Psychiatric Press, 2002: 239–48.
44. Seeman MV. Narratives of twenty to thirty year outcomes in schizophrenia. Psychiatry 1998; 61: 249–61.
45. Fitzgerald P, Seeman M. Women and Schizophrenia – Treatment Implications. In: Castle D, McGrath J, Kulkarni J, eds. 1st edn. London: Cambridge University Press, 2000.
46. Soares CN. Practical strategies for diagnosing and treating depression in women: menopausal transition. J Clin Psychiatry 2008; 69: e30.
47. Seeman M. Neuroleptic prescription for men and women. Soc Pharmacol 1989; 3: 219–36.
48. Chlebowski RT, Col N, Winer EP, et al. American Society of Clinical Oncology technology assessment of pharmacologic interventions for breast cancer risk reduction including tamoxifen, raloxifene, and aromatase inhibition. J Clin Oncol 2002; 20: 3328–43.
49. Furniss K. The Women's Health Initiative. Implications for practice. Adv Nurse Pract 2002; 10: 53–5.
50. Nickelsen T, Lufkin EG, Riggs BL, Cox DA, Crook TH. Raloxifene hydrochloride, a selective estrogen receptor modulator: safety assessment of effects on cognitive function and mood in postmenopausal women. Psychoneuroendocrinology 1999; 24: 115–28.
51. McEvoy JP, Meyer JM, Goff DC, et al. Prevalence of the metabolic syndrome in patients with schizophrenia: baseline results from the Clinical Antipsychotic Trials of Intervention Effectiveness (CATIE) schizophrenia trial and comparison with national estimates from NHANES III. Schizophr Res 2005; 80: 19–32.
52. Seeman MV. Gender differences in the prescribing of antipsychotic drugs. Am J Psychiatry 2004; 161: 1324–33.

53. Seeman M. Sex differences in the prediction of neuroleptic response. In: Gaebel W, Awad A, eds. Prediction of Neuroleptic Treatment Outcome in Schizophrenia. Wien: Springer-Verlag, 1994: 51–64.

54. Seeman M. Schizophrenic men and women require different treatment programs. J Psychiatr Treat Eval 1983; 5: 143–8.

55. Casey DE. Neuroleptic drug induced extrapyramidal syndromes and tardive dyskinesia. Schizophr Res 1991; 4: 109–20.

56. Yassa R, Jeste D. Gender differences in tardive dyskinesia: A critical review of the literature. Schizophr Bull 1992; 18: 701–15.

57. Morgenstern H, Glaser W. Identifying risk factors for tardive dyskinesia among long term outpatients maintained with neuroleptic medication. Arch Gen Psychiatry 1993; 50: 723–33.

58. Services DoHaH. Guideline for the Format and Content of the Clinical and Statistical Sections of New Drug Applications. In: Public Health Service FaDA, ed. Washington DC: Department of Health and Human Services, 1988.

59. Chaves AC, Seeman MV. Sex selection bias in schizophrenia antipsychotic trials. J Clin Psychopharmacol 2006; 26: 489–94.

60. Yonkers KA, Kando JC, Cole JO, Blumenthal S. Gender differences in pharmacokinetics and pharmacodynamics of psychotropic medication. Am J Psychiatry 1992; 149: 587–95.

61. Kulkarni J, Gurvich C, Gilbert H, et al. Hormone modulation: a novel therapeutic approach for women with severe mental illness. Aust NZ J Psychiatry 2008; 42: 83–8.

62. Yassa R JD. Gender differences in tardive dyskinesia: a critical review of the literature. Schizophr Bull 1992; 18: 701–15.

63. Haack S, Seerunger A, Thurmann P, Becker T, Kirchheiner J. Sex-specific differences in side-effects of psychotropic drugs: genes or gender? Pharmacogenomics 2009; 10: 1511–26.

64. Zimmet P, Alberti KG, Shaw J. Global and societal implications of the diabetes epidemic. Nature 2001; 414: 782–7.

65. Petty RG. Prolactin and antipsychotic medications: mechanism of action. Schizophr Res 1999; 35(Suppl): S67–73.

66. Clevenger CPT. Prolactin as an autocrine/paracrine factor in breast tissue. J Mammary Gland Biol Neoplasia 1997; 2: 59–68.

67. Tworoger SS, Hankinson SE. Prolactin and breast cancer etiology: an epidemiological perspective. J Mammary Gland Biol Neoplasia 2008; 13: 41–53.

68. Maus M, Reilly S, Clevenger C. Prolactin as a chemo attractant for human breast cancer. Endocrinology 1999; 11: 5447–50.

69. Seeman MV. Preventing breast cancer in women with schizophrenia. Acta Psychiatr Scand 2011; 123: 107–17.

70. Davis S, Papalia M-A, Norman RJ, et al. Safety and efficacy of a testosterone metered-dose transdermal spray for treating decreased sexual satisfaction in premenopausal women: a randomized trial. Ann Intern Med 2008; 148: 569–77.

71. Davis SR, McCloud P, Strauss BJ, Burger H. Testosterone enhances estradiol's effects on postmenopausal bone density and sexuality. Maturitas 2008; 61: 17–26.

72. Seeman MV. Antipsychotic-induced amenorrhea. J Ment Health 2011; 20: 484–91.

73. Newcomer JW. Second-generation (atypical) antipsychotics and metabolic effects: a comprehensive literature review. CNS Drugs 2005; 19(Suppl 1): 1–93.

74. Jin H, Meyer JM, Mudaliar S, Jeste DV. Impact of atypical antipsychotic therapy on leptin, ghrelin, and adiponectin. Schizophr Res 2008; 100: 70–85.

75. Zhang ZJ, Yao ZJ, Liu W, Fang Q, Reynolds GP. Effects of antipsychotics on fat deposition and changes in leptin and insulin levels. Magnetic resonance imaging study

of previously untreated people with schizophrenia. Br J Psychiatry 2004; 184: 58–62.

76. Haupt DW, Luber A, Maeda J, et al. Plasma leptin and adiposity during antipsychotic treatment of schizophrenia. Neuropsychopharmacology 2005; 30: 184–91.

77. Kulkarni J, Inglis RJ. Road testing the newer antipsychotic agents. Aust Fam Physician 2006; 35: 96–9.

78. Goldstein JM. Gender differences in the course of schizophrenia. Am J Psychiatry 1988; 145: 684–9.

79. Lewine R. Sex differences in schizophrenia: timing of subtypes? Psychol Bull 1981; 90: 423–44.

80. Chaves AC, Addington J, Seeman M, Addington D. One-year stability of diagnosis in first-episode nonaffective psychosis: influence of sex. Can J Psychiatry 2006; 51: 711–14.

81. Long CG, Fulton B, Dolley O, Hollin CR. Dealing with Feelings: the effectiveness of cognitive behavioural group treatment for women in secure settings. Behav Cogn Psychother 2011; 39: 243–7.

82. van der Gaag M, Stant AD, Wolters KJ, Buskens E, Wiersma D. Cognitive-behavioural therapy for persistent and recurrent psychosis in people with schizophrenia-spectrum disorder: cost-effectiveness analysis. Br J Psychiatry 2011; 198(Suppl 1): 59–65.

83. Notman M, Nadelson C. Psychoanalytic Perspectives. In: Romans S, Seeman M, eds. Ontario, Canada: Lippincott, Williams & Wilkins, 2006.

84. Haas G, Glick I, Clarkin J, Spencer J, Lewis A. Gender and schizophrenia outcome: A clinical trial of inpatient family intervention. Schizophr Bull 1990; 16: 277–92.

85. Glick I, Spencer J, Clarkin J, et al. A randomised clinical trial of inpatient family intervention. IV. Follow up results for subjects with schizophrenia. Schizophr Res 1990; 3: 187–200.

86. Seeman MV. Intervention to prevent child custody loss in mothers with schizophrenia. Schizophr Res Treat 2012; doi: 10.1155/2012/796763.

87. Seeman MV. Single-sex psychiatric services to protect women. Medscape Womens Health J 2002; 7: 4.

88. Johnson M. National patient safety report. J Adult Prot 2006; 8: 36–8.

89. Opjordsmoen S. Long-term clinical outcome of schizophrenia with special reference to gender differences. Acta Psychiatr Scand 1991; 83: 307–13.

90. Nimgaonkar V, Ward S, Agarde H, Weston N, Ganguli R. Fertility in schizophrenia: results from a contemporary US cohort. Acta Psychiatr Scand 1997; 95: 364–9.

91. Phillips MR, Yang G, Li S, Li Y. Suicide and the unique prevalence pattern of schizophrenia in mainland China: a retrospective observational study. Lancet 2004; 364: 1062–8.

92. Goldstein J, Faraone S, Chen W, Tsuang M. Genetic heterogeneity may in part explain sex differences in the familial risk for schizophrenia. Biol Psychiatry 1995; 38: 808–13.

93. Goldstein JM, Seidman LJ, Goodman JM. Are there sex differences in neuropsychological functions among patients with schizophrenia? Am J Psychiatry 1998; 155: 1358–64.

94. Seeman MV. Menstrual exacerbations of schizophrenia symptoms. Acta Psychiatr Scand 2012; doi: 10.1111/j.1600-0447.2011.01822.x.

chapter 14

Schizophrenia in later life

Nicola Lautenschlager, Peter Rabins, and David J. Castle

There are two broad groups of elderly people with schizophrenia, namely those with an early-onset illness who have grown old (sometimes called "graduates"), and those who have had their onset in later life. The latter group is particularly fascinating as the onset of schizophrenia in the later years seems difficult to reconcile with the neurodevelopmental model that pervades our understanding of the younger-onset form of the illness (1). There are some researchers (e.g., the International Late-Onset Schizophrenia Group) (2) who propose that there are at least two subtypes of late-onset schizophrenia (LOS), namely those with onset between 40 and 60 years of age (which they term "late-onset schizophrenia") and those with an onset after the age of 60 ("very-late-onset schizophrenia-like psychosis"). Studies have often not differentiated these different putative groups, and nosological and other issues make the literature on LOS patients complex to negotiate. This chapter takes a pragmatic view and focuses on the clinical issues pertinent to elderly people with schizophrenia. For ease, we use the term "late-onset schizophrenia" (LOS) broadly and without prejudice, but delineate where relevant, very late-onset patients.

Epidemiology and risk factors

It is beyond doubt that a form of forms of schizophrenia can onset in late life. Harris and Jeste (3) in a review of the literature, computed weighted means (based on a sample size) of 23.5% of schizophrenia patients having an onset after age 40, of whom 57.5% had their onset in the fifth decade, 30.2% in the sixth decade, and 12.3% after 60: this represents around 13%, 7%, and 3% of all schizophrenia patients, respectively.

There are but few competent prevalence and incidence studies of LOS, in part because of the difficulty in case ascertainment and diagnosis, and in part due to the difficulties in excluding individuals who exhibit psychotic symptoms as part of a dementing process (see below). Of the *prevalence studies*, Kua et al. (4) used the GMS-AGECAT in a Singaporean sample of 612 community-dwelling individuals over the age of 60, and reported an incidence of 0.5% for schizophrenia/paranoia. However, using the same diagnostic criteria in

Liverpool, United Kingdom, Copeland et al. (5) found an incidence of schizophrenia of only 0.12% among 5222 elderly individuals ascertained through general practitioner lists. In the Liverpool study, the *incidence rate* was estimated at 3.0 per 100,000 per year. Castle and Murray (6) used the comprehensive Camberwell Psychiatric Case Register (SE London, United Kingdom) to ascertain all cases of nonaffective psychosis over 20 years from the mid-1960s, irrespective of age at onset, and found 28% had an onset after age 44 years, and 12% after age 60 years; relevant incidence rates for DSM-IIIR defined schizophrenia were 12.6 per 100,000 after age 44 years. Henderson and Kay (7) have reviewed the epidemiology of LOS and related disorders, and provide a useful summary, as shown in Box 14.1.

In terms of *risk factors*, some genetic loading for schizophrenia has been described in most studies that have ascertained this, and there is a suggestion in some studies that the later onset "breeds true," albeit data regarding this are modest (8–11). This is a methodologically difficult area not least due to lack of reliable informant information, but it is reasonable to conclude that the genetic loading for schizophrenia is rather lower than in the early-onset cases. Howard et al. (12) also found an increased family risk for affective disorders in probands with LOS, but this has not been consistently found in other studies. Other potential risk factors, with varying consistency of support in the literature, are shown in Box 14.2 (9,13,14): of course, some of these associations might be a reflection of the illness itself rather than simply a causal factor (e.g., social isolation). Presumably a number of these factors co-aggregate to "produce" the illness in susceptible individuals. The aging brain would be part of this process. Of interest,

---

Box 14.1   Summary of the epidemiology of late-onset schizophrenia.

- Rates are low compared to the dementias
- The prevalence is probably lower than the expected 1%, possibly due to selective mortality
- Among the elderly, there is a suggestion of increasing prevalence with age
- Few studies have ascertained both prevalent and incident cases
- Psychotic symptoms are much more common in the elderly, than diagnoses
- Rates are universally higher in women, markedly so in the very late-onset group
- Reported rates are likely underestimates due to underreporting and other methodological problems
- Impaired hearing and vision are associated with late-onset psychosis
- Social isolation is an associated feature
- Physical health is reportedly poor
- There is almost certainly substantial unmet treatment need among this group

Source: From Ref. 7

> **Box 14.2** Risk factors for late-onset schizophrenia.
>
> - Family history of schizophrenia (fairly consistent)
> - Family history of affective illness (few studies)
> - Female gender (very consistent and very pronounced in very late onset)
> - Sensory impairment (uncorrected vision, hearing difficulties)
> - Social isolation (consistent, but may in part reflect illness process)
> - Poor premorbid social adjustment (fairly consistent)
> - Reasonable premorbid occupational adjustment (reasonably consistent)

for example, are findings that LOS patients show larger brain ventricular volumes than controls, and larger thalamic volumes than early-onset schizophrenia patients, suggesting a role for disruption in thalamocortical circuitry (15).

Symptoms

The syndrome of schizophrenia is characterized by at least four relatively distinct elements: positive symptoms, disorganization, negative symptoms, and cognitive symptoms (16). The positive symptoms are hallucinations and delusions. Disorganization is characterized by formal thought disorder, disorganized behavior, and inappropriate affect. The negative symptoms include loss of initiative, decline in occupational and social function, asocial behavior, and decline in social status and restriction of affect. The cognitive symptoms encompass a set of impairments that are included in the syndrome of impaired executive function. The question of whether LOS-like psychosis is the same syndrome as that of the early-onset condition rests on which characteristics of this syndrome one requires (8,9,17). Table 14.1 summarizes the differences between early and LOS in terms of phenomenological and other domains.

Positive Symptoms

Delusions, fixed, false idiosyncratic beliefs, are prominent in LOS. These are characteristically persecutory or "paranoid" in nature and often consist of the belief that neighbors, government officials or, family members are unfairly accusing the patient of misdeeds. The delusion that objects are being stolen from the patient is also common. These stolen items are often inconsequential and include taking sugar or salt from the table or moving objects in the kitchen so that it is harder for the patient to find them.

It is sometimes difficult to establish whether these strongly held and incorrigible (i.e., the patient cannot be talked out of them) beliefs are truly false. Examples include the claim that money, clothing, or other objects have been stolen or that the person has been abused or neglected in some way. These

Table 14.1 Comparison of early and late-onset schizophrenia

	Early onset	*Late onset*
Sex ratio	~1:1	~7:1 F:M
Premorbid personality	Greater prevalence of schizoid/schizotypal traits than population	Greater prevalence of schizoid/schizotypal traits than population
Hallucinations	Predominantly auditory First-rank tactile experiences common	Auditory common Nonauditory (olfactory, tactile, visual) common
Delusions	Complex persecutory delusions common	Complex persecutory delusions common
Thought disorder	Common	Rare
Negative symptoms	Prominent on long-term follow-up	Less common but long-term follow-up data lacking
Imaging	Enlarged 3rd ventricle, temporal lobe atrophy	Enlarged 3rd ventricle, temporal lobe atrophy

beliefs are often stated with such conviction and in such a way that it is difficult to disprove them; it is thus important for the clinician to be open minded to the possibility that abuse is possible; sometimes there is no support for the belief, for example claims of physical abuse without bruises or other evidence supporting the claim; claims that large sums of money have been taken when the person is not likely to have such resources; or preposterous content that could not possibly be true. When such a claim is made in the presence of other delusions that are clearly false it is much more likely that that claim, also, is false, but delusions and abuse can co-occur. The requirement that delusions be "bizarre" is not always useful. Patients can frame clearly false ideas in a fashion as to make them plausible. For example, the claim that the secret police or government agents are out to harm a person is highly likely to be untrue but whether it is bizarre is a matter of opinion and thus not a useful descriptor.

A common delusion is the belief that someone is repeatedly breaking into a person's home or apartment. This may seem plausible when it is claimed that a person such as an apartment manager who might have a key must be the person carrying out the act, but the claim that this is repeatedly happening, that the objects being stolen or moved are inconsequential, or have occurred in different places greatly diminish their plausibility and convince the clinician that these are delusional beliefs.

The characteristic *hallucinations* in schizophrenia are in the *auditory* realm and auditory hallucinations are prominent in patients with LOS. These are usually "first rank" in nature. That is, they often consist of one or several voices that patients locate as coming from outside their head and through their ears. These voices frequently talk about the person in the third person and may comment on their actions. One characteristic of the auditory hallucinations in LOS that is unusual in early-onset schizophrenia is that the hallucinations are sometimes described as indistinct noises or tappings. These are often located by the patient as coming from the ceiling, roof or the other side of a wall. They might be ascribed to mice.

Nonauditory hallucinations are more common in LOS than in classic schizophrenia. *Olfactory* hallucinations, commonly the belief that gas is being pumped into a person's living quarters, are common and raise the possibility of temporal lobe/complex partial seizures. *Tactile* hallucinations are also common. These often have the characteristics of so-called passivity experiences, in which the person has the experience that something is being done to them. The belief that a machine or other source is sending rays or electronic sensations into the patient's body is an example. These often have an intense and distressing tactile component, and are often described as targeting sexual organs.

A common characteristic of these multimodal hallucinations is captured in the term "partition experiences." This refers to the fact that hallucinations in many modalities are described as coming through the walls. For example, the person may claim that they are hearing neighbors and voices on the other side of a wall or coming through the floor or ceiling from another apartment. The same is true for the tactile experiences, visual hallucinations, and delusions, for example, when a person is described as having the ability to pass through walls, ceilings, or floors and carrying out the undesirable act.

Disorganization

Thought disorder is extremely uncommon in LOS (9). This fact is sometimes used as evidence that the illness is different from schizophrenia of early onset. However, it is of note that many individuals with young-onset schizophrenia do not have thought disorder and it is further noted that it has been difficult to establish clinician reliability for the identification and specification of thought disorder.

Nonetheless, the fact that thought disorder is so uncommon in persons with LOS suggests that if the disease starts after the neurobiologic system that underlies speech and language is established then this symptom will not develop. This could be cited as one piece of evidence of a different etiology but other explanations are plausible.

Negative symptoms

The term "paraphrenia" was introduced by Emil Kraeplin to include a subgroup of individuals who had the positive symptoms of dementia praecox or schizophrenia but lacked the social deterioration and dilapidation that he identified as characteristic of the illness. However, in the last edition of his textbook, published in 1919, he noted that his student Mayer had found high rates of social dilapidation in long-term follow-up of a proportion of individuals who had this "paraphrenic" presentation.

Case series of persons with LOS describe intact personality and lack of social dilapidation as characteristic. Since many of these studies describe individuals relatively close to the onset of the disease, and since social deterioration may be a later manifestation of the disease no matter at what age it starts, it remains unclear whether negative symptoms are truly less common in the last-onset condition or not present at onset. Having said this, the relative preservation of affect suggests that the LOS patients have less "core" negative symptomatology that their early-onset counterparts (9). Functional and social decline have been found in longer term follow-up studies (17), but whether the rates are the same as in younger individuals has yet to be established.

Because many individuals with LOS have either never worked or have retired, it can be more difficult to discern whether there has been occupational impairment or dysfunction induced by the illness. Likewise, elderly individuals often lose friends and relatives to death or become less socially active because of the imposition of physical impairments. Thus, decline in social function can also be difficult to establish or may be attributable to non-disease factors. Thus, it is useful to distinguish between the description of social decline (whether it is present or not) and to note that it may be attributed to environmental or physical factors unrelated to the primary psychiatric illness.

Cognitive symptoms

The cognitive impairments found in persons with LOS present a clinical challenge, since dementia due to a neurodegenerative process is often in the differential diagnosis. Roth's (18) initial delineation of what he called "late paraphrenia" rested largely on the fact that the majority of these patients do not dement. This finding has largely been replicated (17), albeit there is other evidence to show that at least a proportion of them do show cognitive decline in certain domains, as they age. For example, Harvey et al. (19) found that around 30% of 126 elderly schizophrenia patients who had evidence of cognitive dysfunction at baseline showed further deterioration in Clinical Dementia Rating scores at a 30-month follow-up. Risk factors for deterioration included lower levels of education, older age, and more severe positive symptoms.

In the clinical setting, it is crucial to exclude organic factors in an elderly person presenting for the first time with psychotic symptoms. Delirium can be chronic and is often missed if not specifically look for. If the pattern of neuropsychological impairments suggests Alzheimer disease—that is, prominent memory impairment plus aphasia, apraxia, or agnosia—then it is likely that Alzheimer disease is the source of the cognitive disorder and, if the clinical course suggests concomitant onset of positive symptoms and cognitive symptoms, the cause of the positive symptoms. Likewise, if a brain imaging investigations reveal evidence of stroke (not just white matter hyperintensities) and the clinical examination supports a diagnosis of vascular dementia, then schizophrenia should not be diagnosed. Visual hallucinations, mild parkinsonism, and a cognitive impairment pattern including visuospatial impairment suggest dementia with Lewy bodies.

More challenging clinically is the presence of impairments in executive function without prominent abnormalities in other realms of cognition. Such abnormalities are compatible with schizophrenia, although they can be found in frontotemporal lobar dementia, behavioral subtype, focal injury to the frontal lobes, or other disease that preferentially impair frontal-subcortical brain systems.

Management

As in general in old age psychiatry the usual aim of a management plan is to help the patient live as long as possible independent in the community. The management of schizophrenia in later life is complex as the clinical picture and the psychiatric history can be variable (20–22). Many elderly patients with schizophrenia are socially isolated and many have few family contacts. An additional challenge is that collateral information is often not available since patients frequently do not have a regular family doctor. Therefore, a frequent clinical scenario is that treatment needs to be initiated without detailed knowledge about the patient's premorbid state, past psychiatric history, or available social supports. Another important practical factor is the frequent need to build rapport and trust gradually by clinical outpatient teams where patients live because they live isolated lives and lack insight. This often requires a slow and gradual approach that differs somewhat from that adopted with younger individuals with schizophrenia. The "shared care" model is the preferred approach to older schizophrenia patients living in the community with the family doctor, the specialist team, and family members and friends (if available) sharing the responsibility to work toward realizing the management plan. In this context a multidisciplinary team approach has proven to be effective to improve outcomes and to reduce acute episodes which require emergency treatment.

A specific challenge occurs when the patient is in need of residential care due to increasing frailty. Patients with schizophrenia often have difficulties settling into main stream residential care facilities because the staff members rarely have the specific training needed to establish trust and avoid exacerbating symptoms. Some countries, therefore, developed specific psychogeriatric nursing homes with specifically trained staff and access to psychogeriatricians.

Almost all older patients with schizophrenia have prominent physical health problems that they have not attended to, in part because of their schizophrenia (chap. 6). In the case of individuals with early-onset schizophrenia who have grown old, this is frequently due to an unhealthy lifestyle over many decades, limited primary care access, and long-term side effects of pharmacological treatment. Therefore, a thorough medical workup that can identify medical problems and initiate or optimize treatment should be an essential component of the management plan. This may necessitate the treatment team advocating that the patient's medical needs to be addressed by the care system concomitantly with the treatment of the psychiatric symptoms. Older patients with schizophrenia should be encouraged to adhere to a healthy lifestyle that includes engaging in physical activity, eating a healthy diet, undergoing regular checkups with the family doctor and avoiding smoking and excess alcohol or illicit substance use. Specific factors relevant to the occurrence of schizophrenia in late life (see above) including uncorrected sensory disturbance (visual, hearing) need to be addressed.

Pharmacological management

The optimal pharmacological management of patients with early-life schizophrenia grown old may differ from that for those with late- or very-late-onset schizophrenia (21–24). Any changes to the pharmacologic treatment regimen of individuals with chronic, life-long schizophrenia should be approached cautiously since the current treatment might have been devised after many "trial and error" treatment trials in the past; changing it might destabilize the patient. Therefore, changing medication should be done under close clinical observation, perhaps in a hospital environment. A common challenge is that individuals with chronic schizophrenia need a change of their antipsychotic medication regimen because of worsening side effects associated with growing older, even when the medication has been tolerated well for a long time. For example, increasing age might necessitate a downtitration of the dosage because of age-related metabolic changes, medication interactions, or the presence of other illnesses.

For LOS the aim should be to try atypical antipsychotics as first-line treatment due to their lower risk of tardive dyskinesia. However, the lack of antipsychotic trials in the elderly makes evidence-based treatment recommendations difficult. When selecting the antipsychotic medication clinicians should be particularly mindful of side effects that are more problematic in older people, such as for example anticholinergic potential, impaired glucose tolerance and diabetes, metabolic syndrome, parkinsonian symptoms, and falls. The current "black box" warning of increased mortality associated with antipsychotic medication use pertains to individuals with dementia, but the prescription of antipsychotic medications in patients with concomitant cerebrovascular disease and schizophrenia should also be done with caution and the potential risks explained to such patients and their family members (25).

Box 14.3 Summary of management issues risk for late-onset schizophrenia.

- Management is complex and a multidisciplinary team is helpful
- Often slow and gradual approach best in the community
- Shared care model is recommended
- Residential care placements need to be selected carefully
- Management should include a thorough medical workup
- Carefully approach medication changes for old patients with early-life schizophrenia
- If possible aim for using atypical antipsychotics
- Consider black box warnings in relation to cognitive impairment

There is little evidence to guide choosing between atypical antipsychotics other than considering the individual side-effect profile and the medical and psychiatric history of the patient. In general, polypharmacy should be avoided; dosages should be titrated carefully with, if possible, a simple and clear psychotropic regimen and frequent assessments for treatment response and presence of side effects are recommended.

Treatment response is not easy to predict on an individual level and often several treatment trials may be required to determine the optimal drug and dosage. Patients with poor treatment adherence or nonresponse may be treated with a depot antipsychotic agent, but the starting dose should be very low (26). At least a third of patients with late-onset or very-late-onset schizophrenia will not benefit from antipsychotic treatment and less than a half will reach complete remission. Good prognostic indicators include a well-adjusted premorbid personality, an existing social network and adherence to treatment. There is some limited evidence that the additional use of antidepressants can be helpful for the management of negative symptoms in some patients (chap. 3). Box 14.3. summarizes some recommendations for an optimal management plan.

Conclusions

A substantial minority of schizophrenia patients have their first manifestation of their illness in later life. They are joined by patients with an early-onset illness, who have grown old, to enter the realm of late-life psychotic disorders. These individuals have specific needs in terms of treatment, reflective of their age, isolation, and physical health problems. Services need to be responsive to these needs and patients treated in a holistic manner in conjunction with the multidisciplinary care team, inclusive of the general practitioner.

References

1. Murray RM, O'Callaghan E, Castle DJ, Lewis SW. A neurodevelopmental approach to the classification of schizophrenia. Schizophr Bull 1992; 18: 319–32.
2. Howard R, Rabins PV, Seeman MV, et al. Late-onset schizophrenia and very-late-onset schizophrenia-like psychosis: an international consensus. Am J Psychiatry 2000; 157: 172–8.
3. Harris JM, Jeste DV. Late onset schizophrenia: an overview. Schizophr Bull 1988; 14: 39–55.
4. Kua EHA. Community study of mental disorders in elderly Singaporean Chinese using the GMS-AGECAT package. Aust NZ J Psychiatry 1992; 26: 502–6.
5. Copeland JRM, Dewey ME, Scott A, et al. Schizophrenia and delusional disorder in older age: community prevalence, incidence, comorbididty and outcome. Schizophr Bull 1998; 24: 153–61.
6. Castle DJ, Murray RM. The epidemiology of late onset schizophrenia. Schizophr Bull 1993; 19: 691–700.
7. Henderson AS, Kay DWK. The epidemiology of functional psychoses of late onset. Eur Arch Psychiatry Clin Neurosci 1997; 247: 176–89.
8. Roth M, Kay DWK. Late paraphrenia: a variant of schizophrenia manifest in late life or an organic clinical syndrome? A review of recent evidence. Int J Geriatr Psychiatry 1998; 13: 775–84.
9. Howard R, Castle D, Wessely S, Murray R. A comparative study of 470 cases of early-onset and late-onset schizophrenia. Br J Psychiatry 1993; 163: 352–7.
10. Kay DWK, Roth M. Environmental and hereditary risk factors in the schizophrenias of old age (late paraphrenia) and their bearing on the general problem of causation in schizophrenia. J Ment Sci 1961; 107: 649–86.
11. Van Os J, Howard RM, Takei N, Murray RM. Increasing age is a risk factor for psychosis in the elderly. Soc Psychiatr Psychiatr Epidemiol 1995; 30: 161–4.
12. Howard RJ, Graham C, Sham P, et al. A controlled family study of late-onset non-affetcive psychosis (late paraphrenia). Br J Psychiatry 1997; 170: 511–14.
13. Pearlson GD, Kreger L, Rabins PV, et al. A chart review study of late-onset and early-onset schizophrenia. Am J Psychiatry 1989; 146: 1568–674.
14. Palmer BW, McClure FS, Jeste DV. Schizophrenia in late life: findings challenge traditional concepts. Harvard Rev Psychiatry 2001; 9: 51–8.
15. Corey-Bloom J, Jernigan T, Archibald S, et al. Quantitative magnetic resonance imaging of the brain in late-life schizophrenia. Am J Psychiatry 1995; 152: 447–9.
16. Liddle P, Carpenter WT, Crow T. Syndromes of schizophrenia. Br J Psychiatry 1994; 165: 721–7.
17. Rabins PV, Lavrisha M. Long-term follow-up and phenomenologic differences distinguish among late-onset schizophrenia, late life depression, and progressive dementia. Am J Geriatr Psychiatry 2003; 11: 589–94.
18. Roth M. The natural history of mental disorders in old age. J Ment Sci 1955; 101: 281–301.
19. Harvey PD, Silverman JM, Mohs RC, et al. Cognitive decline in late-life schizophrenia: a longitudinal study of geriatric chronically hospitalized patients. Biol Psychiatry 1999; 45: 32–40.
20. Cohen CI, Vahia I, Reyes P, et al. Schizophrenia in later life: clinical symptoms and social well-being. Psychiatr Serv 2008; 59: 232–4.
21. Jeste DV, Eastham JH, Lacro JP, et al. Management of late-life psychoses. J Clin Psychiatry 1996; 57: 39–45.
22. Wynn Owen PA, Castle DJ. Late-onset schizophrenia: epidemiology, diagnosis, management and outcomes. Drugs Aging 1999; 15: 81–9.

23. Sciolla A, Jeste DV. Use of antipsychotics in the elderly. Int J Psychiatry Clin Pract 1998; 2: S27–34.
24. Salzman C, Tune L. Neurolept treatment of late-life schizophrenia. Harvard Rev Psychiatry 2001; 9: 77–83.
25. Gareri P, De Fazio P, De Fazio S, et al. Adverse effects of atypical antipsychotics in the elderly: an overview. Drugs Aging 2006; 23: 937–56.
26. Massand PS, Gupta S. Long-acting injectible antipsychotics in the elderly: guidelines for effective use. Drugs Aging 2003; 20: 1099–110.

chapter 15

Family interventions in schizophrenia

Christine Barrowclough, Alison Ram, Chris Fassnidge, and Til Wykes

Families play an essential role in supporting people with long-term mental illness in the community. Over 60% of those with a first episode of a major mental illness return to live with relatives (1), and this would seem to reduce by only 10–20% when those with subsequent admissions are included (2). However, the carer role is often not an easy one and may be associated with considerable personal costs. In schizophrenia, estimates from different studies suggest that up to two-thirds of family members experience significant stress and subjective burden as a consequence of their caregiver role (3), with one recent study suggesting that positive symptoms represent the greatest strain on family members (4). Not only is such stress likely to affect the well being of the relatives and compromise their long-term ability to support the patient, but it may also have an impact on the course of the illness itself and on outcomes for the patient. Hence one of the most important advances in the treatment of schizophrenia in the last 25 years has been the development of family-based intervention programs. The efficacy of this form of treatment is now well established, with many randomized controlled trials having demonstrated the superiority of family intervention over routine care in terms of patient relapse and hospitalization outcomes (5,6). This chapter outlines the background to this area of work, summarizes the research findings to date, and draws attention to important areas for future development.

Background to family interventions in schizophrenia

The development of multifactorial models of the processes determining risk and relapse in schizophrenia provided the general rationale for the development of family interventions: these have been usefully reviewed by Clements and Turpin (7). These "stress–vulnerability" models emphasized the contribution of psychological and socioenvironmental stressors to the illness course and thereby opened up the way to psychological interventions. In particular, family interventions found much of their initial impetus in the research on expressed emotion (EE). High EE is assessed on the basis of a critical, hostile, or overinvolved attitude toward the patient on the part of a relative living in the same household. Early studies (8,9) found that when patients with schizophrenia were discharged home after being hospitalized for a relapse, their risk of subsequent relapse in the short term was greatly increased if one or more family members were assessed to be "high EE." These results have been replicated many times and a meta-analysis of 27 studies (10) confirmed the elevated risk of relapse for patients in high-EE households. This is supported by more recent research by Aguilera and colleagues (11) who extended this idea and identified that certain cultural aspects can mediate the way family factors relate to the course of schizophrenia. Thus, within the context of stress–vulnerability models, an individual's home (influenced by culture) may be viewed as an environment capable of influencing the illness for better or worse. If attributes of certain households are responsible for precipitating relapse, then they might be identified and modified with a resulting reduction in relapse rates. Throughout the last three decades a series of studies testing this theory have been reported: these are described next.

Family intervention studies

There have been several descriptive reviews of schizophrenia family intervention studies (12–16). Typically, the controlled trials in this area recruited families at the point of hospitalization of a relative for an acute episode of schizophrenia and began the family intervention when the patient was discharged back home. The intervention period lasted from 6 to 12 months, at the end of which patient relapse rates were compared between those who received the family intervention as an adjunct to routine care with those who received routine care only. Routine care included the use of prophylactic medication. A series of interventions were developed which differed on some important dimensions including the following:

- Location of the family sessions (home vs hospital base)
- Number of sessions offered
- Extent of the patient's involvement
- Precise content of the sessions
- Mode of delivery

Since there was no clear understanding of the mechanisms of patient relapse in the home environment, determining the content involved making assumptions about the kinds of problems associated with high-EE families which might contribute to stress. In practice, all of these studies assumed that families had inadequate knowledge or misunderstanding regarding the illness and placed an emphasis on educating relatives about schizophrenia as an essential

Table 15.1   Common goals for successful family therapy
Build up an alliance with relatives who care for the schizophrenic member
Reduce adverse family atmosphere
Enhance the problem-solving capacity of relatives
Decrease expressions of anger and guilt
Maintain reasonable expectations of patient performance
Set limits safeguarding relatives' own well being
Achieve changes in relatives' behavior and beliefs

Source: From Ref. 19.

component, to the extent that some reviewers have subsumed all family interventions under the category "psychoeducation." The other common area targeted was helping the family members to cope with symptom-related difficulties either by a specific problem-solving approach (17) or through the assessment of individual problems and the application of appropriate cognitive behavioral techniques (18). Despite differences in approaches, Mari and Streiner (19) have provided a useful summary of the common "ingredients" or "overall principles" of the treatments (Table 15.1).

Modifications to family interventions

Family interventions have been adapted to accommodate different needs and formats and this is discussed in detail.

First-episode families
Intervention at an early stage is important given that the onset of psychosis is associated with high levels of stress in relatives (20) and that this is a time when there are many concerns, yet families have less knowledge of psychosis to draw on. It is also an opportune time to engage families who are receptive to information and support (21,22). However, it is unclear whether early intervention treatments have long-term positive effects (23). The reader is also referred to chapter 17 for a detailed discussion of first-episode schizophrenia.

Substance use and psychosis
Levels of substance use in people with psychosis are high and this "dual diagnosis" presents many challenges to families. Specialist approaches to helping such families have been described elsewhere (24–26). The latter approach reported good outcomes when used alongside individual work with the patient in an RCT (27). The reader is referred to chapter 7 for a more detailed discussion of dual diagnosis.

Group family work

Group interventions for families have the advantage of allowing relatives to share experiences. Family groups were reported to have better outcomes than individual family work (28,29), although a meta-analysis (30) challenged this conclusion. Suffice to say that some individuals seem to gain particular assistance and solace from the ability to address their family issues in a group context.

Results from the studies

A number of meta-analytic reviews of family intervention studies in schizophrenia have been published (6,19,30–32). A review of 13 studies confirmed the findings from earlier descriptive accounts, concluding that family intervention as an adjunct to routine care decreases the frequency of relapse and hospitalization; and that these findings hold across the wide age ranges, sex differences, and variability in the length of illness found in the different studies. Moreover, the analysis suggested that these results generalize across care cultures where health systems are very different—trials from the United Kingdom, Australia, Europe, the People's Republic of China, and the United States were included. A more inclusive review (32) examined 25 studies spanning 20 years (1977–1997) and again this meta-analysis confirmed the superiority of family-treated patient relapse rates over control groups. The overall effect size was 0.20, corresponding to a decrease in relapse rate of 20% in patients where families received an intervention. Although this treatment effect may seem relatively modest, one must bear in mind that this analysis included studies where the intervention was extremely brief and with little resemblance to the intensive programs in the original studies where effect sizes were generally greater. For example, the studies of Falloon et al., Leff et al., and Tarrier et al. (Table 15.2) (33–35) demonstrated decreased relapse rates for family-treated patients of approximately 40%. The absence of treatment fidelity measures in many of these studies makes it difficult to judge quality control within or between studies. More recently, studies conducted in India, China, and Malaysia concluded that there was a significant improvement in patient symptoms and family functioning after family intervention was provided (36–38).

Further comparison analyses within the Pitschel-Walz et al.'s review (32) draw attention to some of the wide variations in the content and duration of programs in recent years. Longer-term interventions were more successful than briefer interventions, while more intensive family treatments were superior to more limited approaches (e.g., where relatives are offered little more than brief education sessions about schizophrenia). When families are provided with an effective "dose" in terms of duration and intensity of intervention there is evidence of the long-lasting effects from family treatment. Several studies (Table 15.2) found a significant difference remaining between the intervention and control groups at

2 years, and the 5- and 8-year follow-up data of Tarrier et al. (40) and McWilliams et al. (42) demonstrated how durable these effects can be. However, it must be emphasized that all the studies show that relapses increase with the number of years from termination of the intervention. The more recent meta-analysis (30) had conclusions in line with previous reviews: the efficacy of family interventions for reducing relapse was confirmed, although the effect of family interventions has generally decreased over the years. These authors suggest that, in part, this may be explained by the increased use of group formats.

One of the criticisms of family intervention studies has been its narrow focus on reductions in patient relapse and hospitalizations. Pitschel-Walz and colleagues (32) suggest that there are some indications that family interventions have an impact over a wide range of outcomes. *For carers*, these include a reduction in carer burden; a change from high to low EE status; and an improved knowledge about schizophrenia. *For patients* there is some evidence of better medication adherence (this effect would seem to be independent of the effect of family intervention) (39,43); improved quality of life; and better social adjustment. Several studies have also demonstrated that these improved outcomes are achieved with reduced costs to society (17,44,41).

Pilling et al. (30) note that the benefits for family members themselves (such as reduced stress and burden) have received relatively little attention. A recent trial (45) which focused primarily on improving carer outcomes did not produce encouraging results. These authors conclude that there is still uncertainty about the most effective interventions for improving well being in carers of people with psychotic disorders. More recent work has focused on validating a self-administered questionnaire that measures the quality of life of caregivers. This could be useful in improving the health of patients and the quality of life of caregivers, maintaining their ability to care and shift the focus to their health status (4).

Dissemination of family interventions

There have been attempts to disseminate the benefits of family intervention in schizophrenia into routine service delivery. This has been largely through training programs designed to provide clinicians, mainly community psychiatric nurses, with the knowledge and skills required to implement the family work (see Ref. (46) for a review of dissemination programs). Despite the solid evidence base for the efficacy of family-based psychological treatment programs in schizophrenia, and the efforts of the training programs, the implementation of family work in routine mental health services has been at best patchy. In particular, some clinicians in the United States are skeptical of the benefits of family therapy. This means patients are likely to receive family therapy more in the United Kingdom, and less so in the United States, due to U.K. clinicians having more faith in its efficacy (47).

Table 15.2   Controlled studies comparing family intervention with standard/alternative treatment for patients with schizophrenia (minimum 6 months' intervention)

Study	Treatment conditions	N	Type of family intervention	Duration of treatment	Relapse
Kottgen et al. 1984	1. FI, high EE. 2. RC, high EE. 3. Low EE	49	Psychodynamic groups	Up to 2 yr	2 yr: FI equal to RC either high or low EE families
Falloon et al. 1982 (33), 1985	1. Behavioral FI + individual patient treatment. 2. Individual pt treatment	36	Home-based behavioral FI	2 yr	2 yr: behavioral FI superior to individual management
Leff et al. 1982 (34), 1985	1. FI. 2. Routine care	24	Groups + individual sessions. High EE learning from low EE	9 mo	2 yr: FI better than RC
Hogarty et al. 1986, 1987 (39)	1. FI. 2. Social skills. 3. Combined FI + SS. 4. RC	180	Behavioral FI	Up to 2 yr	2 yr: FI better than RC or SS
Tarrier et al. 1988 (35), 1989, 1994 (40)	1. Cognitive–behavioral enactive and symbolic. 2. Education only. 3. RC	83	Cognitive behavioral FI (families' choice of home or clinic)	9 mo	2 yr: FI better than education or RC. Education and RC equal
Leff et al. 1990	1. Multiple-family psychoeducation and support. 2. Single family psychoeducation and support	23	Multiple-family groups in the clinic. single family sessions at home	1 yr	16 mo: conditions equal

Study	Interventions	N	Description	Duration	Outcome
Mingyuan et al. 1993 (70)	1. Multiple-family psychoeducation and support. 2. RC	3092	Clinic-based lectures and discussions	1 yr	1 yr: multiple FI better than RC
Randolph et al. 1994 (71)	1. Behavioral FI. 2. RC	39	Clinic-based behavioral FI	1 yr	2 yr: behavioral FI better than RC
Xiong et al. 1994 (41)	1. Behavioral FI. 2. RC	63	Clinic-based psychoeducation, skills training, medication/ symptom management	18 mo	18 mo: behavioral FI better than RC
Zhang et al. 1994 (72)	1. Multiple and single family. 2. Psychoeducation and support	78	Multiple-family clinic-based psychoeducation counseling, medication/symptom management	1 yr	18 mo: family education and support better than RC
Zastowny et al. 1992 (73)	1. Behavioral FI. 2. Single family psychoeducation and support	30	Hospital-based behavioral FI. Hospital-based single family psychoeducational advice	1 yr	16 mo: conditions equal
McFarlane et al. 1995 (28)	1. Multiple-family psychoeducation and support. 2. Single family psychoeducation and support	172	Multiple-family groups or single family sessions in the clinic	2 yr	2 yr: multiple family conditions better than single family condition
Linszen et al. 1996 (74)	1. Behavioral FI + individual patient treatment. 2. Individual patient treatment	76	Hospital- and home-based behavioral FI	1 yr	1 yr: conditions equal
Schooler et al. 1997 (75)	1. Intensive behavioral FI. 2. Supportive family management	313	Home-based behavioral FI. Supportive family management = clinic-based family groups	2 yr	2 yr: conditions equal

Abbreviations: EE, expressed emotion; FI, family intervention; RC, routine care.

The consensus view in the literature is that the implementation of family interventions faces complex organizational and attitudinal difficulties (48–51), and insufficient attention has been paid to these in dissemination programs. In discussing the factors which might make the transference from research to practice difficult, Mari and Streiner (19) suggested that the requirements of durable service-oriented interventions differed from those based on time-limited research models. The need for changing the clinical practice of the whole service rather than training individuals is underlined in the work of Corrigan and colleagues (52–54). However, difficulties arise not only from staff but also from carer reluctance to engage in family work. Several studies (55,56) of community samples have shown that carer participation in family intervention is relatively low, with only 50% or so of carers taking up the offer of either a support service or family intervention (56), with possibly higher rates when help is offered at a time of crisis (44). Alternatives to professionally led interventions have been suggested (57) such as the psychoeducation groups led by carers (58). Other possibilities include the potential to deliver psychoeducation programs to families in remote communities via telepsychiatry, helping to overcome some of the practical problems faced such as infrastructure, lack of expertise, time constraints, location, and weather (59).

Conclusions

In summary, a number of important conclusions can be drawn concerning family intervention studies. First, while there is robust evidence for the efficacy of family interventions in schizophrenia, it is also clear that short education or counseling programs do not affect relapse rates: "a few lessons on schizophrenia" are simply not sufficient to substantially influence the relapse rate (32).

Second, the quality of interventions needs to be enhanced and monitored to ensure that families are offered the intensity of help likely to give them substantial benefits. It is suggested that care giver involvement in policy making should be considered in order to achieve the greatest benefit from the services provided (60). Successful family interventions require considerable investment in time, skill, and commitment; and as for many patients the effect is to delay rather than to prevent relapse, many patients and families will need long-term and continuing intervention. Work with relatives of recently diagnosed schizophrenia patients indicates that this help needs to begin from the first onset of the psychosis (61,62).

Third, although family interventions improve patient outcomes, there has been little progress in understanding how best to improve the well being of carers. If these data were available, it may be possible to increase engagement of family members as it may significantly impede the progress of the intervention. This is now a globally recognized issue, with research from the World

Federation of Mental Health (63) suggesting that caregivers will play an ever-increasing role in the support of individuals with mental health problems, particularly as social service and health care systems experience greater demands on their resources.

Finally, dissemination and engagement issues need to continue to be addressed and new ways found to assist more families. Although many patients and families benefit greatly from the intervention programs, a substantial number of families are hard to engage, and the implementation of family programs within services presents many challenges.

References

1. Macmillan JF, Gold A, Crow TJ, et al. The Northwick Park Study of first episodes of schizophrenia: IV Expressed emotion and relapse. Br J Psychiatry 1986; 148: 133–43.
2. Gibbons JS, Horn SH, Powell JM, et al. Schizophrenia patients and their families. A survey in a psychiatric service based on a district general hospital. Br J Psychiatry 1984; 144: 70–7.
3. Barrowclough C, Tarrier N, Johnston M. Distress, expressed emotion and attributions in relatives of schizophrenic patients. Schizophr Bull 1996; 22: 691–701.
4. Caqueo-Urízar A, Gutiérrez-Maldonado J, Miranda-Castillo C. Quality of life in caregivers of patients with schizophrenia: a literature review. Health Qual Life Outcomes 2009; 7: 1–5.
5. Girón M, Fernández-Yañez A, Mañá-Alvarenga S, et al. Efficacy and effectiveness of individual family intervention on social and clinical functioning and family burden in severe schizophrenia: a 2-year randomized controlled study. Psychol Med 2010; 40: 73–84.
6. Pharoah FM, Mari JJ, Streiner DL. Family intervention for people with schizophrenia (Cochrane Review). In: The Cochrane Library. Issue 4 Oxford, UK: Update Software, 1999.
7. Clements K, Turpin G. Innovations in the Psychological Management of Schizophrenia. Chichester: John Wiley & Sons, 1992.
8. Brown GW, Birley JLT, Wing JK. Influences of family life on the course of schizophrenic disorders: a replication. Br J Psychiatry 1972; 121: 241–8.
9. Vaughn C, Leff J. The influence of family and social factors on the course of psychiatric illness. Br J Psychiatry 1976; 129: 125–37.
10. Butzlaff RL, Hooley JM. Expressed emotion and psychiatric relapse: a meta-analysis. Arch Gen Psychiatry 1998; 55: 547–52.
11. Aguilera A, Lopez SR, Breitborde NJK, Kopelowicz A, Zarate R. Expressed emotion and sociocultural moderation in the course of schizophrenia. J Abnorm Psychol 2010; 119: 875–85.
12. Barrowclough C, Tarrier N. Psychosocial interventions with families and their effects on the course of schizophrenia: a review. Psychol Med 1984; 14: 629–42.
13. Lam DH. Psychosocial family intervention in schizophrenia: a review of empirical studies. Psychol Med 1991; 21: 423–41.
14. Kavanagh D. Family interventions for schizophrenia. In: Kavanagh DJ, ed. Schizophrenia: An Overview and Practical Handbook. London: Chapman & Hall, 1992.
15. Dixon LB, Lehman AF. Family interventions for schizophrenia. Schizophr Bull 1995; 21: 631–43.
16. Penn DL, Mueser KT. Research update on the psychosocial treatment of schizophrenia. Am J Psychiatry 1996; 153: 607–17.

17. Falloon I, Boyd J, McGill C. The Family of Care of Schizophrenia. London: Guilford, 1984.
18. Barrowclough C, Tarrier N. Families of Schizophrenic Patients: Cognitive Behavioural Intervention. London: Chapman & Hall, 1992.
19. Mari JJ, Streiner DL. An overview of family interventions and relapse in schizophrenia: meta-analysis of research findings. Psychol Med 1994; 24: 565–78.
20. Martens L, Addington J. Psychological well-being of family members of individuals with schizophrenia. Soc Psychiatry Psychiatr Epidemiol 2001; 36: 128–33.
21. Addington J, Addington D, Jones B, Ko T. Family intervention in an early psychosis program. Psychiatr Rehabil Skills 2001; 5: 272–86.
22. Addington J, Collins A, McCleery A, Addington D. The role of family work in early psychosis. Schizophr Res 2005; 79: 77–83.
23. Gafoor R, Nitsch D, McCrone P, et al. Effect of early intervention on 5-year outcome in non-affective psychosis. Br J Psychiatry 2010; 196: 372–6.
24. Mueser KT, Gingerich SL, Rosenthal CK. Educational family therapy for schizophrenia: A new treatment model for clinical service and research. Schizophr Res 1994; 13: 99–107.
25. Barrowclough C. Issues in the dissemination of family intervention for psychosis. World Psychiatry 2003; 2: 31–2.
26. Mueser KT, Glynn SM, Cather C, et al. Family intervention for co-occurring substance use and severe psychiatric disorders: Participant characteristics and correlates of initial engagement and more extended exposure in a randomized controlled trial. Addict Behav 2010; 34: 867–77.
27. Barrowclough C, Haddock G, Tarrier N, et al. Randomised controlled trial of cognitive behavioral therapy plus motivational intervention for schizophrenia and substance use. Am J Psychiatry 2001; 158: 1706–13.
28. McFarlane WR, Lukens E, Link B, et al. Multiple family groups and psychoeducation in the treatment of schizophrenia. Arch Gen Psychiatry 1995; 52: 679–87.
29. Tsiouri I, Gena A, Mouzas O. A group psychoeducational intervention for parents of individuals with schizophrenia. Eur Psychiatry 2011; 26: 1516.
30. Pilling S, Bebbington P, Kuiipers E, et al. Psychological treatments in schizophrenia: I. Meta-analysis of family intervention and cognitive behaviour therapy. Psychol Med 2002; 32: 763–82.
31. Mari JJ, Streiner DL. Family intervention for people with schizophrenia (Cochrane Review). In: The Cochrane Library. Issue 1 Oxford, UK: Update Software, 1996.
32. Pitschel-Walz G, Leucht S, Bauml J, Kissling W, Engel RR. The effect of family interventions on relapse and rehospitalisation in schizophrenia – a meta-analysis. Schizophr Bull 2001; 27: 73–92.
33. Falloon IRH, Boyd JL, McGill CW, et al. Family Management in the prevention of exacerbrations of schizophrenia. N Engl J Med 1982; 306: 1437–40.
34. Leff JP, Kuipers L, Berkowitz R, Eberlein-Fries R, Sturgeon D. A controlled trial of intervention with families of schizophrenic patients. Br J Psychiatry 1982; 141: 121–34.
35. Tarrier N, Barrowclough C, Vaughn C, et al. The community management of schizophrenia: A controlled trial of behavioural intervention with families to reduce relapse. Br J Psychiatry 1988; 153: 532–42.
36. Devaramane V, Pai NB, Vella SL. The effect of a brief family intervention on primary carer's functioning and their schizophrenic relatives levels of psychopathology in India. Asian J Psychiatry 2011; 4: 183–18.
37. Chan S, Yip B, Tso S, Cheng BS, Tam W. Evaluation of a psychoeducation program for Chinese clients with schizophrenia and their family caregivers. Patient Educ Couns 2009; 75: 67–76.

38. Paranthaman V, Satnam K, Lim J, et al. Effective implementation of a structured psychoeducation programme among caregivers of patients with schizophrenia in the community. Asian J Psychiatry 2010; 3: 206–21.
39. Hogarty GE, Anderson CM, Reiss DJ. Family psychoeducation, social skills training, and medication in schizophrenia: the long and short of it. Psychopharmacol Bull 1987; 23: 12–13.
40. Tarrier N, Barrowclough C, Porceddu K, Fitzpatrick E. The Salford Family Intervention Project for Schizophrenic relapse prevention: five and eight year accumulating relapses. Br J Psychiatry 1994; 165: 829–32.
41. Xiong W, Phillips MR, Hu X, et al. Family based intervention for schizophrenic patients in China: a randomised controlled trial. Br J Psychiatry 1994; 165: 239–47.
42. McWilliams S, Hill S, Mannion N, et al. Schizophrenia: a five-year follow-up of patient outcome following psycho-education for caregivers. Eur Psychiatry 2011; 27: 56–61.
43. Sellwood W, Barrowclough C, Tarrier N, et al. Needs based cognitive behavioural family intervention for carers of patients suffering from schizophrenia: 12 month follow up. Acta Scand Psychiatr 2001; 104: 346–55.
44. Tarrier N, Barrowclough C, Bamrah JS. Prodromal signs of relapse in schizophrenia. Soc Psychiatry Psychiatr Epidemiol 1991; 26: 157–61.
45. Szmukler G, Kuipers E, Joyce J, et al. An exploratory randomised controlled trial of a support programme for carers of patients with a psychosis. Soc Psychiatry Psychiatr Epidemiol 2003; 38: 411–18.
46. Tarrier N, Barrowclough C, Haddock G, McGovern J. The dissemination of innovative cognitive-behavioural psychosocial treatments for schizophrenia. J Ment Health 1999; 8: 569–82.
47. Kuller AM, Ott BD, Goisman RM, Wainwright LD, Rabin R. Cognitive behavioral therapy and schizophrenia: a survey of clinical practices and views on efficacy in the United States and United Kingdom. Community Ment Health J 2010; 46: 2–9.
48. Hughes I, Hailwood R, Abbati-Yeoman J, et al. Developing a family intervention service for serious mental illness: clinical observations and experiences. J Ment Health 1996; 5: 145–59.
49. Fadden G. Implementation of family interventions in routine clinical practice following staff training programs: a major cause for concern. J Ment Health 1997; 6: 599–612.
50. McFarlane WR, Dixon L, Lukens E, Lucksted A. Family psychoeducation and schizophrenia: a review of the literature. J Marital Fam Ther 2003; 29: 223–45.
51. Wei SJ, Cooke M, Moyle W, Creedy D. Health education needs of family caregivers supporting an adolescent relative with schizophrenia or a mood disorder in Taiwan. Arch Psychiatr Nurs 2010; 24: 418–28.
52. Corrigan VA, McCracken SG. Psychiatric rehabilitation and staff development: educational and organisational models. Clin Psychol Rev 1995a; 15: 1172–7.
53. Corrigan VA, McCracken SG. Refocussing the training of psychiatric Rehabilitation staff. Psychiatr Serv 1995b; 46: 1172–7.
54. Corrigan VA, McCracken SG, Edwards M, et al. Collegial support and barriers to behavioural programs for severely mentally ill. J Behav Ther Exp Psychiatry 1997; 28: 193–202.
55. McCreadie RG, Phillips K, Harvey JA, et al. The Nithscale schizophrenia surveys VIII Do relatives want family intervention- and does it help? Br J Psychiatry 1991; 158: 110–13.
56. Barrowclough C, Tarrier N, Lewis S, et al. Randomised controlled effectiveness trial of a needs–based psychosocial intervention service for carers of people with schizophrenia. Br J Psychiatry 1999; 174: 505–11.
57. Mairs H, Bradshaw T. Implementing family intervention following training: what can the matter be? J Psychiatr Ment Health Nurs 2005; 12: 488–94.

58. Dixon L, Lucksted A, Stewart B, et al. Outcomes of the peer-taught 12-week family-to-family education program for severe mental illness. Acta Psychiatr Scand 2004; 109: 207–21.
59. Haley C, O'Callaghan E, Hill S, et al. Telepsychiatry and carer education for schizophrenia. Eur Psychiatry 2011; 26: 302–4.
60. Chan SW. Global Perspective of Burden of Family Caregivers for Persons With Schizophrenia. Arch Psychiatr Nurs 2011; 25: 339–49.
61. Kuipers E, Raune D. The early development of expressed emotion and burden in the families of first- onset psychosis. In: Birchwood M, Fowler D, Jackson C, eds. Early Intervention in Psychosis: A Guide to Concepts, Evidence & Interventions. Chichester: John Wiley & Sons, 2000.
62. Amminger PG, Henry LP, Harrigan SM, et al. Outcome in early-onset schizophrenia revisited: findings from the Early Psychosis Prevention and Intervention Centre long-term follow-up study. Schizophr Res 2011; 131: 112–11.
63. World Federation of Mental Health (WFMH). Caring for the Caregiver: Why Your Mental Health Matters When You are Caring for others. Woodbridge VA: WFMH, 2010.
64. Kottgen C, Soinnichesen I, Mollenhauer K. Results of the Hamburg Camberwell Family Interview study, I–III. Int J Family Psychiatry 1984; 5: 61–94.
65. Falloon IRH, Boyd JL, McGill CW, et al. Family management in the prevention of morbidity in schizophrenia: Clinical outcome of a 2 year longitudinal study. Arch Gen Psychiatry, 1985; 42: 887–96.
66. Leff JP, Kulpers L, Sturgeon D. A controlled trial of social intervention in the families of schizophrenic patients. Br J Psychiatry 1985; 146: 594–600.
67. Hogarty GE, Anderson CM, Reiss DJ, et al. Family psycheducation, social skills training and maintenance chemotherapy in the after care treatment of schizophrenia. One year effects of a controlled study on relapse and expresses emotion. Arch Gen Psychiatry 1986; 43: 633–42.
68. Tarrier N, Barrowclough C, Porceddu K, et al. The Salford Family Intervention Project for Schizophrenic relapse prevention: five and eight year accumulating relapses. Brit J Psychiatry 1994; 165: 829–32.
69. Leff JP, Berkowitz R, Shavit A, et al. A trial of family therapy versus relatives' groups for schizophrenia. Brit J Psychiatry 1990; 157: 571–7.
70. Mingyuan Z, Heqin Y, Chengde Y, et al. Effectiveness of psychoeducation of relatives of schizophrenic patients: a prospective cohort study in five cities of China Int J Men Health 1993; 22: 47–59.
71. Randolph ET, Eth S, Glynn SM, et al. Behavioral family management in schizophrenia: outcome of a clinic based intervention. Brit J Psychiatry 1994; 164: 501–6.
72. Zhang M, Wang M, Li J, et al. Randomised control trial family intervention for 78 first episode male schizophrenic patients: an 18 month study in Suzhou, Japan. Brit J Psychiatry 1994; 65(Suppl 24): 96–102.
73. Zastowny RR, Lehman AF, Cole RE, et al. Family management of schizophrenia: a comparison of behavioral and supportive family treatment. Psychiatry Q 1992; 63: 159–86.
74. Linszen D, Dingemans P, Vander Does JW, et al. Treatment, expressed emotion and relapse in recent onset schizophrenia disorders. Psychological Medicine 1996; 26: 333–42.
75. Schooler NR, Keith SJ, Severe JB, et al. Relapse and rehospitalisation during maintenance treatment of schizophrenia. The effects of dose reduction and family treatment. Arch Gen Psychiatry 1997; 54: 453–63.

chapter 16

Models of care in schizophrenia

Tom Burns

Mental health care planning and policy have been heavily influenced by schizophrenia care—too much so in the opinion of some psychiatrists who believe this focus has drawn us too far from our medical roots (1). However, services that meet the needs of this paradigm mental illness have demonstrated themselves to be fit for other disorders while the opposite has generally not been the case. The multidisciplinary community mental health team (CMHT) is the focus of this chapter (2). It is not the only important component of community care of severe and psychotic illnesses but it is the cornerstone. Increasingly our evidence, both direct and indirect, confirms it as the necessary condition for the effective functioning of other parts of the system (day hospitals, vocational services, sheltered accommodation etc.). Research has predominantly focused on *which type* of CMHT rather than on understanding how CMHTs work and, most importantly, what contributes to effectiveness. An exaggerated belief in major differences in effectiveness and practice between different CMHTs is held by service commissioners and planners, which has resulted in endless reorganizations and instability (the last thing a schizophrenia patient needs). CMHTs are more alike than they are different, with identifiable common core practices. Ironically our understanding of these has been advanced by the very research aimed to demonstrate proposed differences.

Outpatient clinics and acute inpatient wards are a feature of all services, taken for granted, and largely unresearched. Hospital admission is the commonest outcome measure for randomized controlled trials (RCTs) of community care (3) but rarely researched as a treatment itself. Some attempts to establish alternatives have been described (4) but none has been taken off. The enormous variation in availability and practice in the other essential components of care such as supervised accommodation, day care, and vocational rehabilitation reflects local context and will not be addressed in this chapter.

Evolution of the CMHT

Multidisciplinary care of psychotic patients in the community evolved in response to the closure of the large mental hospitals. No individual professional has all the skills or capacity to meet the complex needs of such patients. As with deinstitutionalization itself, CMHTs evolved at different times and followed different trajectories in different countries. The magnitude of their success is often underestimated—the fall in inpatient beds by two-thirds in the United Kingdom and United States, for example, needs to be adjusted for population growth over the period. We now have in effect only a tenth of the beds we had in the 1950s. Sectorization and CMHT care developed first in France (5) and the United Kingdom (6) in the early 1960s while the United States made a false start with their ill-fated Community Mental Health Centres. Progress stalled in France but progressed steadily in the United Kingdom, in some parts of Europe, and in the wider English-speaking world. The size and sophistication of CMHTs has increased as the threshold for admission rose. Franco Basaglia's *Psichiatria Democratica* with its famous "Law 180" came late to the scene in 1978 with the most radical of the reforms, effectively closing mental hospitals simultaneously with establishing sector CMHTs (7).

Assertive community treatment and the era of mental health services research

This slow evolution abruptly changed with Stein and Test's 1980 RCT of intensive community support (8). Initially called "Training in Community Living," but soon renamed Assertive Community Treatment (ACT), they had an enormous impact on both the clinical and the research communities. They found an enormous advantage for ACT and described their service model very clearly (Box 16.1), initiating an era of evidence-based medicine approaches to service models. Over the ensuing three decades over 90 studies of ACT were published and it became mandated in most of the United States, much of Australasia and the United Kingdom and is now spreading in Europe. The ACT "mobile" team established the model for other equally carefully described teams, in particular Early Intervention Services for first-episode psychosis and for Crisis teams (referred to in the United Kingdom as Crisis Resolution Home Treatment teams) to reduce hospital admission. The United Kingdom totally reformed its mental health services (9) by requiring the introduction of these teams based essentially on two influential meta-analyses demonstrating the superiority of ACT (10) over case management (11).

ACT is the only mental health community care model to have really extensive experimental research evidence. There are currently no RCTs of Crisis teams and only two of Early Intervention Services (EIS) are available (12,13), but neither of which provides the convincing evidence generally attributed to

---

Box 16.1   ACT principles and practice.

Assertive Community Treatment (ACT) Program principles
- Provision of material resources for patients
- Fostering patient coping skills
- Supporting patient motivation to persevere
- Freeing patient from pathological dependency relationships
- Support and education for those involved with the patient

ACT core components
- Assertive follow-up
- Small caseloads (1:10)
- Increased frequency of contact (weekly to daily)
- *In vivo practice* (treatment delivered at home and in the neighbourhood)
- Emphasis on medication
- Emphasis on engagement
- Support for family and carers
- Provision of services within the team where possible
- Liaison with other services when necessary
- Crisis stabilization and availability 24 hr a day, 7 d a week

Source: Adapted from Ref. 2.

them. Detailed descriptions of these service models are provided by their practitioners, ACT (14), EIS (15,16), and CRHT (17). Of course designing services is not dependent exclusively on RCT evidence and there are several other considerations such as satisfaction with services, ability to recruit staff, and attention to wider clinical and social outcomes. However, the variation in practice and outcomes in the body of ACT research has been a powerful tool in identifying what does and does not work in CMHTs.

Drawing more generalizable principles for service models

Understanding differences in outcome became important in Europe because local studies (18,19) failed to replicate reductions in bed usage. Using metaregression (a powerful form of meta-analysis) it has been demonstrated that the main reason for the outcome differences is that the routine services used as controls had very low admission practices (20). More surprisingly, however, high staffing and low caseloads had no impact on results although the team processes did (Fig. 16.1). In short, multidisciplinary CMHTs were equally good, whether they were highly engineered and expensive ACT teams (21) or routine sector CMHTs (22).

Another examination of these studies illuminates these processes. Over 60 investigators provided descriptions using 20 operationalized characteristics of their experimental services for psychotic individuals (23). Six features recurred regularly, of which two were independently associated with reducing admissions (Fig. 16.2).

Multidisciplinary working is important. A successful practice usually requires a minimum of three different professions (usually medical, nursing, and social work but in some instances psychology or occupational therapy).

Home-based care featured in two forms, policy and practice. Visiting patients at home is a declared policy and fundamental of practice; it is not just for

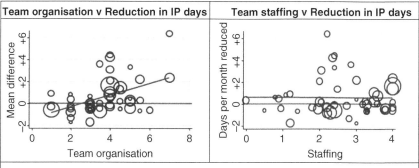

Figure 16.1   *Metaregression results for reduction in hospitalization. Source: Adapted from Ref. 20.*

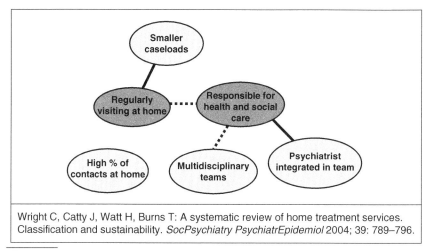

Figure 16.2   *Associations between common service components. Source: Adapted from Ref. 23.*

emergencies. The high percentage of contacts in the home exceeded clinic contacts in the care of schizophrenia patients.

Smaller caseloads refer to caseloads of 20 or fewer per full-time case manager. A limited caseload size with an agreed ceiling (usually around 20–25) has generally now been adopted across many CMHTs albeit in some jurisdictions caseloads are rather higher. Active management of caseloads follows from this with balanced intake and discharge thresholds so case managers focus their time and attention on the most needy patients.

Psychiatrist integrated in the team means that the psychiatrist was a routine member of meetings and reviews. Two questions were asked about psychiatrists. Psychiatric time (calculated as hours per 100 patients) demonstrated remarkable variation and seemed to have little bearing. Working as an integrated member occurred regularly but not acting as an independent resource for complex medical opinions.

Lastly, teams were *responsible for health and social care,* meaning that patients could access both without needing a referral. Responsibility for health and social care and a policy of home visits were the two components independently associated with reduction in hospitalization.

What does not help?

Two features missing from this list continue to be recommended but are neither justified nor useful. A *24-hour cover* by individual teams appears in documents but not in practice. Commissioners, pressurized by carer groups, often continue to insist on this. In a study visit to nine high-profile ACT teams in the United States in the 1990s, I observed that no one operated a meaningful 24-hour service (all officially claimed to). Most patched their phones through to the local duty team or emergency room. This makes eminent clinical sense and most mature teams adopt it. The *whole-team approach* is an imprecise term. If it means that schizophrenia patients should have input from several members of their team, fine. Interpreted rigidly to preclude having a primary case manager it is neither practical nor humane. I only observed it being implemented in one of the nine ACT teams I visited. Its origins are in 1970s misconceptions about parental contribution to psychosis (Box 16.1) and it should be dismissed.

Continuity of care vs specialization

The discussion until now has drawn on evidence. What follows draws on clinical consensus which is neither fixed nor necessarily stable. I will attempt to provide a balanced overview but where my own prejudices (for continuity, simplicity, and structure) intrude, I hope, they will be obvious and can be adjusted for by the reader.

Most of medicine has experienced a massive upsurge in super-specialization. There are understandable pressures for highly targeted and specialized service models based either on function (e.g., ACT, EIS, and CRHT teams mentioned earlier) or diagnosis (e.g., schizophrenia team, bipolar team, depression team, and so on). The judgment should be a pragmatic one.

In favor of specialization is the development of appropriate and sophisticated skills and the maintenance of focus. Against it is the reality of discontinuity that is always experienced and is particularly disliked by patients and carers. It is also disliked by many nonmedical staff who value establishing therapeutic relationships as a core skill. In addition to this that most of the professional time is devoted to "atypical" cases and the scope for boundary disputes can outweigh any hard-gained efficiency. There is also the risk of slipping into a rather mechanical, even dehumanized, approach if only working with very similar, highly dependent individuals. There are areas of specialization that no one now questions—child and adolescent psychiatry, for instance, or old age services or eating disorder services. But is the degree of specialization between standard CMHTs and rehabilitation services for schizophrenia productive? Is the separation of inpatient and community responsibility better? These will surely depend on a whole range of factors and vary from place to place. Given the overwhelming importance in schizophrenia care of personal knowledge of each patient, the presumption must be for continuity until the advantage of a division has been established. The individual decision depends on circumstances and imposed uniformity should be avoided.

Size and composition of CMHTs

CMHTs have steadily increased in size from 4–5 members of staff in the 1970s to 20 plus now. There is enormous variation both within and between healthcare systems. It is certainly difficult to sustain effective care with fewer than about six full-time members, covering sickness and annual leave, responding to emergencies, and readily providing for joint visiting when safety is an issue. On the other hand, when teams get larger than about 12–15, communication and information transfer starts to become a significant burden. This can be exacerbated if many staff members are either sharing responsibilities or part timers. Larger teams can often offer a broader range of specialized skills (e.g., a dual diagnosis worker, a vocational specialist) but the energy integrating them and keeping them informed, plus patients' undoubted resistance to being referred on, need to be balanced against the gains.

There is a constant discussion about the composition of teams. With schizophrenia, medical and nursing memberships are clearly essential and probably also social work. Administrative arrangements for integrating social workers can be Byzantine but it is the personal availability that is vital as indicated earlier. There are striking cultural variations in the role allocated to psychologists, occupational therapists and even, in Scandinavian teams, physiotherapists. Whether all these members should carry an individual "generic" caseload or restrict themselves to specialized input remains disputed. In successful ACT teams there is usually an emphasis on the primacy of generic working but in most CMHTs it is the other way round. An excessive generic approach is probably rather wasteful but ensures shared understanding and builds invaluable team spirit.

The balance between trained professionals and support workers is also vexed. The evidence above suggests that there is no substitute for a proper range of trained professionals in a team, both to deliver skilled interventions and to enrich assessments. Well-selected, trained, and supported support staff can undoubtedly make a major contribution but there is a risk in too rigid a hierarchy of tasks. A regular observation in working with psychosis patients is how their evaluation and respect for us often derives from the "nonprofessional" input. The genuinely kind act that is not dependent on my doctor role will be remembered long after a clever diagnosis.

There is an emerging international consensus on individual and team caseload sizes. Few developed secondary services would expect a full-time case manager to coordinate for more than 20–25 patients. If they don't need contact at least once a month do they need specialist care or should they be referred back to their family doctor? Of course this would not hold if there is no effective primary care provision for psychotic patients. Multidisciplinary working pools several perspectives to understand and address patients' problems. Those contributing need to be familiar with the specifics of the case. In effect this means that total caseloads of more than 200–250 are impractical. In the U.K. context these numbers include a significant proportion of simpler, nonpsychotic patients, many of whom are seen solely by doctors in outpatient departments. In a team focusing predominantly on psychosis or schizophrenia the caseload should probably be more like 100–150.

Managing caseloads

There is an extensive literature on case-mix and on developing criteria and threshold assessment instruments for referral to CMHTs. None of it has caught on in routine practice. However, effective caseload management is vital for teams. Two things have to be achieved. First, keeping the team's resources focused on the most needy patients and therefore having to discharge recovered patients; and second, making sure that the clinical burden is fairly evenly shared so that the staff members are not overburdened and patients not short-changed. Setting up a system that achieves this is much better than trying to micromanaging it. Three things are needed: (*i*) fixed individual caseloads, (*ii*) fixed maximum times for patient acceptance, and (*iii*) consistent assessment process (Box 16.2). In practice this means staff members are required broadly to take on new patients at the same rate and therefore must make clinical judgments about

---

Box 16.2   Clinical focus trio.

1. Single point of entry assessment
2. Fixed maximum waits for assessment
   - Routine – one month
   - Urgent – one week
   - Emergency – same day
3. Fixed maximum individual caseloads

---

who should be discharged to make room. Most staff members prefer to do this themselves in discussion with the team and only when really stuck is direction necessary. This will not be appropriate occasionally but if interventions are frequently required it usually indicates team dysfunction.

Assessments and reviews

There are conflicting opinions on whether all new patient assessments should be by a doctor, with cogent arguments on both sides. CMHTs have a long tradition of sharing and informality and prize skill sharing, role blurring and a flattened hierarchy, all of which mitigate against it. Some crisis teams simply do not have doctors. My position has changed on this based on experience and observation of varying practices. On balance I think that all new assessments should be by a psychiatrist, alone or jointly with another team member (my preferred option). I will give my reasons and the reader can decide. First, assessment is a core psychiatric skill, and no other profession gets the same drilling in diagnosis and assessment. Second, medical assessments are taken more seriously outside the CMHT—GPs will accept a referral back from a trained psychiatrist but may question one from a nonmedic. Third, it is what people clearly insist on when they have a choice—always so in private practice and for influential individuals in public services. Who sees your relative? Why should it be different for the powerless schizophrenia patient? Also it speeds up decision making. This is particularly obvious in crisis teams where patients are repeatedly visited, sometimes for considerable periods, before a comprehensive assessment is finally obtained. It establishes a consistent threshold for deciding that the team accepts the patient for specialist care. Last, it clarifies roles within the CMHT and facilitates focused clinical discussion. When the doctor actually knows the patient for whom he or she takes clinical responsibility less time is spent in speculative and futile discussion. However, there are alternative views.

Patients should be reviewed with the team in at least four instances (Box 16.3). All should have a full review when *newly assessed* to obtain input from the whole team and ensure appropriate allocation and devise a care plan. They should also

---

Box 16.3   CMHT reviews.

1. New assessment
   - Full initial history and mental state
   - Construct care plan
2. Routine periodic assessment [every 6 or 12 months]
   - Full history and mental state
   - Structured assessments (HoNOS, BPRS etc.)
   - Refresh care plan
3. Crisis or management change
   - Brief, focused
   - Record in notes or in care plan
4. Discharge
   - Structured history
   - Assessment of treatment goals/outcome

---

be reviewed if there is a *crisis* or a need to change management. This may need to be quite brief depending on how familiar team members are. They should be routinely reviewed at *agreed intervals*. Most schizophrenia patients in long-term care are reviewed this way every 3, 6, or 12 months and this may be the time for structured recording of clinical needs and updating proposed interventions in the care plan. Lastly, all patients should be reviewed at *discharge* not only to keep a balance of clinical demand in the team but also as a vital learning opportunity. Many teams have "allocation meetings" when the referral information is considered to determine assessment. It is difficult to see what this achieves; if the information is accurate the patient can be easily triaged by a senior clinician. If it is inaccurate it will only be obvious after the assessment. Either way the time seems wasted.

Routine periodic reviews are often the major opportunity to engage the patient's family and other involved agencies. Some formal recording of these reviews (e.g., the Care Plan Approach (24)) is the norm and often this can be the time to complete structured clinical assessments to track slow change over time; for example, the Health of the Nation Outcome Scale (HoNOS) (25), Brief Psychiatric Rating Scale (BPRS) (26), and PSP (27). Whether a disorder-specific instrument such as PSP or BPRS or a generic one such as HoNOS is preferable is hotly debated. However, the value of *some* structured assessment is undoubted. They track patient progress, but presenting them in reviews encourage rigor in assessment and provides a common clinical vocabulary and establishes greater consistency in assessment across team members. The same advantages can also be true for structured reviews of the team's functioning. Regular treatment audits can be highly revealing, for instance indicating whether trials of clozapine or carer support really are being delivered or are they simply pious policy statements.

Team meetings

Multidisciplinary work requires lots of information exchange. Imaginative use of white boards can streamline much of this—for example for "zoning" patients, managing clozapine blood tests, and setting up joint visits (14). However, making sure that meetings do not erode time for patient care is a constant challenge. Most teams have abandoned a "shift" system precisely because the time taken up swapping information and the disruption of care outweighed the advantages. Flexible evening working and perhaps a skeleton presence at weekends for vital routine contacts is much more efficient. In the long term it is usually more acceptable to staff. Similarly most mature teams abandon fixed duty rotas other than perhaps having a named contact for crises. Rapid easy assessments soon put paid to most crises.

ACT teams aim for brief daily meetings but most CMHTs make do with one long (2–3 hours) formal team meeting a week for reviews, supplemented by one or two briefer handovers for crises. Time has to be found for a management meeting, some form of team development, and an educational slot. Whether these can be rotated on the end of the main team meeting will depend on team style and workload. A habit of starting and finishing the day in the team base is generally very good for morale and safety but may not be practical if distances to visits are great.

The future

Multidisciplinary team care of serious mental illness is now well established and, despite multiple reorganizations, remarkably durable. It is about having to adapt to a much more risk-averse culture and one demanding a much more intensive, bureaucratic governance. It has maintained its core structures and values and now manages to incorporate evidence-based practice and to generate an evidence base of its own. We have to remind ourselves that it is the treatments (not the team structures or processes) that get patients better. To deliver these we need stability despite powerful forces for change and legitimate development. Further subspecialization will be inevitable but needs to reflect genuine differences in skill sets, not the ambitions of clinical enthusiasts or the seduction of easy organizational change for managers and policy makers. Our litmus test should not be how good it looks on paper or in an organizational diagram but how well it delivers effective treatments to our patients in a respectful, sustainable and acceptable form.

References

1. Craddock N, Antebi D, Attenburrow MJ, et al. Wake-up call for British psychiatry. Br J Psychiatry 2008; 193: 6–9.

2. Burns T. Community Mental Health Teams, A Guide to Current Practices. Oxford: Oxford University Press, 2004.

3. Burns T. Hospitalisation as an outcome measure in schizophrenia. Br J Psychiatry Suppl 2007; 191(Suppl 50): s37–41.

4. Johnson S, Gilburt H, Lloyd-Evans B, et al. In-patient and residential alternatives to standard acute psychiatric wards in England. Br J Psychiatry 2009; 194: 456–63.

5. Kovess V, Boisguerin B, Antoine D, Reynauld M. Has the sectorization of psychiatric services in France really been effective? Soc Psychiatry Psychiatr Epidemiol 1995; 30: 132–8.

6. Johnson S, Thornicroft G. The sectorisation of psychiatric services in England and Wales. Soc Psychiatry Psychiatr Epidemiol 1993; 28: 45–7.

7. Tansella M. Editorial: the Italian experience and its implications. Psychol Med 1987; 17: 283–9.

8. Stein LI, Test MA. Alternative to mental hospital treatment. I. Conceptual model, treatment program, and clinical evaluation. Arch Gen Psychiatry 1980; 37: 392–7.

9. Department of H. Modern Standards and Service Models: National Service Framework for Mental Health. London: Department of Health, 1999.

10. Marshall M, Lockwood A. Assertive community treatment for people with severe mental disorders (Cochrane Review). Cochrane Library 1998.

11. Marshall M, Gray A, Lockwood A, Green R. Case management for severe mental disorders (Cochrane Review). Cochrane Library 2001.

12. Craig TKJ, Garety P, Power P, et al. The Lambeth Early Onset (LEO) team: randomised controlled trial of the effectiveness of specialised care for early psychosis. BMJ 2004; 329: 1067–70.

13. Petersen L, Jeppesen P, Thorup A, et al. A randomised multicentre trial of integrated versus standard treatment for patients with a first episode of psychotic illness. BMJ 2005; 331: 602.

14. Burns T, Firn M. Assertive Outreach in Mental Health: A Manual for Practitioners. Oxford: Oxford University Press, 2002.

15. Birchwood M, McGorry P, Jackson H. Early intervention in schizophrenia. Br J Psychiatry 1997; 170: 2–5.

16. Edwards J, McGorry PD, Pennell K. Models of early intervention in psychosis: an analysis of service approaches. In: Birchwood M, Fowler D, Jackson C, eds. Early Intervention in Psychosis: A Guide to Concepts, Evidence and Interventions. New York: John Wiley & Sons, 2000: 281–314.

17. Smyth MG, Hoult J. The home treatment enigma. Br Med J 2000; 320: 305–9.

18. Burns T, Creed F, Fahy T, et al. Intensive versus standard case management for severe psychotic illness: a randomised trial. UK 700 Group. Lancet 1999; 353: 2185–9.

19. Thornicroft G, Wykes T, Holloway F, Johnson S, Szmukler G. From efficacy to effectiveness in community mental health services. PRiSM Psychosis Study 10. Br J Psychiatry 1998; 173: 423–7.

20. Burns T, Catty J, Dash M, et al. Use of intensive case management to reduce time in hospital in people with severe mental illness: systematic review and meta-regression. BMJ 2007; 335: 336.

21. Killaspy H, Bebbington P, Blizard R, et al. The REACT study: randomised evaluation of assertive community treatment in north London. BMJ 2006; 332: 815–20.

22. Burns T. End of the road for treatment-as-usual studies? Br J Psychiatry 2009; 195: 5–6.

23. Wright C, Catty J, Watt H, Burns T. A systematic review of home treatment services. Classification and sustainability. Soc Psychiatry Psychiatr Epidemiol 2004; 39: 789–96.

24. The Care Programme Approach for people with a mental illness referred to the Special Psychiatric Services, 1990.

25. Trauer T, Callaly T, Hantz P, et al. Health of the nation outcome scales. Results of the Victorian field trial. Br J Psychiatry 1999; 174: 380–8.
26. Overall JE, Gorham DL. Brief Psychiatric rating scale. In: William G, ed. ECDEU Assessment Manual of Psychopharmacology. Rockville: ECDEU, MD: 1976: 157–69.
27. Morosini PL, Magliano L, Brambilla L, Ugolini S, Pioli R. Development, reliability and acceptability of a new version of the DSM-IV Social and Occupational Functioning Assessment Scale (SOFAS) to assess routine social functioning. Acta Psychiatr Sand 2000; 101: 323–9.

chapter 17

A treatment approach to the patient with first-episode schizophrenia

Shon Lewis and Richard Drake

There has been considerable recent research and clinical interest in early intervention in schizophrenia, underpinned by the idea that the earlier the intervention, the better the potential outcome. This begs the question as to how early is early, as it is clear that many people with schizophrenia have a long-standing (probably largely inherited) brain vulnerabilities which manifest in nonspecific ways until the evolution of frank psychotic symptoms. This vulnerability may transition through a phase of nonspecific symptoms and behaviors, including social withdrawal, and anxiety and depression. The nonspecific nature and poor-positive predictive value of these types of symptom mitigate against pharmacological intervention until frank psychosis intervenes, although some researchers have used antipsychotics, antidepressants, omega-3 fatty acids, and cognitive–behavioral therapy (CBT) in those at particularly "high risk" (Box 17.1) to try to "prevent" the evolution to frank psychosis. Observational evidence suggests selective serotonin reuptake inhibitors (SSRIs) may be less efficacious (1). There may also be more specific subtle perceptual and experiential changes long studied in Germanic psychiatry, the "basic symptoms" (2). These have similar predictive value but might be more predictive if they co-occur with other symptoms (3). Combinations of substance misuse, paranoia, bizarre ideation, family history of psychosis, and social dysfunction may be relatively predictive too (1).

The "high risk" strategy remains controversial and requires a careful balancing of risks and potential benefits after discussion with each individual patient. A prodromal syndrome may be included in DSM V, but some argue that it is currently insufficiently specific to be of clinical utility, since some data suggest decreasing predictive value over time in specialist clinics and the benefits of various management strategies are not yet well evidenced (5).

Box 17.1 Characteristics of people at "high risk" for psychosis. Two most predictive (4,2) sets of criteria, or most related to psychosis, (3) in help-seeking adults

1. Yung et al. (2004) (4) Ultra High-Risk Mental State
   - Attenuated (subthreshold) Psychotic Symptom(s) over 1 week–5 years
   - Trait (Schizotypal Disorder or first-degree relative with schizophrenia plus decrement of at least 30 points in GAF over 1 month–5 years)
   - Brief Limited Intermittent Psychotic Symptoms (BLIPS): at least one psychotic symptom for under 1 week in the past year

   Any one of the following moderately predicts psychosis within 12 months:
   - Trait + Attenuated
   - Trait or Attenuated >5 years
   - Trait or Attenuated or BLIPS *and* GAF <40
   - Trait or Attenuated or BLIPS *and* poor attention
2. Klosterkötter et al. (2001) (2) Highest Risk Basic Symptom Criteria
   Any one of the following weakly to moderately predicts psychosis within 9.6 years:
   - Thought interference, perseveration, pressure, or block
   - Receptive dysphasia
   - Difficulty distinguishing ideas and perception; or fantasy and memory
   - Vague ideas of reference
   - Derealization
   - Subtle visual and auditory abnormalities

What is better established is the early treatment of frank psychotic symptoms once they evolve, and there have been attempts through health promotion and early recognition strategies to reduce the duration of untreated psychosis (DUP). Determining the DUP is necessary at presentation to confirm presence of the temporal diagnostic criteria: one month for ICD 10 schizophrenia or DSM IV schizophreniform disorder; or for DSM IV schizophrenia, one month's psychosis (possibly less if treated) and 6 months of social dysfunction with prodromal or residual symptoms. Most patients present with a DUP of a few weeks; but for some it will be months and for a few, years. Median DUPs in Europe, Canada, and Australia are usually 2–6 months; but mean and median values from the United States are often longer. Not only does longer DUP predict worse symptomatic outcome but recent studies have found this after adjustment for insidious onset or premorbid disability. The period of untreated psychosis is thus believed to be associated with accumulating symptomatic as well as social and interpersonal harm. It has been suggested that neurotoxic processes during this time can lead to cumulative long-term damage. Thus, shortening DUP may be of long-term benefit, apart from reducing distress.

Clinical assessment

A number of potential differential diagnoses need to be considered in the assessment of a patient with the first manifestation of psychotic symptoms: these are as shown in Table 17.1. A thorough history must be obtained from the patient and corroborating information sought from any other sources. These may include primary care staff; carers and family; and perhaps police or social services. In some countries or communities community authority figures or traditional healers may have been consulted. A family history of psychotic disorder, history of substance use, and life events should be sought. Information from schools (or school leavers' reports in some countries) may be relevant.

A physical, including neurological, examination is essential. Investigations are as listed in Table 17.2. Appropriate blood tests include full blood count; ESR; electrolytes, urea and calcium; liver function tests; thyroid function tests, and others as indicated, such as TPH. Since illicit substance use is widespread a urine drug screen is mandatory in most countries. Patients need an electro-encephalogram and CT or an MRI scan if there is any indication from the other information, for example if any neurological abnormality is suspected or the history is atypical. Some argue that these investigations are appropriate in all cases. In some areas a lumbar puncture for cerebrospinal fluid (CSF) is routine, depending on the type and severity of an endemic infectious disease.

Careful symptom rating allows the tracking of clinical change over time. It is an increasingly important function in service and treatment evaluation. Outcomes for first episode schizophrenia can be measured in terms of severity of symptoms, or social outcomes, or by related constructs such as quality of life or patient satisfaction. A variety of validated rating scales are available to the clinician, as outlined in chapter 19. Attention should also be given to tracking of physical health parameters, as discussed in chapter 6.

Initial management: Antipsychotic drugs

As discussed in chapter 1, antipsychotics are the mainstay of management in first episodes as much as later ones: since the evidence base is larger in established disease this may offer a guide to treatment where the evidence in first episodes is lacking or unclear.

Individuals in their first episode of schizophrenia are more susceptible to the motor side effects of antipsychotics, which makes atypical antipsychotics an attractive option. However, in first episodes the evidence for superior efficacy of these agents is mixed. A major open trial comparing several antipsychotics, European First-Episode Schizophrenia Trial (EUFEST) (6), found time to discontinuation was significantly longer for olanzapine, amisulpride, and ziprasidone than haloperidol, but this may have been influenced by prescribers' expectations; indeed, secondary outcomes such as Positive and

Table 17.1 Differential diagnoses of ICD10 schizophrenia

ICD-10 disorders	Specific causes
Nonaffective psychoses	
Acute psychotic disorders	
Schizoaffective disorder	
Persistent delusional disorder	
Induced or "other persistent" delusional disorders	
Affective psychoses	
Manic, mixed, or depressive episodes with psychosis	
Drug-induced psychoses	
Acute intoxication, withdrawal with delirium, drug-induced psychotic disorder, flashbacks	*Alcohol, illicit drugs, medications, lead, mercury*
Organic secondary psychoses (organic delusional disorder or delirium)	
Epilepsy	Partial seizures, partial complex status, peri-ictal or interictal psychoses
Intracranial lesions	Tumors, cysts, abscesses, malformations, hemorrhages (rarely stroke)
Connective tissue disorder	Esp. SLE
Infections	Syphilis, HIV, HSV encephalitis, new variant Creutzfeldt-Jakob disease (CJD), TB meningitis
Metabolic disorders	Calcium, Wilson's disease; vitamin B_{12}, folate, and niacin deficiency; metachromatic leukodystrophy, Nieman–Pick's, etc.
Endocrine disorders	Thyroid, glucocorticoid etc.
Genetic causes	Huntingdon's, velocardiofacial syndrome etc.

(Continued)

Table 17.1 Differential diagnoses of ICD10 schizophrenia (*Continued*)

	ICD-10 disorders	Specific causes
Dementias	Alzheimer's, vascular	E.g., Pick's, Lewy-body disease, CJD
Personality disorders	Paranoid, schizoid, borderline type	
Schizotypy	Schizotypal disorder	
Developmental disorders	Autism, Asperger's syndrome, other pervasive developmental disorders	Subacute sclerosing panencephalitis, some metabolic disorders
Neuroses	Dissociative disorders, PTSD, obsessive–compulsive disorder, hypochondriacal disorder, adjustment disorder	
Feigning	Malingering, factitious disorder	

Table 17.2 Screening investigations in first-episode schizophrenia

First line	*Second line*
Neurological examination	CT/MRI scan
Complete blood cell count, ESR	Autoantibodies
Routine blood biochemistry, calcium	Syphilis serology
Thyroid function	HIV serology
Liver function	Chromosome studies
Electroencephalogram	Serum copper
Drug screen: urine or hair	Arylsulfatase A
	CSF examination

Negative Symptom Scale (PANSS) and adherence scores indicated no differences between agents. Haloperidol caused more motor side effects and olanzapine more weight gain. Vasquez-Barquero's group found no significant differences in acute efficacy in a double-blind comparison of haloperidol, olanzapine, and risperidone in 172 first episodes (7). Schooler et al. (8) found risperidone delayed the relapse better in 555 participants randomized to risperidone or haloperidol; but at outcome both groups had the same level of symptoms. Lieberman and colleagues (9) reported that olanzapine reduced symptoms slightly better than haloperidol by most measures in a double-blind trial with 263 participants.

Thus, it is the lower burden of extrapyramidal effects that leads to many clinicians advocating the use of non-clozapine atypical antipsychotics in first-episode patients. There are also suggestions that these agents have benefits over the typical antipsychotics in the amelioration of negative and cognitive symptoms (chap. 3 and 4): they have been linked to better cognition in some trials in first-episode sufferers (10), although this did not translate into better social function and the EUFEST trial found no significant advantages in cognitive outcomes (11).

People in their first episode of schizophrenia are likely to respond to lower doses of antipsychotics than later episodes, just as they are more sensitive to motor side effects. Mean modal doses in trials have been about 3 mg of risperidone; 9–12 mg of olanzapine; 375 mg of quetiapine; and 2–5 mg haloperidol or 150–400 mg chlorpromazine. Notably, in EUFEST (6) substantial proportions (26–61% depending on the drug) received maximum permitted doses: 4 mg haloperidol, 800 mg amisulpride, 20 mg olanzapine, 750 mg quetiapine, and 160 mg ziprasidone.

There are emerging concerns about metabolic side effects of some second-generation antipsychotics (perhaps clozapine and olanzapine most saliently) in first-episode patients (chap. 1 and 6). There are, however, suggestions that a longer-term effect on weight gain is more similar than short-term effects in first-episode patients (12). Many antipsychotics that are potent D2 blockers, including the atypicals risperidone and amisulpride, cause hyperprolactinemia and sexual side effects (chap. 1). Again these need to be assessed and require appropriate interventions should they intervene.

Antipsychotics in practice

From all such confusing findings one may draw several conclusions. There is some evidence that atypical antipsychotics are superior and their use for first-line treatment is preferred for reasons of tolerability. As outlined in chapter 1 and shown in Figure 1.1, a typical initial dose of 0.5 mg risperidone or 2.5–5 mg olanzapine, increasing to an initial treatment dose of 2 mg risperidone or 7.5 mg olanzapine, is relatively well evidenced. Recent evidence (13) implies that if absolutely no clinical response is seen to the treatment dose by a further 2 weeks or so, response is unlikely. This may prompt incremental increases toward the higher end of the treatment range, provided the medication is well tolerated (e.g., about 4 mg risperidone or 20 mg olanzapine). If the drug is not well tolerated a switch may be made to a second-line drug. It is clear that about 70% saturation of limbic D2 receptors is sufficient for treatment and motor side effects can often be avoided by appropriate dosing. In that case anticholinergic drugs can be avoided, though in the certain situations in the early stages it may well be prudent to prescribe them "as required" to avoid motor side effects, including dystonias and oculogyric crises (Table 1.1), which can affect attitudes to medication and, later, adherence. Clearly there is a balance to be struck between safe treatment and minimizing risk of side effects.

Other side effects should be closely monitored, including blood lipids and considering the possibility of developing diabetic ketoacidosis. In part on the basis of concerns about motor, sexual, and metabolic side effects, some clinicians use alternatives such as quetiapine (increasing to an initial treatment dose of about 400 mg, although somnolence may be a problem at first), amisulpride (increasing to an initial treatment dose of 200 mg), or aripiprazole (initial treatment dose of 5 mg, going up to 10 mg) first line.

The use of mixtures of antipsychotics or adjunctive agents has been subjected to very little rigorous scientific scrutiny in first-episode patients. There is some evidence from patients with established illness that a regular adjunctive sodium valproate is beneficial when patients are violent.

Acute agitation

The management of acute agitation in schizophrenia is discussed in detail in chapter 8. In first-episode patients special care needs to be taken in these scenarios, given the potential for the distressing nature of any events to make later engagement with service providers difficult.

In terms of medication, benzodiazepines are often used as relatively safe short-term or "as required" adjuncts for agitation or catatonic symptoms.

An approach favored in the past was to use higher doses of oral typical antipsychotics, particularly those with antihistaminic properties. This is less safe and should be avoided as far as possible; as discussed in chapter 8 atypical agents are being used more and more in these situations, with good effect.

For the very acute situation requiring rapid tranquillization, either oral benzodiazepines (e.g., lorazepam or clonazepam) plus a quickly absorbed atypical antipsychotic can be used. Commonly used alternatives, of similar efficacy (14), for parenteral antipsychotic have been olanzapine and haloperidol; increasing numbers of clinicians favor the former. Lorazepam cannot be used simultaneously with the olanzapine because of respiratory depression, and there is a risk of hypotension. Haloperidol has a risk of motor side effects and therefore, parenteral anticholinergics should be prescribed (or the sedative anticholinergic antihistamine namely promethazine (14)); but there is no difficulty with additional parenteral benzodiazepines (e.g., lorazepam or midazolam). Recent evidence of ventricular arrhythmias associated with haloperidol has prompted some countries to mandate an EKG where practical, though the arrhythmias are not always predicted by long QTc. Zuclopenthixol acetate should not be used generally in first-episode patients, because of delayed onset, extended duration of action, and propensity to extrapyramidal side effects. For a more detailed exposition of these matters, the reader is referred to chapter 8 and in particular Figure 8.1.

Psychosocial and family interventions

Patients will need appropriate monitoring and support either in the community or hospital, depending on their symptoms, environment, ability to cooperate and other risk-related behavior. Their carers need appropriate support too, especially if the patient stays in the community. Assessment of the resources available from their support network, its reliability and members' needs is a key part of initial assessment and must continue throughout. Finding the appropriate support and setting may obviate the need for higher doses of antipsychotics.

The usual form of structured support for the family is by psychoeducation and behavioral problem solving (15), where possible with the involvement of a family support worker. It is particularly indicated in those with over 35 hours per week exposure to their carers. Key features include involvement of carers and patients; and sufficient durations of therapy. Chapter 15 provides a comprehensive overview of family-based treatments in schizophrenia.

As symptoms remit, vocational and wider social functioning should be assessed. As outlined elsewhere in this book, interventions including occupational therapy, social skills training, cognitive remediation, and vocational intervention have been advocated, with varying degrees of success, in established schizophrenia. Packages including elements of these interventions form key parts of some of the complex interventions and services discussed next.

A large proportion of first-episode psychosis sufferers abuse alcohol and illicit drugs, which worsens every type of outcome. The sequence of engagement in services, persuasion, and support to give up and then maintain abstinence is critical. Specific interventions by specialist services may be needed, including motivational interviewing and pharmacotherapy (chap. 7). There is early evidence that cognitive–behavioral interventions can be beneficial in established schizophrenia (16). Some have advocated fully integrated services for both psychosis and substance misuse but in practice sharing care between services is a common option. CBT for those without substance dependence but with established schizophrenia can reduce residual psychopathology and there is some evidence of reduction in symptoms after first episodes (17).

Psychodynamic psychotherapy at the acute stage probably worsens symptoms. Long-term supportive dynamic therapy may be beneficial but less so than assertive psychoeducational approaches (18).

Management of initial uncertainty

Clinical uncertainty is not uncommon in the first episode. In some cases it is unclear whether the patient is fully psychotic or merely has a mental state putting them at risk of frank psychosis. In other cases it is unclear whether they have an acute self-limiting or drug-induced psychosis. In prodromal patients the long-term benefits of antipsychotics are uncertain, especially when compared with CBT or SSRIs. Acute psychotic disorders and drug-induced psychoses subside rapidly in most cases. On the other hand, delaying definitive treatment for schizophrenia seems to be harmful. How to resolve this dilemma?

One approach is to discriminate on the basis of consequences and likelihood. The more mild the symptoms, the more typical the picture of an "at-risk" or drug-induced state or acute psychosis (often with a very short DUP and clear precipitant), the more likely one would wait and see. The more severe the symptoms, the less acute and the less typical of the above, the more likely one would treat and see. In the latter case, very rapid recovery would argue against schizophrenia but one might remain uncertain. Those who appear to have drug-induced psychosis but later achieve diagnoses of primary psychosis are more likely to have poor insight or a family history at presentation (19). This is probably indicative of an underlying "psychosis proneness" and the terms "drug precipitated" psychosis might be apposite in such individuals.

Course and further treatment

Recovery from the first episode of positive symptoms is usual and 15–20% will not have another. Relapse, often with increasing disability and negative symptoms, is the common pattern. At presentation certain factors can be identified that predict outcome, as shown in Box 17.2.

Box 17.2 Predictors of poor outcome following first-episode psychosis.

- Being young at first onset
- Being male
- Having a low IQ
- Manifesting severe negative symptoms at onset
- Exhibiting poor premorbid social adjustment
- Having a long duration of untreated psychosis
- Experiencing an insidious onset of symptoms
- Having a family history of schizophrenia

Recovery in the full sense of vocational and social rehabilitation, as well as symptom remission, should be the goal of treatment. However, evidence about how to achieve this in first-episode sufferers is only just emerging. Following remission, because of the high chance of relapse, long-term treatment and monitoring is indicated. Robinson et al. (20) found relapse occurring up to 5 years after presentation and so antipsychotic prophylaxis may be considered as long as this, although most clinical guidelines suggest a period of at least 1–2 years.

One-third to one-half of first-episode patients are nonadherent to prescribed medications during a follow-up (21). Poor adherence with treatment is if anything is more problematic than at later stages of illness because placebo controlled trials show greater benefits of antipsychotics in first-episode treatment and first relapse prevention. Robinson and colleagues (20) found that nonadherence increased the odds of relapse five-fold. Attention and time paid to therapeutic alliance at this stage may be returned later on. A particular feature of insight—the recognition that treatment has produced benefit—may have a particular importance for longer-term outcomes (22). As discussed in chapter 10, compliance therapy, an intervention aimed at improving medication adherence based on motivational interviewing, showed early promise but replication has proved problematic (23).

There have, therefore, been efforts to find effective alternatives to long-term, full-dose antipsychotics that patients might find more acceptable. Studies show low-dose antipsychotics consistently lead to much more frequent relapse. One study attempted discontinuation after recovery and only in those who appear to stabilize, it found about half could not do so (24). However, 20% of patients succeeded without relapse over 18 months. Comparing those trying to discontinue to those on continuous treatment, symptoms at follow-up were no worse and social function better if anything, though relapse rates were twice as high (20% compared with 40%). Relapses are associated with continuous illness and increased risk of suicide, as well as being disruptive, so this is not a trivial cost. Other studies demonstrate that intermittent treatment works better after first episodes than later ones; but only if patients are ready to restart medication at the first sign of symptoms, even if they are nonspecific ones preceding psychosis. Therefore, this may indicate a suitable approach for some of those not agreeing to the safer option of full prophylaxis.

If patients fail to respond to a full dose of the initial antipsychotic for at least 6 weeks or cannot tolerate it then an alternative, preferably from a different class, should be substituted. The diagnosis should be reviewed, as should overall management, including psychosocial interventions. Factors such as illicit drug use and adherence should be reconsidered. A depot antipsychotic formulation might be appropriate, or supervision and rapidly dissolving formulations. Adjunctive agents such as lithium (particularly for excitement or affective symptoms) should be considered. About 85% of patients respond in some way by this stage. If there is no response, despite the lack of evidence of superior efficacy of clozapine as first-line therapy (25), there is clear evidence for prescription of this drug third line in those likely to agree and adhere to it (26) (chap. 1). One notable algorithm in consenting patients used trials of two antipsychotics consisting of "low dose" non-clozapine atypicals for 2 weeks (e.g., olanzapine 5–10 mg, risperidone 2–3 mg, quetiapine 300–400 mg), escalating if there was no evidence of response to "full doses" for 2 weeks (olanzapine 12.5–20 mg, risperidone 4–6 mg, quetiapine 425–800 mg) and high doses for 2 weeks (olanzapine 22.5–30 mg, risperidone 6.5–10 mg, and quetiapine 850–1200 mg) before clozapine (26); this is compatible with the approach outlined in Figure 1.1. The efficacy of second-line antipsychotics was relatively poor and the question of clozapine as second line was raised, though this one could also support switching to a different class of agent and considering depot formulations.

Treating depression and anxiety

Though around a quarter of first-episode sufferers meet criteria for depression, many will recover and there is no evidence that antidepressants will help during active illness. Atypical antipsychotics may have some efficacy against mood symptoms. However, for those who develop depression after their first episode or remain depressed after other symptoms have remitted antidepressants may be indicated (e.g., SSRIs). They may affect serum antipsychotic levels. CBT may be appropriate but there is no specific evidence for efficacy in this population. A full discussion of these issues can be found in chapter 5.

As discussed in chapter 5, anxiety symptoms are common in schizophrenia, and can be disabling. In first-episode patients, particular attention should be paid to social anxiety symptoms, as this is a time of life when young people learn to socialize and to establish their social networks.

Settings and services

Phase-specific first episode or early intervention services allow staff to accumulate specialist experience and the service can be tailored to respond rapidly, diagnose appropriately, and meet the needs of a group that includes a high proportion of young adults in the process of individuation and sensitive to stigma. Some first-episode services have been sited in shopping centers or have close ties with youth organizations and social services, in order to improve accessibility and reduce stigma.

First-episode services need to pay particular attention to engagement. This may mean making the services discrete from generic mental health services, and this has been adopted in some settings, although there is no evidence that such separation is crucial to efficacy. What appears to be most important is the offering of a series of high fidelity interventions targeting the needs of the individual, and being respectful of their particular developmental and social contexts (as outlined below). The needs of carers and relatives also need to be met, including provision of education and support.

There is accumulating evidence of benefit, at least over the shorter term, from these services. Uncontrolled studies from Melbourne, Australia found instituting such a service improved a range of outcomes, though most were still hospitalized (27). The specific role of early detection has been evaluated in a controlled prospective study comparing different areas in Scandinavia, one of which instituted a public education campaign and adapted services to shorten DUP. Results showed that reduced DUP could be achieved, from a median of 12 weeks to 4 weeks, but the evidence that this translated into improved quality of life (28) or reduced symptoms was lacking or inconsistent at 1-year follow-up. Results at 2 years showed long-term reduction in negative symptoms, but the clinical impact of the modest reductions achieved, is questionable, and interpretation of this design was difficult because there was no blind rating and allowing for differences between areas was difficult (29). Two randomized trials of full early intervention services are noteworthy. A randomized, controlled trial in Copenhagen (30) (OPUS) found benefits in symptom reduction and other outcomes with an enhanced first-episode service. This offered a wider range of treatments than the usual service, actively delivered. The Lambeth Early Onset (LEO) randomized, controlled trial in 144 first and second episodes in London (31) found an early intervention service improved service and reduced readmission rates at 18 months. Odds of relapse were halved but this was not significant, perhaps due to the sample size. However, there is as yet no evidence that early intervention alters the long-term course of illness for most patients, and a substantial proportion continues to have a poor illness trajectory (32).

There are some arguments against discrete first-episode services (32). These include that they fragment care for what may be a life-long illness requiring continuing care: indeed, the transition to "adult" services can be very difficult for the young person. Also, such services can divert resources from other services, sometimes even ones that this patient group will use later on. Staff in generic services can become de-skilled in the area of early episode psychosis management, and arguably end up with the "residue" of patients who don't get better. Also, most first-episode services target the young, and do not usually cater for older sufferers such as those presenting with "late-onset" schizophrenia and many first episodes of delusional disorder. These patients may have quite different psychosocial needs and, certainly adults over 60 may need lower doses of medication still. Whatever the form of service offering care for first episodes, the accumulating evidence from first-episode service research does offer some guide to what are appropriate approaches to individual patients.

Conclusions

The first-episode movement has gained a major following among clinicians and researchers. While no one could argue against attempts to provide optimal care to people in this phase of illness, the evidence base for long-term benefits is lacking, and many patients continue to require concerted management. It is this group whose management is considered in the following chapter.

References

1. Cannon TD, Cadenhead K, Cornblatt B, et al. Prediction of psychosis in youth at high clinical risk: a multisite longitudinal study in North America. Arch Gen Psychiatry 2008; 65: 28–37.
2. Schltze-Lutter F, Klosterkötter J, Picker H, et al. Predicting first episode schizophrenia by basic symptom criteria. Clin Neuropsychiatry 2007; 4: 11–22.
3. Ruhrmann S, Schultze-Lutter F, Salokangas RK, et al. Prediction of psychosis in adolescents and young adults at high risk: results from the prospective European prediction of psychosis study. Arch Gen Psychiatry 2010; 67: 241–51.
4. Yung AR, Phillips LJ, Yuen HP, McGorry PD. Risk factors for psychosis in an ultra high-risk group: psychopathology and clinical features. Schizophr Res 2004; 67: 131–42.
5. Drake RJ, Lewis SW. Valuing prodromal psychosis: what do we get and what is the price? Schizophr Res 2010; 120: 38–41.
6. Kahn RS, Fleischhacker WW, Boter H, et al. Effectiveness of antipsychotic drugs in first-episode schizophrenia and schizophreniform disorder: an open randomised clinical trial. Lancet 2008; 371: 1085–97.
7. Crespo-Facorro B, Perez-Iglesias R, Ramirez-Bonilla M, et al. A practical clinical trial comparing haloperidol, risperidone, and olanzapine for the acute treatment of first-episode nonaffective psychosis. J Clin Psychiatry 2006; 67: 1511–21.
8. Schooler N, Robinowitz J, Davidson M, et al. Risperidone and haloperidol in first-episode psychosis: a long-term randomized trial. Am J Psychiatry 2005; 162: 947–53.
9. Lieberman JA, Tollefson G, Tohen M, et al. Comparative efficacy and safety of atypical and conventional antipsychotic drugs in first-episode psychosis: A randomized double-blind trial of Olanzapine vs Haloperidol. Am J Psychiatry 2003; 160: 1396–404.

10. Harvey PD, Rabinowitz J, Eerdekens M, Davidson M. Treatment of cognitive impairment in early psychosis: a comparison of risperidone and haloperidol in a large long-term trial. Am J Psychiatry 2005; 162: 1888–95.
11. Davidson M, Galderisi S, Weiser M, et al. Cognitive effects of antipsychotic drugs in first-episode schizophrenia and schizophreniform disorder: a randomized, open-label clinical trial (EUFEST). Am J Psychiatry 2009; 166: 675–82.
12. Perez-Iglesias R, Crespo-Facorro B, Martinez-Garcia O, et al. Weight gain induced by haloperidol, risperidone and olanzapine after 1 year: findings of a randomized clinical trial in a drug-naive population. Schizophr Res 2008; 99: 13–22.
13. Leucht S, Busch R, Hamann J, et al. Early-onset hypothesis of antipsychotic drug action: a hypothesis tested, confirmed and extended. Biol Psychiatry 2005; 57: 1543–9.
14. Raveendran NS, Tharyan P, Alexander J, et al. Rapid tranquillisation in psychiatric emergency settings in India: pragmatic randomised controlled trial of intramuscular olanzapine versus intramuscular haloperidol plus promethazine. BMJ 2007; 335: 86.
15. Lenior ME, Dingemans PM, Linszen DH, et al. Social functioning and the course of early-onset schizophrenia: five-year follow-up of a psychosocial intervention. Br J Psychiatry 2001; 179: 53–8.
16. Haddock G, Barrowclough C, Tarrier N, et al. Cognitive-behavioural therapy and motivational intervention for schizophrenia and substance misuse. 18-month outcomes of a randomised controlled trial. Br J Psychiatry 2003; 183: 418–26.
17. Tarrier N, Lewis S, Haddock G, et al. Cognitive-behavioural therapy in first-episode and early schizophrenia. 18-month follow-up of a randomised controlled trial. Br J Psychiatry 2004; 184: 231–9.
18. Rosenbaum B, Valbak K, Harder S, et al. Treatment of patients with first-episode psychosis: two-year outcome data from the Danish National Schizophrenia Project. World Psychiatry 2006; 5: 100–3.
19. Caton CL, Hasin DS, Shrout PE, et al. Stability of early-phase primary psychotic disorders with concurrent substance use and substance-induced psychosis. Br J Psychiatry 2007; 190: 105–11.
20. Robinson D, Woerner MG, Alvir JMJ, et al. Predictors of relapse following response from a first episode of schizophrenia or schizoaffective disorder. Arch Gen Psychiatry 1999; 56: 241–7.
21. Verdoux H, Lengronne J, Liraud F, et al. Medication adherence in psychosis: predictors and impact on outcome. A 2-year follow-up of first-admitted subjects. Acta Psychiatr Scand 2000; 102: 203–10.
22. Drake RJ, Dunn G, Tarrier N, et al. Insight as a predictor of the outcome of first-episode nonaffective psychosis in a prospective cohort study in England. J Clin Psychiatry 2007; 68: 81–6.
23. McIntosh AM, Conlon L, Lawrie SM, Stanfield AC. Compliance therapy for schizophrenia. Cochrane Database Syst Rev 2006; 3: CD003442.
24. Wunderink A, Nienhuis FJ, Sytema S, et al. Targeted treatment revisited: results of an RCT in first episode psychosis. Schizophr Res 2006; 81(Suppl): 255.
25. Lieberman JA, Phillips M, Gu H, et al. Atypical and conventional antipsychotic drugs in treatment-naive first-episode schizophrenia: a 52-week randomized trial of clozapine vs chlorpromazine. Neuropsychopharmacology 2003; 28: 995–1003.
26. Agid O, Remington G, Kapur S, et al. Early use of clozapine for poorly responding first-episode psychosis. J Clin Psychopharmacol 2007; 27: 369–73.
27. Power P, Elkins K, Adlard S, et al. Analysis of the initial treatment phase in first-episode psychosis. Br J Psychiatry Suppl 1998; 172: 71–6.
28. Melle I, Haahr U, Friis S. Reducing the duration of untreated first-episode psychosis – effects on baseline social functioning and quality of life. Acta Psychiatr Scand 2005; 112: 469–73.

29. Melle I, Larsen TK, Haahr U, et al. Prevention of negative symptom psychopathologies in first-episode schizophrenia: two-year effects of reducing the duration of untreated psychosis. Arch Gen Psychiatry 2008; 65: 634–40.
30. Petersen L, Jeppesen P, Thorup A, et al. A randomised multicentre trial of integrated versus standard treatment for patients with a first episode of psychotic illness. BMJ 2005; 331: 602.
31. Craig TK, Garety P, Power P, et al. The Lambeth Early Onset (LEO) Team: randomised controlled trial of the effectiveness of specialised care for early psychosis. BMJ 2004; 329: 1067.
32. Bosanac P, Patton G, Castle DJ. Early intervention in psychotic disorders: Faith before facts? Psychol Med 2010; 40: 275–84.

chapter 18

Treatment-resistant schizophrenia

William D. Spaulding, Robert W. Johnson, Jeffrey R. Nolting, and Amanda Collins Messman

In the clinical and scientific literature, "treatment-resistant schizophrenia" almost universally means not responsive to antipsychotics.* However, the meaning of "not responsive" varies widely, ranging from "having no measurable impact on the illness" to "suboptimal symptom reduction" (1). People are usually deemed to have treatment-resistant schizophrenia even if they are responsive to clozapine or drugs not usually used to treat schizophrenia (e.g., anticonvulsant/mood stabilizers), if they are unresponsive to non-clozapine antipsychotics. There is no universally accepted theoretical rationale for linking treatment resistance to one class of drugs. Current terminological conventions reflect historical precedent (had atypical antipsychotics been discovered first, they would not be termed atypical).

The meaning of being "resistant" to one particular class of drug is further obscured by the tendency of psychiatric drugs to produce benefits across diagnostic boundaries (e.g., the mood stabilizing effects of some antipsychotics and the antipsychotic effects of some mood stabilizers), and by findings that suggest non-clozapine atypicals are not superior to typicals for the reduction of psychotic symptoms (2). Response to pharmacotherapy in schizophrenia is multidimensional, involving individually unique combinations of negative symptoms, positive symptoms, affective dysregulation, cognitive impairment, and other aspects of sociobehavioral functioning (3). Nevertheless, especially

---

*The terms "treatment resistant" and "refractory" are used synonymously in the clinical and scientific literature on schizophrenia. In late 2011, an unconstrained PubMed scan of the National Library of Medicine for "treatment-resistant schizophrenia" yielded 1239 citations. "Refractory schizophrenia" yielded 812 hits. Constraining the scan to appearance in titles yielded 220 and 178 instances, respectively. "Treatment refractory" is technically redundant, because "not responsive to treatment" is one definition of "refractory." Since "treatment resistant" is used more frequently, it is used in this chapter.

in controlled studies (1,4), individuals are generally identified as treatment resistant based on diagnosis plus the presence of specific positive or negative psychotic symptoms, as measured by standardized structured interviews, after one or more formal trials of non-clozapine antipsychotics. Inevitably, arbitrary cutoff points must be used to determine the level of severity that serves as the criterion for inclusion in the resistant group. Also, individuals sometimes show large differences in their responses to different antipsychotics, for reasons not well understood. Failing only one or two drug trials is therefore not a perfectly reliable criterion (5). These are manageable methodological problems when the research question is narrowly about whether one drug produces better outcome than another, but they are significant impediments to a more complete understanding of the nature of treatment resistance. Perhaps most importantly, the methodological conventions of comparative drug trials can promote an implicit presumption that drug response (and, inversely, non-response) is a unidimensional "either-or" dichotomy, when in fact it is a multiplicity of continuous dimensions, for both typical and atypical antipsychotics (and for treatment in general, including psychosocial treatment).

Moreover, it is generally acknowledged that schizophrenia itself is a heterogeneous category, probably not unified by a single set of causes. There are numerous etiological processes that operate in variable combinations to produce the many presentations of illness within the schizophrenia spectrum. Research to articulate relationships between these factors and drug response is underway, but still in its early stages (6,7). Our perception of "treatment resistance" reflects in part our inability to treat all possible processes and combinations. In addition, there are probably other biological factors, remote from the etiology of the illness itself, for example alleles, which affect pharmacokinetics (8) that contribute to treatment resistance in some individuals.

Considering the conceptual and methodological ambiguities, it should not be surprising that the actual prevalence of treatment-resistant schizophrenia has been difficult to ascertain. Although estimates vary widely, the proportion of people with schizophrenia who do not respond to antipsychotic medication at all is at least 20% (9) and those with minimal response may be as high as 60% (10). Naturally occurring subpopulations, for example patients with extended inpatient histories, are expected to include higher concentrations of treatment-resistant patients (11). Estimates of the effectiveness of clozapine range from 30% to 50% for people whose illness is resistant to typicals (12). However, the clinical benefits are reduced by the number of patients who tolerate it poorly (e.g., drowsiness, weight gain, and related metabolic side effects) and by the risk of lethal blood dyscrasia. Even with clozapine in the formulary, the proportion of people with significant and persistent symptoms is estimated to be as high as two-thirds (13).

In partially controlled trials it is possible to demonstrate improvement with non-clozapine atypicals in patients with previous medication failure (14), but such studies are generally designed to compare different atypicals. Without active placebo controls, clinical benefits of previously nonresponsive patients can be attributed to trial conditions, like precise measurement of symptoms, extra attention to tolerance, heightened expectations, and so forth. Fully controlled trials may eventually detect population differences in response to specific agents. However, population differences do not necessarily inform clinical decision making. Trial groups based on diagnosis include too much heterogeneity to reveal much about individual differences in treatment response. It appears more likely that new research paradigms addressing *personalization* (matching treatments to individual characteristics) will guide us more directly toward maximizing treatment response in the real world (15).

The evidence that valproic acid enhances the effectiveness of antipsychotic medication is sufficient that the FDA has approved that agent for such use. There is accumulating evidence for lamotrigine as well (16). Mood stabilizers act on components of the neurophysiological system (e.g., ion channels) that are separable from those acted upon by antipsychotics (e.g., D2 receptors). Augmentation of antipsychotic effects by mood stabilizers may, therefore, actually be treatment of a separate but comorbid etiological process. Arguably this is different from overcoming a treatment-resistant illness, although the practical outcome is the same. Other non-antipsychotic biological treatments reported to benefit treatment-resistant and/or clozapine-resistant patients include clonidine (17) and electroconvulsive therapy (18).

As treatment for schizophrenia expands beyond pharmacotherapy and other biological approaches, the implications of being refractory specifically to *biological* treatment are changing. There is no longer any doubt that psychosocial treatment substantially improves outcome beyond that achieved with medication alone ((19); chap. 2, 3, 11, and 12). Among people whose illness is resistant to typical antipsychotics, clozapine enhances their chances of benefiting from psychosocial treatment (20) but this does not mean that psychosocial interventions are always dependent on successful pharmacological treatment. Specialized types of cognitive–behavioral therapy (CBT) can help with medication-resistant hallucinations and delusions (21,22) (chap. 2). The putative benefits of the atypical risperidone for cognitive functioning (relative to typicals) appear to be overwhelmed and obscured by the benefits of a comprehensive psychiatric rehabilitation program (23) (chap. 4). Intensive psychiatric rehabilitation is effective for people for whom medication has been ineffective or insufficient (24,25) (chap. 16). Silverstein et al. (25) propose that these findings indicate that the proportion of people diagnosed with schizophrenia who are treatment resistant is substantially smaller than generally believed, because "resistant" has meant resistant to only pharmacotherapy. Eventually, it will become necessary to revise the concept of treatment-resistant schizophrenia itself to reflect our expanding armamentarium (26).

Another imperative for revising the basic concept of treatment resistance comes from the *recovery movement*, a world-wide consumerist mental health reform movement. The recovery movement rejects traditional assumptions about the nature of mental illness, framing it not as a disease to be cured but as a *disability to be overcome*. This view comports with the reality that no "cure" for severe mental illness (SMI) exists, but more importantly it challenges prevailing treatment priorities on diagnostic signs and symptoms rather than the functional consequences of the illness. "Recovery" means recovery of functional abilities to live independently, to work productively, to have social relationships, to participate in community life and so on. Recovery also has subjective dimensions, including self-respect, a sense of well being and hope for the future. Inspired by a presidential commission report (27), *recovery-oriented mental health service systems* have become a national aspiration in the United States and elsewhere. The recovery concept challenges the *importance* of resistance to drug treatment, as opposed to resistance to other treatments that address functional disabilities and promote well-being. It is clear to all that people whose diagnostic symptoms respond well to pharmacological (or other) treatment may nevertheless fail to recover social functioning and subjective well-being. This type of treatment resistance is at least as important as resistance to pharmacological treatment.

Thus, for both conceptual and practical purposes, treatment resistance needs to incorporate more than just medication response, and it needs to include dimensions of personal and social functioning beyond those typically of interest in antipsychotic drug trials. Most importantly, it needs to give clinicians solutions more helpful than waiting for the research to generate better medications. With the proliferation of treatment targets brought by holistic recovery models of schizophrenia, it will soon be easier to make subgroups according to treatment *responsiveness* rather than resistance. Our theoretical concepts would be brought more in line with our clinical judgment and decision making by replacing the general concept of treatment resistance in patient subgroups with quantitative dimensions of treatment responsiveness associated with specific treatments for specific individuals.

Meanwhile, it is useful to identify specific clinical tools and the types of treatment resistance for which they may be helpful. That is the organizational scheme for the remainder of this chapter. Most of the tools discussed elsewhere in this book are potentially effective for drug treatment-resistant schizophrenia. The tools listed here (summarized in Box 18.1) are ones that are

---

Box 18.1   The seven tools used in treatment resistance.

- Medication algorithms
- Neuropsychological therapy and environmental engineering
- Contingency management
- Cognitive–behavioral therapy for treatment-resistant psychotic symptoms
- Systematic, expanded, and individualized assessment of pharmacotherapy
- Therapeutic jurisprudence
- Risk assessment and risk management

especially important for directly addressing treatment resistance, and for making other treatments accessible to patients whose illnesses are otherwise treatment resistant.

Seven clinical tools for managing treatment-resistant schizophrenia

Medication algorithms

Research criteria for identifying medication resistance are generally unhelpful in clinical practice (4). *Medication algorithms* (28) are proposed as alternative tools for determining optimal medication regimens for people whose illness does not respond well to initial treatment attempts (chap. 1). Even after considerable development, it is difficult to be confident that medication algorithms will impact clinical outcome (29). On the other hand, there are persistent concerns that in real-world practice treatment resistance is determined prematurely because of inadequate clinical trials (5). Algorithms could indirectly benefit outcome by encouraging more systematic and rigorous evaluation of all medication effects.

Considering existent algorithms in the context of current trends, it is likely that the steps toward identifying medication resistance will approximate this sequence ("trials" means trials of sufficient time, with titration to maximum dose, which are often difficult to accomplish in clinical practice; the reader is also referred to Figures 1.1 and 1.2 in chapter 1 for treatment algorithms and Tables 1.2 and 1.3 for details of different medications, including recommended doses.

1. Trials of first recourse agents, including one or more atypical D2 antagonists (risperidone, paliperidone, olanzapine, ziprasidone, quetiapine, asenapine, etc.) and a D2 partial agonist (e.g., aripiprazole)
2. A trial of atypical antipsychotic augmented by a mood stabilizer
3. A trial of an injectable depot preparation of an atypical (this step may come earlier when adherence is a suspected factor: see also chap. 1 for details of available depots and chap. 10 for a broader discussion of adherence)
4. Trials of combinations of atypical antipsychotics
5. A trial of typical antipsychotic (some practitioners would forego this step, as discussed in chap. 1);
6. A trial of clozapine (see chap. 1 for details of clozapine);
7. Trials of typical/atypical combinations (chap. 1).

Steps 4 and 7 will probably generate the most controversy as algorithms evolve. Polypharmacy is a recognized problem (5,9) and algorithms are designed to avoid it. There is no widely accepted theoretical model for selecting antipsychotic combinations, nor even agreement about whether a rational/theoretical approach will be better than a strictly empirical or even intuitive approach. An empirical test of antipsychotic polypharmacy is monumentally difficult, but a large multi-center trial is under way and may eventually provide the first empirical support for this approach to treatment resistance (13).

Neuropsychological therapy and environmental engineering

Even when pharmacotherapy is effective in reducing the cognitive disorganization of acute psychosis, stabilized and optimally medicated patients often have significant residual neurocognitive impairment. In this sense, all or most postacute impairment is treatment resistant. Such impairment is a strong limiting factor in rehabilitation success. A number of neuropsychological approaches to directly treating the neurocognitive impairments of schizophrenia have been recently developed (chap. 4). These approaches are sometimes termed "cognitive remediation," but controversially so, because the connotations of "remediation" are unclear. "Therapy" describes the type of activity without connotation, and "neuropsychological" describes the level of functioning the treatment addresses, and the scientific and technical origins of the techniques. They range from computer-based tasks that exercise basic attention and memory to group-format techniques that enhance social perception and problem solving. Outcome measures that have shown effects of neuropsychological therapy range from social competence to psychotic symptoms to work performance (chap. 11 and 12). A meta-analysis of 17 controlled neuropsychological therapy trials (30) supports the approach's effectiveness. A number of distinct types of therapy have evolved, targeting a range of cognitive impairments and accommodating a variety of subpopulations and settings (31). This type of therapy appears to benefit patients across the spectrum of severity, treatment resistant or not, but for treatment-resistant patients it could be a crucial determinant of further recovery.

A similar approach, based on operant learning principles, has proven effective in helping people with severe neurocognitive impairment (32,33). In this approach, individuals are systematically reinforced with tokens as they successively approximate motor behaviors prerequisite to group participation, such as appropriate motor orientation, eye contact, disregard of ambient distraction, and performance of elemental group-related tasks. This approach is thought to be important, especially for people who have the most severe disabilities and functional limitations and may otherwise be treatment resistant to conventional skill training.

There is some overlap between techniques that address neuropsychological functioning and techniques used in CBT and social skills training (discussed in chap. 12). Integrated packages sometimes include evidence-based techniques from multiple domains. For example, since the 1980s, social skills training materials have incorporated the CBT technique of structured problem solving, and have included strategies for doing social skills training with people having neurocognitive impairments. *Integrated Psychological Therapy* (IPT) (34,35) is an evidence-based exemplar that integrates all three techniques in a group skills training format. Meta-analysis (31) suggests that IPT is more effective than standard treatment for symptom reduction, psychosocial functioning, and neurocognition in adults with schizophrenia. The benefits appear across multiple outcome measurement domains, including psychological testing, self-report, and clinician ratings, and are independent of treatment setting (inpatient vs. outpatient, academic vs. nonacademic) and stage of illness (acute vs. chronic). Moreover, the benefits appear to increase or accumulate over time (36). The neuropsychological components of IPT contribute uniquely to overall outcome (37). *Cognitive Enhancement Therapy* is a package similar to IPT, with empirical evidence of effectiveness (38).

High-intensity psychiatric rehabilitation programs such as the one described by Spaulding et al. (37) and Silverstein et al. (25) have nonspecific benefits for neuropsychological functioning, even without components that explicitly target cognitive impairment. People with treatment-resistant illnesses disproportionately find themselves in such programs, so nonspecific treatment effects on neurocognitive impairment should be expected to be an important factor for success in moving to less intensive and less restrictive settings.

Neurocognitive impairments that do not respond to treatment can nevertheless be managed through specialized environmental engineering that provides compensatory supports (39–41) (chap. 4). This approach involves environmental modifications, ranging from sound proofing (to reduce auditory distraction) to packaging wardrobe elements for daily use (to compensate for disinhibition and deficits in executive cognition). Such interventions have been shown to enhance routine daily functioning and adherence to treatment, both of which provide a demonstrable contribution to rehabilitation progress and recovery. However, it is important to exercise caution when employing these solutions to ensure that they are not being used when a rehabilitative approach would reestablish more normal cognitive and behavioral functioning and greater independence.

Related compensatory approaches aim to create environmental supports that reduce cognitive burdens, stress, and requirements for functioning while providing for the individual's needs and quality of life (42). In a sense, broader approaches such as *assertive community treatment* (ACT) and *supported employment* (chap. 16 and 12 respectively) are examples of compensatory environmental engineering. Although they are not based on neuropsychological considerations, they do aim to compensate for deficits in behavioral functioning with prosthetic environmental features.

Contingency management

Contingency management is a genre of techniques that evolved from learning and social-learning theories in the 1960s. They are especially important in nonacute psychiatric inpatient and residential settings, where people with treatment-resistant conditions are disproportionately represented (43). In fact, in many modern mental health systems, such settings are populated *solely* by people with conditions that are resistant to pharmacotherapy. The consistent effectiveness of contingency management in these settings makes this approach especially important for treatment-resistant schizophrenia.

The earliest applications of contingency management for schizophrenia, in the form of *token economies* in psychiatric hospitals, provided strong empirical evidence of effectiveness in promoting adaptive behavior (44). In a 7-year controlled clinical outcome trial (45) described at the time as "the largest outcome trial in the history of psychiatry," a social learning-based rehabilitation program that included contingency management was vastly superior to psychiatric treatment as usual. It was also superior to an enriched version of *therapeutic community*, a psychosocial approach that was popular in psychiatric and substance abuse settings in the 1960s and 1970s. Replication studies and an accumulation of case studies and institutional experience continues to support the effectiveness of contingency management in replacing inappropriate behavior (including psychotic symptoms), with adaptive behavior and increasing participation in treatment and rehabilitation (24,25,46). In its modern form, contingency management is a more highly individualized and targeted treatment than in the early token economies. In addition, it typically involves extensive interaction between the identified patient and therapist(s), with negotiations and contracts to link specific rewards and other consequences to specific desired behaviors (47). Highly individualized contingency management interventions are often termed *behavior management programs*.

As psychiatric rehabilitation has evolved, the role of contingency management in enhancing engagement in therapeutic activities has become increasingly important (48). The original goal of promoting adaptive behavior can now be more extensively operationalized, in terms of engagement and participation in social skills training, occupational/vocational activities, and the various other psychosocial modalities discussed in this book. In this sense, contingency management addresses and compensates for what may be the most malignant and pervasive consequence of resistance to pharmacotherapy, failure to engage in psychosocial treatment and rehabilitation. When combined with other social-learning modalities, contingency management has been shown to be specifically effective with two of the most troublesome and drug-resistant problems encountered in mental health settings, namely aggression (49,50); and see chapter 8 for a discussion of treatment of aggression in schizophrenia) and polydipsia (51). Most recently, contingency management is being applied to co-occurring substance abuse, frequently a barrier to recovery from SMI (52,53).

CBT for treatment-resistant psychotic symptoms

As outlined in Chapter 2, specialized forms of CBT show robust effects on drug treatment-resistant hallucinations (54). Delusions, which are generally more resistant to psychopharmacotherapy, can also be effectively resolved.

In real-world clinical settings the efficacy of these approaches may often be compromised by other common features of treatment-resistant psychosis, most notably, inability or unwillingness to engage in therapeutic activities. Depending on the underlying causes, responsiveness to CBT may be dependent on other treatments, most notably neuropsychological therapy and contingency management.

The focus of CBT on the person's perceptions and beliefs is producing a convergence with two other important developments in services for people with treatment-resistant SMI. The first is *motivational interviewing* (55), a dyadic therapy technique designed to clarify the person's values and desires in a way that motivates the person toward positive change. Mental illness is highly compatible with CBT and other psychiatric rehabilitation approaches, and has been demonstrated to be helpful for people with SMI by enhancing engagement in substance abuse treatment (56) and adherence to and maintenance of a rehabilitation regimen (57). Substance abuse and adherence are significant factors in treatment-resistant schizophrenia and are covered in more detail in chapters 7 and 10 respectively.

The second converging factor is as promoted by the recovery movement. In the recovery perspective, the very notion of treatment resistance is an artifact of a flawed paradigm overly dependent on medical treatment. Convergence of CBT and mental illness techniques with recovery concepts could in the near future produce a new, holistic approach to treatment resistance in which the identified patient gains a greater degree of personal control over the illness and its disabilities, transcending limitations of pharmacology and other treatment technologies (58). This would transform the meaning, much less the treatment, of treatment-resistant schizophrenia, even beyond the transformation envisioned by Silverstein et al. (25) and Quintero (26).

Systematic, expanded, and individualized assessment of psychopharmacotherapy

Ordinarily, prescription of antipsychotic medication is based on a relatively brief clinical interview, sometimes with corroborating information from the patient's social environment. The data produced by this approach can be so unreliable that it prevents an accurate assessment of drug effects, or even of the target symptoms themselves. In the terminology of experimental design, this creates a low power test, vulnerable to *type 2 errors* (failing to detect an effect when it is in fact present). A type 2 error creates in turn the appearance of treatment resistance. Once an illness is perceived to be drug resistant, prescribing practice becomes driven by the prescriber's liability management and related factors, if it is rational at all. This often leads to the pervasive problem of polypharmacy (9) which further obscures drug effects. Increasing the measurement power of the drug trial prevents this cascade and helps discriminate between true treatment resistance and drug effects that are subtle, unusual, outside the usual domains of psychopharmacological assessment, or otherwise difficult to detect.

The power of psychopharmacological assessment should first be increased by expanding the database beyond subjective report and historical records. This requires resources not common in real-world mental health settings, but people with drug-resistant psychosis often find themselves in environments where expanded, milieu-based assessment is more feasible, such as inpatient and residential settings. In such settings, where there are high proportions of people with drug-resistant psychosis, investment in expanded assessment capabilities is well justified. Expansion should include the use of standardized measures that quantify the information a prescriber would normally collect anecdotally, such as the Brief Psychiatric Rating Scale (59). Outside the consulting room, standardized observational measures such as the Nurses Observational Scale for Inpatient Evaluation (60) provide quantitative data on the patient's behavior in the ambient environment, often quite different from behavior in a structured interview. The Time-Sample Behavioral Checklist (TSBC) (61) is a related observational measure that provides even more precise behavioral data relevant to evaluation of medication effects. Further refinement of TSBC data such as rates of aggressive behavior, which are inadequately assessed by time-sampling methods, is provided by the Clinical Frequencies Recording System. It is complementary to the type of data yielded by the TSBC and provides a complete picture of discrete program schedule dependent performances, patterns of usage of goods and services, and low frequency critical behaviors.

In treatment settings where staff members are trained to implement contingency management, systematic quantitative observation of highly specific behaviors is routine, and is easily adapted to the purposes of a drug trial. Behavior management programs provide precise data on the frequency and quality of specific target behaviors, including medication-responsive behaviors.

Rehabilitation-oriented treatment settings also generate data in domains not conventionally associated with drug trials, as shown in Box 18.2, and which should be crucial targets for assessing functional responses to treatment. For example, The Independent Living Skills Inventory (62) provides information on a person's ability to perform domain specific skills required for successful community living, such as money management, cooking and occupational

---

Box 18.2 Broader outcomes in rehabilitation settings.

- Following daily routines
- Participating in occupational activities
- Managing personal finances
- Engaging in social activities

skills. Using such data within the context of thoughtfully designed naturalistic drug trials affords more reliable assessment and measurement of the etiology of the resistance and increases the probability of detecting significant drug effects on an individual's functioning, whose illness will otherwise be deemed drug treatment resistant.

Another way to increase the power of a drug trial is to amplify the longitudinal dimension of measurement. All of the clinical measures discussed above are well suited to repeated administration over time. The residential and inpatient settings in which people with treatment-resistant schizophrenia are often treated are usually well suited to frequent longitudinal data collection. Availability of longitudinal data enhances evaluation not only of medication effects but overall progress in rehabilitation. This is crucial to optimizing an individual rehabilitation and recovery plan. An administrative commitment to systematic collection and analysis of longitudinal behavioral data may be one of the most important aspects of treating treatment resistant schizophrenia. Chapter 19 provides further assessment tools that can be used in clinical practice.

Therapeutic jurisprudence

Therapeutic jurisprudence is a set of principles and techniques intended to use the law to benefit and enhance mental health (17). Therapeutic jurisprudence is especially relevant to treatment-resistant schizophrenia, because of the frequency with which the latter is accompanied by legal complications such as civil commitment, issues of competency (Box 18.3) and court-ordered treatment (63,64). It is increasingly necessary for clinicians who treat people with treatment resistant psychosis to be proficient in dealing with legal complications and making good therapeutic use of legal processes and mechanisms. This includes collaborating with

---

Box 18.3 Five steps for assessing competence.

- Patient registers the information provided
- Patient absorbs, retains, and recalls this information
- Patient understands the information is relevant to them in that they appreciate that decisions they make will have certain consequences for them (*cognitive* understanding)
- Patient makes decisions about the consequences of decisions compatible with their own values and beliefs (*evaluative* understanding)
- Patient communicates their understanding and the decisions based on that understanding

Source: Based on Pargiter and Cloverdale, 2001.

- patients, to educate them about their legal status and its relationship to treatment;
- legal authorities and rehabilitation teams, to make optimal clinical use of relevant legal processes and mechanisms;
- legal authorities, consumers, advocates, and policy makers, to make mental health law and its implementation conducive to rehabilitation and recovery and
- legal authorities, to educate consumers, advocates, legal professionals and mental health professionals in therapeutic jurisprudence.

Risk assessment and risk management

People with treatment-resistant schizophrenia are disproportionately found by a legal authority, at some point in time, to be dangerous to themselves and/or others. For a full discussion of these issues, see chapter 9. Safely serving these people in the least restrictive and most integrated settings possible, particularly community settings, requires highly reliable assessment and management of the consequent risks. Historically, mental health professionals' ability to predict dangerousness has been dubious, but the last decade has seen crucial advances in the relevant technology (65). Effective treatment and rehabilitation for treatment-resistant SMI will require the best risk assessment and management that science and technology can provide. This means explicit evaluation of a person's potential for dangerousness, under existing circumstances and under circumstances anticipated in the foreseeable future (it is no longer acceptable to say simply that a person is not dangerous right here and right now (66). This includes review and interpretation of the person's social history, use of appropriate psychometric and actuarial instruments and functional assessment of the person's psychiatric disorder.

Risk management requires a complete risk assessment plus a complete enumeration of the conditions, circumstances, and environments that could precipitate behavior wherein one is considered to be dangerous to oneself or others in the future, and a plan for minimizing those risks.

Treatment resistance, dissemination, and mental health policy

The array of evidence-based tools for treatment-resistant schizophrenia reinforces the idea that, in a very pragmatic sense, treatment resistance is defined by access to effective treatments. It is less a characteristic of the illness than of our treatment technology and availability of it. Dissemination of new treatment methods is increasingly understood to be a bottleneck, especially in mental health, and specifically nonpharmacological treatments (67,68). In this sense, mental health policies that either enhance or limit access to needed treatments are critical factors in the size and morbidity of the "treatment-resistant subpopulation."

Bureaucratic values that favor uniformity in design and regulation of service systems create barriers to serving groups with atypical needs, almost by definition. Similarly, mental health administrators tend to think of services as *commodities*, like iron ore or pork bellies, invariant in quality (69). The idea of specialized services for special need subgroups is antithetical to such a perspective. Nevertheless, the breadth and complexity of the treatment array for treatment-resistant schizophrenia, appropriately defined, demands specialization in order to minimize the size of the recipient population and ultimately the cost of providing treatment. Specialized programs such as those described by Paul and Lentz (45), Spaulding et al. (37), and Silverstein et al. (25), capable of performing personalized data-driven coordination of multiple pharmacological and psychosocial treatments, are cost effective for the treatment-resistant subpopulation, but the "one size fits all" administrative perspective makes it difficult for such programs to survive (70). In addition, such programs require an organizational structure and clinical procedures incompatible with those of traditional "medical model" public institutions, the historical venue for care of people with treatment-resistant schizophrenia. This creates resistance to reform from administrative and professional interests invested in traditional institutional practices (71).

Unfortunately, public psychiatric institutions still attract concentrations of "treatment-resistant" people (72). The attraction is accelerated by persistent use of a treatment approach known to be ineffective for the treatment-resistant population. Without progressive policy and strong leadership, the mental health system itself becomes a major cause of treatment-resistant schizophrenia.

Conclusions

Although good drug response enhances success in psychosocial treatment, the latter is not necessarily dependent on the former for effectiveness. Some specific treatments succeed where pharmacotherapy fails, although this does not mean that the mechanisms of treatment response or the actual outcome is exactly the same. Management of these complications is not an easy task for the treatment team; the use of both medication algorithms *and* more general algorithms for treatment and rehabilitation of schizophrenia (73) is essential. Comprehensive multimodal psychiatric rehabilitation (74,75) is the best available solution for people who have pervasive difficulty with following daily routines and performing the basic activities of daily living, whether or not those difficulties are associated with poor response to pharmacotherapy. Contingency management has been shown to be a highly effective component of rehabilitation, especially in settings where people with drug-resistant illnesses are disproportionately represented. Moreover, those settings can produce enriched data on behaviors not typically associated with drug trials, but which might be crucial targets for assessing treatment response.

Programmatic, multimodal approaches effective for treatment-resistant schizophrenia require a departure from traditional organizational schemes, clinical practices, and interdisciplinary relationships. Progressive mental health policy and strong leadership are required to make needed services available. Otherwise, treatment-resistant schizophrenia is as much a product of the service system as it is a characteristic of the illness.

References

1. Suzuki T, Remington G, Mulsant BH, et al. Treatment resistant schizophrenia and response to antipsychotics: a review. Schizophr Res 2011; 133: 54–62.
2. Lieberman JA, Stroup TS, McEvoy JP, et al. Effectiveness of antipsychotic drugs in patients with chronic schizophrenia. N Engl J Med 2005; 353: 1209–23.
3. Lindenmayer JP. Treatment refractory schizophrenia. Psychiatr Q 2000; 71: 373–84.
4. Brenner H, Roder V, Hodel B, et al. Integrated Psychological Therapy for Schizophrenic Patients. Toronto: Hogrefe & Huber, 1994.
5. Tsutsumi C, Uchida H, Suzuki T, et al. The evolution of antipsychotic switch and polypharmacy in natural practice–a longitudinal perspective. Schizophr Res 2011; 130: 40–6.
6. Molina V, Reig S, Sarramea F, et al. Anatomical and functional brain variables associated with clozapine response in treatment-resistant schizophrenia. Psychiatry Res 2003; 124: 153–61.
7. Gandal MJ, Edgar JC, Klook K, Siegel SJ. Gamma synchrony: towards a translational biomarker for the treatment-resistant symptoms of schizophrenia. Neuropharmacology 2011; 62: 1504–18.
8. Kawanishi C, Furuno T, Kishida I, et al. A patient with treatment-resistant schizophrenia and cytochrome P4502D6 gene duplication. Clin Genet 2002; 61: 152–4.
9. Stahl SM, Grady MM. A critical review of atypical antipsychotic utilization: comparing monotherapy with polypharmacy and augmentation. Curr Med Chem 2004; 11: 313–27.
10. Solanki RK, Singh P, Munshi D. Current perspectives in the treatment of resistant schizophrenia. Indian J Psychiatry 2009; 51: 254–60.
11. Mortimer AM, Singh P, Shepherd CJ, Puthiryackal J. Clozapine for treatment-resistant schizophrenia: National Institute of Clinical Excellence (NICE) guidance in the real world. Clin Schizophr Relat Psychoses 2011; 4: 49–55.
12. McIlwain ME, Harrison J, Wheeler AJ, Russell BR. Pharmacotherapy for treatment-resistant schizophrenia. Neuropsychiatr Dis Treat 2011; 7: 135–49.
13. Nose M, Accordini S, Artioli P, et al. Rationale and design of an independent randomised controlled trial evaluating the effectiveness of aripiprazole or haloperidol in combination with clozapine for treatment-resistant schizophrenia. Trials 2009; 10: 31.
14. Kane JM, Potkin SG, Daniel DG, Buckley PF. A double-blind, randomized study comparing the efficacy and safety of sertindole and risperidone in patients with treatment-resistant schizophrenia. J Clin Psychiatry 2011; 72: 194–204.
15. Spaulding W, Deogun J. A pathway to personalization of integrated treatment: Informatics and decision science in psychiatric rehabilitation. Schizophr Bull 2011; 37(Suppl 2): S129–37.
16. Goff DC. Review: lamotrigine may be an effective treatment for clozapine resistant schizophrenia. Evid Based Ment Health 2009; 12: 111.
17. Dardennes RM, Al Anbar NN, Rouillon F. Successful augmentation of clozapine-resistant treatment of schizophrenia with clonidine. Prog Neuropsychopharmacol Biol Psychiatry 2010; 34: 724–5.

18. Garg R, Chavan BS, Arun P. Quality of life after electroconvulsive therapy in persons with treatment resistant schizophrenia. Indian J Med Res 2011; 133: 641–4.

19. Mojtabai R, Nicholson RA, Carpenter BN. Role of psychosocial treatments in management of schizophrenia: A meta-analytic review of controlled outcome studies. Schizophr Bull 1998; 24: 569–87.

20. Rosenheck R, Tekell J, Peters J, et al. Does participation in psychosocial treatment augment the benefit of clozapine? Department of Veterans Affairs Cooperative Study Group on Clozapine in Refractory Schizophrenia. Arch Gen Psychiatry 1998; 55: 618–25.

21. Rector NA, Beck AT. Cognitive behavioral therapy for schizophrenia: An empirical review. J Nerv Ment Dis 2001; 189: 278–87.

22. Zimmermann G, Favrod J, Trieu V, et al. The effect of cognitive behavioral treatment on the positive symptoms of schizophrenia spectrum disorders: a meta-analysis. Schizophr Res 2005; 77: 1–9.

23. Liberman R, Gutkind D, Mintz M, et al. Impact of risperidone versus haloperidol on activities of daily living in the treatment of refractory schizophrenia. Compr Psychiatry 2002; 43: 469–73.

24. Paul G, Menditto A. Effectiveness of inpatient treatment programs for mentally ill adults in public psychiatric facilities. Appl Prev Psychol 1992; 1: 41–63.

25. Silverstein S, Hatashita-Wong M, Wilkniss SM, et al. Behavioral rehabilitation of the "treatment-refractory" schizophrenia patient: conceptual foundations, interventions and outcome data. Psychol Serv 2006; 3: 145–69.

26. Quintero J, Barbudo del Cura E, Lopez-Ibor MI, Lopez-Ibor JJ. The evolving concept of treatment- resistant schizophrenia. Actas Esp Psiquiatr 2011; 39: 236–50.

27. President's New Freedom Commission on Mental Health. Report to the President (2004). [Cited 2004 Oct 15]. [Available from: http://www.mentalhealthcommission.gov/reports/reports.htm].

28. Chiles JA, Miller AL, Crimson ML, et al. The Texas medication algorithm project: Development and implementation of the schizophrenia algorithm. Psychiatr Serv 1999; 50: 69–74.

29. Crabtree BL, Dostrow VG, Evans CJ, et al. Outcome assessment of an antipsychotic drug algorithm: effects of the Mississippi State Hospital algorithm project. Psychiatr Serv 2011; 62: 963–5.

30. Twamley EW, Jeste DV, Bellack AS. A review of cognitive training in schizophrenia. Schizophr Bull 2003; 29: 359–82.

31. Roeder V, Medalia A, eds. Neurocognition and Social Cognition in Schizophrenia Patients. Basic Concepts and Treatment. Key Issues Ment Health. Vol 177. Basel: Karger, 2010.

32. Silverstein SM, Menditto A, Stuve P. Shaping attention span: an operant condition procedure for improving neurocognitive functioning in schizophrenia. Schizophr Bull 2001; 27: 247–57.

33. Silverstein S, Spaulding W, Menditto A, et al. Attention shaping: a reward-based learning method to enhance skills training outcomes in schizophrenia. Schizophr Bull 2009; 35: 222–32.

34. Roder V, Mueller DR, Mueser KT, et al. Integrated Psychological Therapy (IPT) for schizophrenia: is it effective? Schizophr Bull 2006; 32: S81–93.

35. Roeder V, Brenner H, Mueller D, Spaulding W. Integrated Psychological Therapy for Schizophrenia, 2nd edn. London: Hogrefe, 2010.

36. Bell MD, Bryson GJ, Greig TC, Fiszdon JM, Wexler BE. Neurocognitive enhancement therapy with work therapy: productivity outcomes at 6- and 12-month follow-ups. J Rehabil Res Dev 2005; 42: 829–38.

37. Spaulding WD, Reed D, Sullivan M, et al. Effects of cognitive treatment in psychiatric rehabilitation. Schizophr Bull 1999; 25: 657–76.
38. Hogarty GE, Flesher S, Ulrich R, et al. Cognitive enhancement therapy for schizophrenia: Effects of a 2-year randomized trial on cognition and behavior. Arch Gen Psychiatry 2004; 61: 866–76.
39. Goldberg J. Cognitive retraining in a community psychiatric rehabilitation program. In: Spaulding W, ed. Cognitive Technology in Psychiatric Rehabilitation. Lincoln: University of Nebraska Press, 1994: 67–86.
40. Heinssen R. The cognitive exoskeleton: environmental interventions in cognitive rehabilitation. In: Corrigan P, Yudofsky S, eds. Cognitive Rehabilitation of Neuropsychiatric Disorders. Washington DC: American Psychiatric Press, 1996: 395–424.
41. Velligan D, Bow-Thomas L, Huntzinger C, et al. Randomized controlled trial of the use of compensating strategies to enhance adaptive functioning in outpatients with schizophrenia. Am J Psychiatry 2000; 157: 1317–23.
42. Velligan DI, Bow-Thomas CC. Two case studies of cognitive adaptation training for outpatients with schizophrenia. Psychiatr Serv 2000; 51: 25–9.
43. Corrigan PW, Liberman RP, eds. Behavior Therapy in Psychiatric Hospitals. New York: Springer, 1994.
44. Ayllon T, Azrin NH. The Token Economy. New York: Appleton-Century-Crofts, 1968.
45. Paul GL, Lentz RJ. Psychosocial treatment of chronic mental patients: Milieu vs. social learning programs. Cambridge, MA: Harvard University Press, 1977.
46. Wong S, Massel H, Mosk M, et al. Behavioral approaches to the treatment of schizophrenia. In: Burroughs G, Norman T, Rubenstein G, eds. Handbook of Studies on Schizophrenia. Amsterdam: Elsevier Science Publishers, 1986: 79–100.
47. Heinssen RK. Improving medication compliance of a patient with schizophrenia through collaborative behavioral therapy. Psychiatr Serv 2002; 53: 255–7.
48. Heinssen R, Levendusky P, Hunter R. Client as colleague: Therapeutic contracting with the seriously mentally ill. Am Psychol 1995; 50: 522–32.
49. Beck N, Greenfield S, Gotham H, et al. Risperidone in the management of violent, treatment-resistant schizophrenics hospitalized in a maximum security forensic facility. J Am Acad Psychiatry Law 1997; 25: 461–8.
50. Beck NC, Menditto AA, Baldwin L, et al. Reduced frequency of aggressive behavior in forensic patients in a social learning program. Hosp Community Psychiatry 1991; 42: 750–2.
51. Baldwin L, Beck N, Menditto A, et al. Decreasing excessive water drinking by chronic mentally ill forensic patients. Hosp Community Psychiatry 1992; 43: 507–9.
52. Strong Kinnaman JE, Slade E, Bennett ME, Bellack AS. Examination of contingency payments to dually-diagnosed patients in a multi-faceted behavioral treatment. Addict Behav 2006; 32: 1480–5.
53. Haddock G, Spaulding W. Psychological treatment of psychosis. In: Weinberger D, Harrison P, eds. Schizophrenia, 3rd edn. New York: Wiley-Blackwell, 2011: 666–86.
54. Miller WR, Rollnick S. Motivational Interviewing: Preparing People for Change, 2nd edn. New York: The Guilford Press, 2002.
55. Carey KB, Carey MP, Maisto SA, et al. The feasibility of enhancing psychiatric outpatients' readiness to change their substance use. Psychiatr Serv 2002; 53: 603–8.
56. Kemp R, Kirov G, Everitt B, et al. Randomized controlled trial of compliance therapy: 18-month follow-up. Br J Psychiatry 1998; 173: 271–2.
57. Spaulding W, Nolting J. Psychotherapy for schizophrenia in the year 2030: Prognosis and prognostication. Schizophr Bull 2006; 32: S94–S105.
58. Ventura J, Green M, Shaner A, et al. Training and quality assurance with the BPRS. Int J Methods Psychiatr Res 1993; 3: 221–44.

59. Honigfeld G, Gillis RD, Klett CJ. Nurses' observation scale for inpatient evaluation: a new scale for measuring improvement in chronic schizophrenia. J Clin Psychol 1965; 21: 65–71.

60. Paul GL. ed. Observational Assessment Instrumentation for Service and Research: The Time-sample Behavioral Checklist for Assessment in Residential Settings (part 2). Champaign, IL: Research Press, 1987.

61. Menditto AA, Wallace CJ, Liberman RP, et al. Functional assessment of independent living skills. Psychiatr Rehabil Skills 1999; 3: 200–19.

62. Spaulding W, Poland J, Elbogen E, et al. Therapeutic juripsrudence in psychiatric rehabilitation. Thomas M. Cooley Law Rev 2000; 17: 135–70.

63. Elbogen E, Tomkins A. The psychiatric hospital and therapeutic jurisprudence: applying the law to promote mental health. In: Spaulding W. ed. New Directions for Mental Health Services. The State Hospital in the 21st Century. Vol. 89. San Francisco: Jossey Bass, 1999: 71–84.

64. Bauer A, Rosca P, Khawalled R, et al. Dangerousness and risk assessment: the state of the art. Isr J Psychiatry Relat Sci 2003; 40:182–90.

65. Hunter R, Ritchie AJ, Spaulding W. The Sell decision: implications for psychological assessment and treatment. Prof Psychol Res Pract 2005; 36: 467–75.

66. Lehman A, Steinwachs D, Dixon L, et al. Patterns of usual care for schizophrenia: initial results from the schizophrenia Patient Outcomes Research Team (PORT) client survey. Schizophr Bull 1998; 24: 11–20.

67. Lehman AF, Kreyenbuhl J, Buchanan RW, et al. The Schizophrenia Patient Outcomes Research Team (PORT): updated treatment recommendations 2003. Schizophr Bull 2004; 30: 193–217.

68. Bickman L. Why don't we have effective mental health services? Adm Policy Ment Health 2008; 35: 437–9.

69. Spaulding W, Sullivan M, Poland J, Ritchie AJ. State psychiatric institutions and the left-behinds of mental health reform. Am J Orthopsychiatry 2010; 80: 327–33.

70. Stuve P, Menditto A. State hospitals in the new millenium: rehabilitating the "not ready for rehab" players. In: Spaulding W. ed. The Role of the State Hospital in the 21st century. Vol. 84. San Francisco: Jossey-Bass, 1999: 35–46.

71. Fisher W, Geller J, Pandiani J. The changing role of the state psychiatric hospital. Health Aff 2009; 28: 676–84.

72. Spaulding WD, Johnson DL, Coursey RD. Combined treatments and rehabilitation of schizophrenia. In: Sammons MT, Schmidt NB. eds. Combined Treatments for Mental Disorders. Washington DC: American Psychological Association, 2001: 161–90.

73. Spaulding WD, Sullivan ME, Poland JS. Treatment and Rehabilitation of Severe Mental Illness. New York: Guilford, 2003: 154–6.

74. Liberman RP. Recovery from Disability: Manual of Psychiatric Rehabilitation. Washington DC: American Psychiatric Press, 2008.

75. Daicoff S, Wexler B. Therapeutic jurisprudence. In: Goldstein A. ed. Handbook of Psychology: Forensic Psychology. New York: John Wiley & Sons, 2003: 561–80.

chapter 19

Rating scales in schizophrenia: Clinical applicability

Marc Corbière and Tania Lecomte

Clinicians are increasingly asked to offer evidenced-based practices and to demonstrate their efficiency and efficacy in delivering interventions, therefore necessitating the use of specific measures such as rating scales. Rating scales are also useful for many clinical purposes, such as determining specific patient profiles, deficits, symptoms, needs, and skills. Evaluations in the field of psychiatry are often complex because of the various aspects needing to be considered such as patients' characteristics, behaviors, cognitive deficits, motivations, symptoms, and physical health issues. Furthermore, the patent's mental, physical, and emotional states need to be taken into consideration prior to conducting an assessment, since these might alter the results. For example, it is relevant to evaluate cognitive deficits in order to judge whether the patent can reliably answer a self-report questionnaire or whether it is better to obtain the information through other means (e.g., interview). Indeed, patients with attention deficits or with difficulties with abstract concepts can struggle with choosing an answer on a scale, such as Likert scales, especially if the proposed responses offer subtle differences.

Assessments in mental health typically involve ordinal scales, also known as Likert scales, where a concept is measured from, for example: 1 = not present to 7 = extremely severe. Other scales are dichotomous (1 = yes, 2 = no), continuous (rate from 1 to 100), or use specific intervals or anchor points. The two most important aspects to consider before using rating scales are as follows: (*i*) the context in which the evaluation has to be done, whether it being for assessing needs, skills, change over time, and so on and (*ii*) the psychometric qualities of the scale, that is, its reliability and validity. *Reliability* is the ability of the scale to convey consistent and reproducible information. *Validity* is the degree to which the scale measures what it is supposed to measure in an exact manner (1,2).

The purpose of this chapter is to provide clinicians with a small number of rating scales that may be used to help monitor and assess their patients and other aspects of their practice when working with people with schizophrenia. The scales were specifically selected according to the following points:

- All selected regarding their usefulness for clinical practice—many other measures exist and some are more relevant for research or specific other indications.
- The most important needs, deficits, symptoms, and patient profiles linked to recovery are covered.
- Easy to administer—none of the measures necessitate specific training or lengthy manuals.
- Brief—length of assessment was considered.
- All are easily accessible, with little or no fee involved.
- All have demonstrated adequate psychometric qualities with individuals with schizophrenia.
- Some can be used at various points in time to measure change, if that is the goal.
- Some generate various subscales as well as more general score(s) that are easy to calculate and interpret.
- Some are self-report, others are informant or clinician-report and others have both versions available.

Rating scales assessing symptoms, needs, strengths, skills, and deficits

Tools presented in this section aim at assessing clients' symptoms, needs, strengths, skills, and deficits in order to offer them the most appropriate services. These scales can be used in a multidisciplinary team context to better understand the patients and help them meet their goals.

Symptoms

There exist various scales specifically designed to assess symptoms in individuals with schizophrenia. For example, the Brief Psychiatric Rating Scale (BPRS) (3) and the Positive and Negative Symptom Scale (PANSS) (4) are among the most commonly used scales. Other assessments aim at measuring more specific aspects of symptoms such as the PSYRATS for hallucinations and delusions (5), the SAPS for positive symptoms and the SANS for negative symptoms (6). However, all of these measures necessitate specific training, often involving inter-rater reliability checks, videotape ratings, and regular supervision. Since we only wish to present measures that do not require extensive training, we will not describe the above-mentioned instruments, though they can be clinically useful to assess the impact of medication or other treatments when clinicians are properly trained in administering them.

Brief Symptom Inventory
Description

The Brief Symptom Inventory (BSI; (7)) is a shortened version of the SCL-90 (Symptom Check List-90), and consists of 53 items to assess psychological distress and symptom severity in both patient and non-patient populations. The BSI measures the experience of symptoms in the previous 7 days, and consists of nine scales: Somatization, Obsessive Compulsive, Sensibility, Depression, Anxiety, Hostility, Phobic anxiety, Paranoid Ideation, Psychoticism, and three additional scales to measure global symptom severity, positive symptom distress, and positive symptoms. Psychologists, psychiatrists, physicians, nurses, and other healthcare professionals can use the BSI to assess individual at intake for psychological problems and measure their progress following a treatment. A brief (18 item) version also exists (8).

Scoring

Items are rated on a 5-point rating scale from 0 (no at all) to 4 (extremely). In addition to the nine symptom dimensions, three global indices assess a patient's general psychiatric distress: (*i*) Global Severity Index (GSI), (*ii*) Positive Symptom Distress Index (PSDI) and (*iii*) Positive Symptom Total. For example, the GSI is conceived to quantify a patient's severity of illness or symptom severity. Scores for each subscale are between 0 and 4 except for the global score which has values between 0 and 53. Norms have been established for use in particular settings.

The Behavior and Symptom Identification Scale
Description

The Behavior and Symptom Identification Scale (BASIS-32; (9)) measures symptoms and social functioning with 32 items, which cover five subscales: Psychosis, Impulsivity and Addictive Behavior, Anxiety/Depression, Interpersonal Relations, and Living Skills and Role Functioning. The scale measures the degree of difficulty the person has experienced in the previous 7 days for each item. Since only the past week is assessed, it can also be used at regular intervals to assess change over time; for example, before and after receiving care. The BASIS-32 is more often used for assessing large groups of patients and determining their clinical and social functioning, rather than for specific treatment purposes. A briefer 24-item version is also available (BASIS-24; (10)).

Scoring

The BASIS-32 measures the degree of difficulty experienced by the individual on a five-point scale ranging from 0 = no difficulty to 5 = extreme difficulty. The BASIS-32 is scored using an algorithm that gives an overall score with five subscales mentioned above.

The Calgary Depression Scale

Description

The Calgary Depression Scale for Schizophrenia (CDSS; (11)) is a 9-item structured interview scale specifically developed for the assessment of depression in schizophrenia patients. It is a semistructured goal-directed interview assessing depression, hopelessness, self-depreciation, guilty ideas of reference, pathological guilt, morning depression, early waking, suicide, and observed depression during the interview.

Scoring

The CDSS is a semi-structured interview with specific questions and probes for each of the 9 items, rated from 0 (absent) to 3 (severe). A total score is obtained by adding each of the item scores. Norms and cut-off points are available.

Needs and strengths

With services aiming at helping individuals in their recovery process, assessing patients' goals, needs, and strengths is critical. Qualitative interviews can also serve this purpose but might result in omissions in questioning on certain central aspects of experience, such as spiritual goals, sexual problems, or needing help with raising the children. The following measures either cover many domains or cover them in a fairly comprehensive manner.

The Camberwell Assessment of Needs

Description

The Camberwell Assessment of Needs (CAN; (12)) measures the level of difficulty and level of assistance needed in the previous month for people with mental health problems. The CAN consists of 22 areas of functioning including housing, food, cleaning, hygiene, daily activities, physical health, psychotic symptoms, treatment or illness information, psychological distress, personal security, social security, security of others, alcohol, drugs, social relationships, emotional relationships, sexual life, care of children, education, financial tasks, use of the telephone, and use of public transportation.

Scoring

The patient and their clinician independently rate both the perceived difficulty in functioning and the assistance provided to the respondent in each of the 22 areas (essentially one question per area). The need rating for each area is as follows: (a) *no need* (score of 0) – they have no serious problems in the area, (b) *met need* (score of 1) – they have no or moderate problems in the area due to help given, (c) *unmet need* (score of 2) – a serious problem, irrespective of any help given, and (d) *not known* (no score or missing score) – either not known or not disclosed. Also, when a met or unmet need is identified, further questions are asked to identify how much help the service user is receiving from informal sources (e.g., relatives) and formal sources (e.g., community services), and how much help they need from formal sources.

Client Assessment of Strengths, Interests, and Goals
Description

The Client Assessment of Strengths, Interests, and Goals (CASIG; (13)) is a comprehensive functioning assessment which addresses most psychiatric rehabilitation treatment domains, which are community living skills, cognitive skills, medication practices (adherence and side effects), quality of life and treatment, symptoms, consumer rights, and unacceptable community behaviors. Each scale ends with a goal question pertaining to that domain. The community living skills and symptoms domains are adapted from the *Independent Living Skills Survey (ILSS)* (14) and the *Brief Psychiatric Rating Scale (BPRS;* (15)) respectively. The assessment also elicits goals in five broad areas (residence, financial, relationships, religion/spirituality, and physical and mental health). The CASIG assesses multiple outcomes relevant to clients and clinicians that focus on strengths and skills. It is capable of assessing change over time (can be readministered every 3 months).

Scoring

The domain related to the "goals" is conceived by open questions while all the other sections, including community living skills, medication practices, side effects, symptoms, cognitive difficulties, consumer rights, quality of life, quality of treatment, and unacceptable community behaviors, are built with dichotomous questions (yes-no) and can be added up for each subscale (yes = 1, no = 0). Following each domain, or subscale, a yes-no question is asked to determine whether the respondent wishes to make that domain a personal goal. If yes, a four-point Likert scale (from "none" to "a lot") follows to assess how much help the client believes he/she needs to meet that goal.

Skills and deficits

Various instruments assess skills and deficits, with some comprehensive measures including such scales (e.g., the *CASIG* includes most of the *Independent Living Skills Survey* items). Deficits, especially cognitive deficits, are typically assessed with cognitive tests by trained neuropsychologists, but can also be assessed indirectly through novel techniques, such as the one presented here. For the purpose of brevity, only three essential domains of skills and deficits are presented: social skills training readiness/cognitive deficits, social functioning, and work competence.

Micro-Modules Learning Tests
Description

The Micro-Modules Learning Test (MMLT; (16)) is a measure of three major components of skills training: responsiveness to verbal instructions, ability to learn from watching a modeled behavior, and ability to reproduce behavior in a role-play. In contrast to the Assessment of Interpersonal Problem Solving Skills (AIPSS; (17)), which focuses mostly on problem-solving social situations, the MMLT comes in different versions in order to apply them to any of the UCLA social skills training modules, and does not require any training. It also is highly correlated with measures of cognition, particularly verbal memory and verbal fluency, as well as theory of mind, suggesting that individuals who score poorly on the MMLT could benefit from cognitive remediation prior to taking part in a skills training group (chap. 12).

Scoring
The MMLT comes with verbal instructions, written instructions, a videotape, and a scoring sheet with specific anchor points. Each question contains three levels of difficulty and the participant is rated according to the level achieved (0 if all wrong, to 3 if the most difficult level was correct).

Social Functioning Scale
Description
The Social Functioning Scale (SFS; (18)) is a 78-item scale that assesses social functioning and more particularly abilities and performance of people with schizophrenia in seven areas: Withdrawal/Social Engagement, Interpersonal Communication, Independence Performance, Independence Competence, Recreation, Prosocial, and Employment/Occupation.

Scoring
A scoring scale is provided for each scale and allows identifying problem areas. Each scale is rated in various ways (Likert scales, ratings from 0 to 100, yes/no answers, straight answers (e.g., number of friends?). It covers in detail many aspects of social competence and is designed to assess change over time, particularly following clinical interventions such as family therapy (chap. 15).

Work Behavior Inventory
Description
The Work Behavior Inventory (WBI; (19,20)) is a 36-item vocational situational assessment used to measure work function/performance for people with severe mental illness with the following five subscales: Work Habits, Work Quality, Personal Presentation, Cooperativeness, and Social Skills. Items stem from other measures of work behavior such as the Work Personality Profile (WPP, (21)) and the Minnesota Satisfactoriness Scales (MSS, (22)), and from additional observations and supervision at work sites. The WBI can be very useful for job coaches or vocational rehabilitation specialists wishing to offer precise and useful support to their patients who are working (chap. 11).

Scoring
The items are assessed on a 5-point anchorage with behavioral examples, from 1 to 5, with 1 representing consistently inferior performance, 5 representing

consistently superior performance, and 2, 3, and 4 representing intermediate points on the performance continuum. Each continuum combines frequency and severity of problem behaviors. Each of the five subscales contains seven items and the final item is a global item reflecting overall the work performance. The WBI subscales range from 7 to 35, and the summation of all scores gives the total score.

Recovery Assessment Scale
Description
The Recovery Assessment Scale (RAS; (23)) consists of 41 items assessing mental health recovery in people with severe mental illness (not specifically schizophrenia). From factor analyses (exploratory and confirmatory), most of the items are spread out on five factors: (*i*) personal confidence and hope (9 items); (*ii*) willingness to ask for help (3 items); (*iii*) goal and success orientation (5 items); (*iv*) reliance on others (4 items) and (*v*) no domination by symptoms (3 items).

Scoring
Each item is assessed on a 5-point Likert scale (from 1 = strongly disagree to 5 = strongly agree). Explicit guidelines indicating how to score responses can be availed by contacting the authors of the scale.

Specific mediators and moderators

Even though symptoms, needs, skills, and strengths are important aspects to measure before, during, and after a treatment, other crucial variables or specific mediators and moderators can also be assessed when wishing to better understand the patent's situation or in order to ensure that the treatment is as effective as possible. Such mediators and moderators, when problematic, often become treatment targets. For instance, treatment outcome is directly influenced by treatment adherence, which can be influenced by the relationship between the patient and the therapist, as well as by other factors such as the patient's substance use, self-esteem, and quality of life. Another example: a patient's symptoms might have decreased with the appropriate medication but specific beliefs continue to cause distress and might necessitate a specific treatment, such as cognitive–behavioral therapy.

Social Engagement Scale
Description
The Service Engagement Scale (SES (24)) is a 14-item measure consisting of statements that assess patient's engagement with services.

Scoring
Items are assessed on a four-point Likert scale from "not at all or rarely" to "most of the time." The total score ranges from a minimum of zero to a maximum of 42. Higher scores indicate lower engagement. Four subscales assess availability ("When a visit is arranged, the patient is available"), collaboration ("The patients actively participate in managing their illness"), help-seeking ("The patient seeks help to prevent a crisis") and treatment adherence ("The patient refuses to cooperate with treatment").

Self-Esteem Rating Scale- Short-Form
Description
The Self-Esteem Rating Scale- Short-Form (SERS-SF; (25)) is an abbreviated version of the SERS (26) and involves statements that are linked to social contacts, such as friends, as well as achievements and competency. The SERS-SF consists of two scales, positive and negative self-esteem, which have been documented as being relevant for individuals with schizophrenia (25,27). The SERS-SF taps into multiple aspects of self-evaluation such as overall self-worth, social competence, problem-solving ability, intellectual ability, self-competence, and worth compared with others.

Scoring
The items are rated on a seven-point Likert scale (from 1 = never to 7 = always), 10 scored positively and 10 negatively, with scores ranging from –70 to –10 (negative items) and from 10 to 70 (positive items). Both exploratory and confirmatory factor analyses confirm that the 20-item SERS-SF is highly valid, and is in fact superior in terms of construct validity and parsimony to the original 40-item SERS (25).

Drug/Alcohol Time Line Follow-Back Calendar
Description
Compared with other lengthy addiction self-report instruments that mostly aim at determining a diagnosis of dependence or abuse (e.g., the Addiction Severity Index, the Alcohol Use Scale and the Drug Use Scale) the most clinically useful addiction instrument is probably the Drug/Alcohol Time Line Follow-Back Calendar (TLFBC; (28)). The TLFBC provides a summary of the patient's use of substances over the previous 6 months, has a high accuracy and can help clinicians determine patterns of abuse and change over time.

Scoring
The TLFBC is conceived as a grid that helps go back in time, a month at a time, to determine what the person used, the frequency of use within the month, and the quantities used for each day.

MacArthur-Maudsley Delusions Assessment Schedule
Description

The MacArthur-Maudsley Delusions Assessment Schedule (MADS; (29)) consists of seven dimensions related to delusional beliefs: conviction, negative affect, action, inaction, preoccupation, pervasiveness, and fluidity. The *Conviction subscale* represents patient's certainty about the delusional belief; the *Negative affect subscale* addresses whether the delusional belief makes the individual unhappy, frightened, anxious, or angry; the *Action subscale* calculates the extent to which patients' actions are motivated by the delusional belief; the *Inaction subscale* measures whether a patient has refrained from any actions (e.g., eating, drinking etc.) because of the delusional belief within the previous two months and since the delusions began; the *Preoccupation subscale* assesses the extent to which the patient indicates that their thoughts focus exclusively on the delusion; the *Pervasiveness subscale* reflects the degree to which the delusional belief penetrates all aspects of the patient's experiences; and the *Fluidity subscale* reflects the degree to which the delusional belief changed frequently during the interview, often encompassing new people or contexts as they entered the discussion.

Scoring

Specific questions are asked about the first four dimensions; the last three are rated on anchored scales on the basis of the interviewers' global impressions. The summation of the four *Conviction* items varies from 0 to 8, the summation of the four Negative affects items ranges from 0 to 4. With respect to the Actions subscale, the 13 questions are either specific or open-ended. The *Inaction* subscale comprises eight questions (score from 0 to 8). *Preoccupation* and *Pervasiveness* subscales are respectively one item (either a score from 0 to 3 or a score from 0 to 4). Finally the *fluidity* subscale varies from no variation (score of 0) to frequent changes (score of 2).

Belief About Voices Questionnaire-Revised
Description

The Belief About Voices Questionnaire-Revised (BAVQ-R; (30)) consists of 35 items assessing individuals' beliefs about their auditory hallucinations, as well as their emotional and behavioral reactions to them. Three subscales measure beliefs about the voice, that is, its intent on doing good (benevolence, six items) or on harming (malevolence, six items); and its power (omnipotence, six items). Two further subscales, "resistance" (9 items) and "engagement" (8 items), measure how the person reacts emotionally and behaviorally to their voices.

Scoring

All the items are rated on a 4-point scale ranging from disagree 0 to agree strongly (3). Scores are added according to each of the five subscales, mentioned earlier.

The Working Alliance Inventory
Description
The Working Alliance Inventory (WAI; (31)) is a self-administered questionnaire and reflects the quality of the patient/clinician therapeutic relationship. There are three subscales: The *Bond* subscale reflects the positive relation between the clinician and the patient. The *Task* subscale concerns the behaviors and cognitions that support the agreement between the clinician and the patient on the tasks to be accomplished. The *Goal* subscale concerns the collaboration between the clinician and the patient regarding the goals to be attained.

Scoring
The WAI authors recommended that four scores have to be considered, one from each of the three subscales (i.e. Bond, Task, and Goal), and one overall score (31). The global scale simply represents the sum of all items. All items are assessed on a seven-point Likert-type scale (from 1 = never to 7 = always). The authors initially built the scale with 36 items, holding three 12-item subscale scores - Bond, Task and Goal - as well as one overall score. Subsequently, Tracey and Kokotovic (32) proposed a short-form scale containing 12 items drawn in equal proportion from the three initial subscales. Even though the Bond, Tasks and Goals subscales are distinct components of the alliance, they remain strongly intercorrelated at empirical and statistical levels for people with severe mental illness (33).

Satisfaction with Life Domains
Description
The Satisfaction with Life Domains (SLDS; (34)) comprises 15 life domains: housing, neighborhood, food, clothing, health, roommate, friends, relationships with family members, getting on with other people, job or day programming, activity in spare time, activity for fun, services in the area, economic situation, and living place in comparison with state hospital. Other versions with more items have been developed for specific purposes (e.g., breast cancer).

Scoring
Individuals use a 7-point Likert scale to rate the items. They are asked to indicate their feelings by choosing one of seven faces, gradually changing from a "delighted" face with a large upturned smile (scored 7) to a "terrible" face with a deep frown (scored 1)—thus making the assessment easy to answer for most individuals.

Conclusions

This chapter aims to aid clinicians in the choice and use of rating scales in their practice when working with individuals with schizophrenia. Since many scales and different types of measures exist, we recommend choosing measures that are

Table 19.1 Summary of rating scales proposed

	What it measures	Type of measure	Length of administration	Advantages	Inconveniences
BSI (Derogatis & Melisaratos, (7))	Psychiatric symptoms	Self-rated	15–20 minutes	Assesses various symptoms, not those linked to schizophrenia only	Self-report only, some information might need to be obtained through a more detailed interview or chart
BASIS-32 (Eisen et al., (9))	Symptoms and functioning	Self-rated	15–30 minutes	Validated in multiple countries, with large samples – many norms exist	Not suggested for individual clinical decisions. Scales are statistically derived–not always easy to interpret clinically
CDSS (Addington et al., (11))	Depressive symptoms	Interview	20–30 minutes	Adapted for schizophrenia, truly measures depression and not positive or negative symptoms, or extra-pyramidal side effects of medication. Available in multiple languages	Only one global score, only one version (interview-based)

(Continued)

Table 19.1 Summary of rating scales proposed (*Continued*)

	What it measures	Type of measure	Length of administration	Advantages	Inconveniences
CAN (Phelan et al., (12))	Community functioning needs	Self-rated and clinician-rated	15–60 minutes	Covers many domains. Has two versions and adaptations according to age group. Available in many languages and has many norms	Not in depth, each domain is briefly covered
CASIG (Wallace et al., (14))	Community functioning, goals, needs, quality of life, and more	Self-report (CASIG-SR) and Informant version (CASIG-I)	60 min for the CASIG-SR and 45 minutes for the CASIG-I	Covers many areas. Includes two versions. In depth, useful for planning treatment with clients. Available in paper and CD-ROM	Assessments are long. Questions are mostly dichotomous
MMLT (Silverstein, Wallace & Schenkel, (16))	Readiness for skills training	Interactive, video, questions and answers, role-plays	35–50 minutes	Good screening for cognitive difficulties that might impede on benefiting from skills training. A different version exists for each skills training module	Only linked to the UCLA skills modules. Necessitates equipment (VHS)
SFS (Birchwood et al., (18))	Social competence	Semistructured interview and version for family members	20–30 minutes for each version	Two versions. Covers many aspects	Different rating scales and anchor points—can be a bit confusing to score

WBI (Bryson et al., (19))	Vocational functioning	Observational measure that includes employer/supervisor interview	15 minutes behavioral observation plus a brief interview with employer or supervisor	Real-life observations in work settings	Can only be used if employer is aware of the mental condition of the client
RAS (Corrigan et al., (23))	Recovery	Self-rated	15–20 minutes	Assesses many dimensions of recovery. Validated in multiple studies and countries. Not specific to schizophrenia (severe mental illness)	Does not assess process, only dimensions
SES (Tait et al., (24))	Engagement in services	Clinician report	10–15 minutes	Helps determine profiles of treatment adherence and engagement with services	Only one version— no information is obtained on reasons for difficulties with engagement
SERS-SF (Lecomte et al., (25))	Self-esteem	Self-rated	15–20 minutes	Many aspects of self-esteem are measured, including positive and negative self-esteem. More adapted to schizophrenia and more specific than other measures (i.e., Rosenberg Self-Esteem Scale)	The scoring involves negative scores, at times difficult to interpret

(Continued)

Table 19.1 Summary of rating scales proposed (*Continued*)

	What it measures	Type of measure	Length of administration	Advantages	Inconveniences
TLFBC (Mueser et al., (28))	Substance abuse	Interview	Varies according to addiction patterns—from 10–30 minutes	More accurate than most self-report addiction measures. Accurate profile of use	Does not give scores or norms. Does not determine diagnosis of dependence or abuse
MADS (Taylor et al., (29))	Delusions	Interview	20–45 minutes	In depth. Useful for determining the impact of delusions on person's life	Different scoring for the subscales—can be tedious
BAVQ-R (Chadwick, Lees & Birchwood, (30))	Auditory hallucination	Self-rated	15–20 minutes	Covers various dimensions of voices, and the impact on the person's life	Does not address form or content of hallucination
WAI (Horvath & Greenberg, (31))	Working alliance	Self-rated (client and clinician version) as well as observer-rated (for research or supervisors)	10 minutes	Two versions of the relationship between the client and clinician. Many versions exist (short, long, with or without subscales)	High correlations between subscales
SLDS (Baker & Intagliata, (34))	Quality of life	Self-rated	10–20 minutes	Can be used with individuals with cognitive deficits, because of scale using smiling–frowning faces. Many domains covered	Not in depth, each domain is briefly covered

validated and appropriate for the setting and clientele. The measures proposed here were all selected according to these criteria, as well as others such as necessitating no specific training involved and being quick and easy to administer. Some of the measures have been used for many years and have ample empirical support, whereas others are more recent. For a summary, see Table 19.1. Many other measures could have been presented since the list is not exhaustive.

Individuals with schizophrenia rarely follow a linear path in terms of recovery; rating scales can help the patients as well as the clinicians gain a better understanding of these changes over time and the potential effects of the treatments or services received. Rating scales can be used at various times during treatment or the recovery process, to help gain knowledge and build a working alliance, or to evaluate progress and change, or even to determine the effectiveness of specific services offered by a mental health team. Last but not least, clinical rating scales can help create bridges between research and clinical practice and potentially initiate fruitful collaborations that can help improve services and the recovery process of individuals with schizophrenia.

References

1. Anastasi A. Psychological Testing. New York: Macmillan, 1988.
2. Sajatovic M, Ramirez L. Rating Scales in Mental Health. Cleveland, Ohio: Case Western Reserve University, 2003.
3. Ventura J, Lukoff D, Nuechterlein KH, et al. Appendix 1: Brief psychiatric rating scale (BPRS) expanded version (4.0) scales, anchor points and administration manual. Int J Methods Psychiatr Res 1993; 3: 227–43.
4. Kay SR, Fiszbein A, Opler LA. The positive and negative syndrome scale (PANSS) for schizophrenia. Schizophr Bull 1987; 13: 261–76.
5. Haddock G, McCarron J, Tarrier N, Faragher EB. Scales to measure dimensions of hallucinations and delusions: the psychotic symptom rating scales (PSYRATS). Psycholog Med 1999; 29: 879–98.
6. Andreasen NC, Olsen S. Negative vs positive schizophrenia: definition and validation. Arch Gen Psychiatry 1982; 39: 784–94.
7. Derogatis LR, Melisaratos N. The brief symptom inventory: an introductory report. Psycholog Med 1983; 13: 596–605.
8. Derogatis LR. Brief Symptom Inventory (BSI)-18: Administration, Scoring and Procedures Manual. Minneapolis, MN: NCS Pearson, 2001.
9. Eisen SV, Dill DL, Grob MC. Reliability and validity of a brief patient-report instrument for psychiatric outcome evaluation. Hosp Community Psychiatry 1994; 45: 242–7.
10. Eisen SV, Gerena M, Ranganathan G, Esch D, Idiculla T. Reliability and validity of the BASIS-24 mental health survey for whites, African-Americans, and Latinos. J Behav Health Serv Res 2006; 33: 304–23.
11. Addington D, Addington J, Maticka-Tyndale E, Joyce J. Reliability and validity of a depression rating scale for schizophrenics. Schizophr Res 1992; 6: 201–8.
12. Phelan M, Slade M, Thornicroft G, et al. The Camberwell assessment of need: the validity and relability of an instrument to assess the needs of people with severe mental illness. Br J Psychiatry 1995; 167: 589–95.
13. Wallace CJ, Kochanowicz N, Wallace J. Independant Living Skills Survey. Unpublished manuscript, Mental Health Clinical Research Center to the Study of Schizophrenia,

West Los Angeles VA Medical Center. Los Angeles, CA: Rehabilitation Medicine Service (Brentwood Division), 1985.

14. Wallace CJ, Lecomte T, Wilde J, Liberman RP. CASIG: a consumer-centered assessment for planning individualized treatment and evaluating program outcomes. Schizophr Res 2001; 50: 105–9.

15. Lukoff D, Nuechterlein KH, Ventura J. Manual for expanded brief psychiatric rating scale. Schizophr Bull 1986; 12: 594–602.

16. Silverstein SM, Wallace CJ, Schenkel LS. The micro-module learning tests: work-sample assessments of responsiveness to skills training. Schizophr Bull 2005; 31: 73–83.

17. Donahoe CP, Carer MJ, Bloem WD, et al. Assessment of interpersonal problem solving skills. Psychiatry 1990; 53: 329–39.

18. Birchwood M, Smith J, Cochrane R, Wetton S, Copestake S. The social functioning scale: The development and validation of a new scale of social adjustment for use in family intervention programmes with schizophrenic patients. Br J Psychiatry 1990; 157: 853–9.

19. Bryson G, Bell MD, Lysaker P, Zito W. The work behavior inventory: a scale for the assessment of work behavior for people with severe mental illness. Psychiatr Rehabil J 1997; 20(Suppl 4): 47–55.

20. Lysaker P, Bell M, Bryson G, Zito W. Raters Guide for the Work Behavior Inventory: Rehabilitation, Research, and Development Service. West Haven, CT: Department of Veteran Affairs, 1993.

21. Bolton B, Roessler R. Manual for the Work Personality Profile. Fayetteville, AR: University of Arkansas Research & Training Center in Vocational Rehabilitation, 1986.

22. Gibson DL, Weiss DJ, Dawis RV, Lofquist LH. Manual for the Minnesota Satisfactoriness Scales. Minneapolis, MN: University of Minnesota, 1977.

23. Corrigan P W, Salzer M, Ralph RO, Sangster Y, Keck L. Examining the factor structure of the Recovery Assessment Scale. Schizophr Bull 2004; 30: 1035–41.

24. Tait L, Birchwood M, Trower P. A new scale (SES) to measure engagement with community mental health services. J Ment Health 2002; 11: 191–8.

25. Lecomte T, Corbière M, Laisne F. Investigating self-esteem in individuals with schizophrenia: relevance of the self-esteem rating scale-short form. Psychiatry Res 2006; 143: 99–108.

26. Nugent WR, Thomas JW. Validation of a clinical measure of self-esteem. Res Soc Work Pract 1993; 3(Suppl 2): 191–207.

27. Barrowclough C, Tarrier N, Humphreys L, et al. Self-esteem in schizophrenia: relationships between self-evaluation, family attitudes, and symptomatology. J Abnorm Psychol 2003; 112(Suppl 1): 92–9.

28. Mueser KT, Noordsy DL, Drake RE, Fox L. Integrated Treatment for Dual Disorders: a Guide to Effective Practice. New York: Guilford Press, 2003.

29. Taylor PJ, Garety P, Buchanan A, et al. Delusions and Violence, in Violence and Mental Disorder: Developments in Risk Assessment. Chicago: University of Chicago Press, 1994.

30. Chadwick P, Lees S, Birchwood M. The revised beliefs about voices questionnaire (BAVQ-R). Br J Psychiatry 2000; 177: 229–32.

31. Horvath AO, Greenberg LS. Development and validation of the working alliance inventory. J Couns Psychol 1989; 36(Suppl 2): 223–33.

32. Tracey TJ, Kokotovic AM. Factor structure of the working alliance inventory. Psychol Assess 1989; 1(Suppl 3): 207–10.

33. Corbière M, Bisson J, Lauzon S, Ricard N. Factorial validation of a French short-form of the working alliance inventory. Int J Methods Psychiatr Res 2006; 15(Suppl 1): 36–45.

34. Baker F, Intagliata J. Quality of life in the evaluation of community support systems. Eval Program Plann 1982; 5: 69–79.

Index

T - #1036 - 101024 - C0 - 234/156/17 - PB - 9781842145340 - Gloss Lamination